CALCIUM ANTAGONISTS AND CARDIOVASCULAR DISEASE

Perspectives in Cardiovascular Research
Volume 9

Perspectives in Cardiovascular Research

Series Editor

Arnold M. Katz

Chief, Division of Cardiology
University of Connecticut School of Medicine
Farmington, Connecticut

Calcium Antagonists and Cardiovascular Disease

Perspectives in Cardiovascular Research
Volume 9

Editor

L. H. Opie, M.D., Ph.D.

Professor of Medicine (Cardiac)
University of Cape Town
Cape Town, South Africa
and
Director
Ischemic Heart Disease Research Unit
Medical Research Council of South Africa
Cape Town, South Africa

Sponsored by the Council
of the International Society on Cardiac Metabolism
and Federation of Cardiology

Raven Press ▪ New York

Raven Press, 1140 Avenue of the Americas, New York, New York 10036

Made in the United States of America

Library of Congress Cataloging in Publication Data
Main entry under title:

Calcium antagonists and cardiovascular disease.

(Perspectives in cardiovascular research ; v. 9)
Includes index.
1. Calcium—Antagonists—Therapeutic use—Addresses,
essays, lectures.   2. Heart—Diseases—Chemotherapy—
Addresses, essays, lectures.   3. Calcium—Physiological
effect—Addresses, essays, lectures.   I. Opie, Lionel H.
II. Series.   [DNLM: 1. Calcium—Metabolism.   2. Calcium
channel blockers.   3. Cardiovascular diseases.
W1 PE871AL v.9 / QV 150 C1435]
RC684.C34C335   1984   616.1′061   82-42629
ISBN 0-89004-967-X

The material contained in this volume was submitted as previously unpublished material, except in the instances in which credit has been given to the source from which some of the illustrative material was derived.

Great care has been taken to maintain the accuracy of the information contained in the volume. However, Raven Press cannot be held responsible for errors or for any consequences arising from the use of the information contained herein.

Materials appearing in this book prepared by individuals as part of their official duties as U.S. Government employees are not covered by the above-mentioned copyright.

Preface

Eleven years ago, Professor Peter Harris of the Cardiothoracic Institute in London and I edited a book entitled *Calcium and the Heart*. In those days, calcium was not a "main-line" subject. Only Fleckenstein referred in any detail to the role of specific inhibitors of calcium action and introduced his concept of calcium antagonists in that book. Four of the six major contributors to that book have also participated in the present book—Fleckenstein, Nayler, Katz, and Schwartz. A comparison of that book and the present shows the enormous rate at which our understanding has grown over the last 12 years. Whereas, in 1971, Professor Harris only found one clinical application of calcium therapy (keeping solutions of calcium salts at hand in the coronary care unit), the present widespread use of calcium-antagonist drugs requires a new book, rather than a new edition of an old book.

The basic purpose of this book is to provide practical knowledge on calcium ion movements and calcium antagonists for cardiologists, research physicians, pharmacologists, and postgraduate students. This aim has been immensely facilitated by two sponsored meetings recently held in Cape Town, South Africa. First, the Council on Cardiac Metabolism of the International Society & Federation of Cardiology sponsored the Symposium on Calcium and Calcium-Antagonists. Excellent support was obtained from a variety of sources, listed in the Acknowledgments. Second, Bayer-Miles Pharmaceutical Company sponsored a satellite symposium at the nearby university town of Stellenbosch, focusing on the role of calcium in myocardial ischemia, infarction, arrhythmias, and hypertension, and the appropriate intervention by calcium antagonists. A series of articles based on the contributors to those two symposia form the backbone of this volume.

In addition, a number of critically important contributors who did not attend the Symposia have very generously agreed to contribute chapters. Such contributors merit special mention and are A. Fleckenstein, E. Carafoli, R. Murphy, H. Yasue, A. Scriabine, H. Mayer, J. Traber, P. Henry, N. Sperelakis, and A. Schwartz. Any success there might be for this book will reflect the outstanding qualities of the individual contributors. Of these contributors, one requires special mention—Professor R. Krebs of Bayer Pharmaceutical Company who is also Professor of Pharmacology and Toxicology at the University of Meinz. Professor Krebs not only helped to organize the meeting in Stellenbosch, but agreed to act as section editor for Pharmacology of Calcium Antagonist Drugs.

The title *Calcium Antagonists and Cardiovascular Disease* was chosen for three reasons. First, *calcium antagonists* was the term coined by Fleckenstein, who has written the first chapter of this book. Second, as Scriabine and his group show, calcium antagonists include, as a subdivision, calcium-channel inhibitors. Third, a practical point was that *calcium antagonists* had been the term most widely abstracted at the recent 1982 Meeting of the American Heart Association, winning over the alternate titles.

The contributions of these outstanding authors represent a topical and important book. It is distinguished from other books on calcium antagonists by the careful way in which it probes the role of calcium ion fluxes, the role of calcium in cardiovascular disease, and the pharmacology of calcium-antagonist agents before going on to the clinical application in angina and ischemic heart disease, arrhythmias, and hypertension. This book is offered at a time when clinical interest in calcium antagonists is exceedingly high.

Optimal use of this book requires that the reader should be prepared to delve deeply into physiological, pathological, and pharmacological aspects of calcium metabolism and calcium antagonists, before coming to the clinical application.

Lionel H. Opie

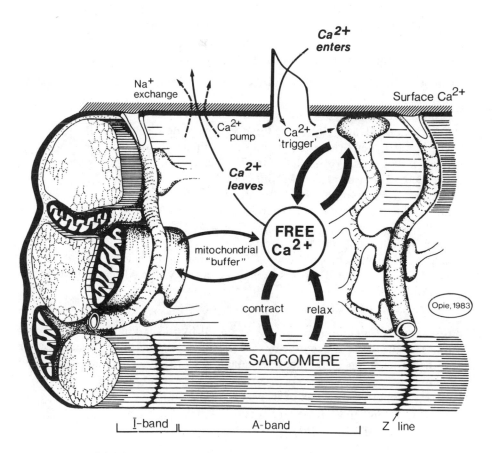

Critical role of calcium in heart muscle contraction.

Acknowledgments

The Council on Cardiac Metabolism of the International Society and Federation of Cardiology wishes to thank the following organizations for help with the two Symposia on Calcium and Calcium Antagonists organized during and after the Southern Africa Cardiac Society Congress:

1. Participants in the meetings organized by the Southern Africa Cardiac Society Congress:
   Prof. F. Bühler, Sandoz Ltd.
   Dr. C. Conti, University of the Orange Free State
   Dr. P. Corr, Leibovicius Trust and Glaxo Pharmaceuticals
   Prof. J. de Leiris, Warner-Lambert Pharmaceuticals
   Dr. D. C. Harrison, Pfizer Laboratories
   Dr. D. Hearse, Hoechst Pharmaceuticals
   Dr. R. Jennings, Council on Metabolism of International Society & Federation of Cardiology
   Prof. W. Nayler, Knoll Pharmaceuticals
   Dr. P. Poole-Wilson, University of Cape Town and Eli Lilly
   Dr. W. Roberts, Medical Research Council of South Africa & Leibovicius Trust
   Dr. J. Willerson, ICI Pharmaceuticals Ltd.

2. Post-Congress Calcium Symposium, organized by Bayer Pharmaceuticals
   Major support has been achieved by courtesy of Bayer Pharmaceuticals, together with participation of the above speakers, and the organizations supporting them.
   Speakers supported in whole or in part by Bayer are:
   Prof. F. Bühler (part support)
   Dr. C. Conti (part support)
   Prof. P. Hugenholtz
   Dr. A. Katz
   Prof. P. Lichtlen
   Prof. A. Maseri
   Prof. C. Rosendorff
   Dr. J. Willerson (part support)

We are particularly indebted to Dr. G. Erdmann of Bayer-Miles Pharmaceutical Ltd. and Mr. Neil Lane for taking on the vast task of organizing the Post-Congress Symposium.

Contents

Pharmacology of Calcium Antagonist Drugs
Section Editor: R. Krebs

Angina and Myocardial Infarction

Arrhythmias

Hypertension

Combination Therapy

Future Perspectives

Contributors

P. Bolli
Department of Research and Department
  of Medicine
University Hospital
Basel, Switzerland

M. R. Bristow
Division of Cardiology
Stanford University
School of Medicine
Stanford, California 94305

M. Buchbinder
Division of Cardiology
Stanford University
School of Medicine
Stanford, California 94305

F. R. Bühler
Division of Cardiology
Kantonsspital
4031 Basel, Switzerland

L. M. Buja
Department of Internal Medicine
  (Cardiovascular Division) and
  Department of Pathology
University of Texas Health Science Center
  and Parkland Memorial Hospital
Dallas, Texas 75235

E. Carafoli
Laboratory of Biochemistry
Swiss Federal Institute of Technology
  (ETH)
8092 Zurich, Switzerland

K. Chien
Department of Internal Medicine
  (Cardiovascular Division) and
  Department of Pathology,
University of Texas Health Science Center
  and Parkland Memorial Hospital
Dallas, Texas 75235

W. T. Clusin
Division of Cardiology
Stanford University
School of Medicine
Stanford, California 94305

C. J. Cohen
Miles Institute for Preclinical
  Pharmacology
New Haven, Connecticut 06509

C. R. Conti
Division of Cardiology
University of Florida
Box J-277 JHM Health Center
Gainesville, Florida 32610

J. B. Conti
Division of Cardiology
University of Florida
Box J-277 JHM Health Center
Gainesville, Florida 32610

P. B. Corr
Cardiovascular Division
Washington University
School of Medicine
St. Louis, Missouri 63110

P. A. Crean
Cardiovascular Unit
Royal Postgraduate Medical School
Hammersmith Hospital
Ducane Road
London W12 OHS, United Kingdom

M. J. Daly
Department of Medicine
University of Melbourne
Austin Hospital
Heidelberg, Victoria, 3084 Australia

J. S. Dillon
Department of Medicine
University of Melbourne
Austin Hospital
Heidelberg, Victoria, 3084 Australia

W. U. Dompert
Neurobiology Department
Troponwerke
D-5000 Cologne 80, Federal Republic of
  Germany

H.-J. Engel
Department of Medicine
Division of Cardiology
Hannover Medical School
Hannover, Federal Republic of Germany

R. L. Feldman
Division of Cardiology
University of Florida
JHM Health Center
Gainesville, Florida 32610

A. Fleckenstein
Physiologisches Institut
Albert-Ludwigs-Universität
D-7800 Freiburg, Federal Republic of
  Germany

W. T. Gerthoffer
Department of Physiology
School of Medicine
University of Virginia
Charlottesville, Virginia 22908

W. Gevers
Muscle Research Unit of South African
  Medical Research Council and University
  of Cape Town Department of Medical
  Biochemistry
Medical School of University of Cape
  Town
Observatory 7925, Cape Town, South
  Africa

C. W. Hamm
MRC-UCT Ischaemic Heart Disease
  Research Unit
Department of Medicine
Groote Schuur Hospital and University of
  Cape Town
Cape Town, South Africa

D. C. Harrison
Division of Cardiology
Stanford University School of Medicine
Stanford, California 94305

D. J. Hearse
The Rayne Institute
St. Thomas' Hospital
London SE 1, United Kingdom

P. D. Henry
Department of Medicine
Baylor College of Medicine
Houston, Texas 77030

J. A. Hill
Division of Cardiology
University of Florida
JHM Health Center
Gainesville, Florida 32610

P. G. Hugenholtz
Department of Cardiology
The Thoraxcenter
University Hospital,
Rotterdam, The Netherlands

U. L. Hulthén
Department of Research and Department
  of Medicine
University Hospital
Basel, Switzerland

C. Izquierdo
Department of Internal Medicine
  (Cardiovascular Division) and
  Department of Pathology
University of Texas Health Science Center
  and Parkland Memorial Hospital
Dallas, Texas 75235

R. A. Janis
Miles Institute for Preclinical
  Pharmacology
New Haven, Connecticut 06509

L. D. Jee
MRC-UCT Ischaemic Heart Disease
  Research Unit
Department of Medicine
University of Cape Town and Hypertension
  Clinic, Groote Schuur Hospital
Cape Town, South Africa

R. B. Jennings
Department of Pathology
Duke University Medical Center
Durham, North Carolina 27710

J. W. de Jong
Department of Cardiology
The Thoraxcenter
University Hospital
Rotterdam, The Netherlands

A. M. Katz
Division of Cardiology
University of Connecticut Health Center
School of Medicine
Farmington, Connecticut 06032

R. Krebs
Bayer AG
Pharma Forschungzentrum
Ressort Medizin
Postfach 101709
D-5600 Wuppertal 1, Federal Republic of
  Germany

G. Kroneberg
Pharmaceutical Research Development
Bayer AG
D-5600 Wuppertal 1, Federal Republic of
  Germany

J. de Leiris
Laboratoire de Physiologie Animale
Université Scientifique et Médicale de
  Grenoble
Grenoble, France

P. R. Lichtlen
Department of Medicine
Division of Cardiology
Hannover Medical School
Hannover, Federal Republic of Germany

A. Maseri
Cardiovascular Unit
Royal Postgraduate Medical School
Hammersmith Hospital
Ducane Road
London W12 OHS, United Kingdom

H. Meyer
Chemical Research Laboratories
Pharmaceutical Division
Bayer AG
Wuppertal-Elberfeld, Federal Republic of
  Germany

A. Mukherjee
Department of Internal Medicine
  (Cardiovascular Division) and
  Department of Pathology
University of Texas Health Science Center
  and Parkland Memorial Hospital
Dallas, Texas 75235

C. A. Muller
MRC-UCT Ischaemic Heart Disease
  Research Unit
Department of Medicine
Groote Schuur Hospital and University of
  Cape Town
Cape Town, South Africa

R. A. Murphy
Department of Physiology
School of Medicine, Box 449
University of Virginia
Charlottesville, Virginia 22908

W. G. Nayler
Department of Medicine
Austin Hospital
Heidelberg, Victoria 3084, Australia

L. H. Opie
MRC-UCT Ischaemic Heart Disease
  Research Unit
Department of Medicine
Groote Schuur Hospital and University of
  Cape Town
Cape Town, South Africa

C. J. Pepine
Division of Cardiology
University of Florida
JHM Health Center
Gainesville, Florida 32610

S. Pestre
Laboratoire de Physiologie Animale
Universite Scientifique et Medicale de
Grenoble
Grenoble, France

P. A. Poole-Wilson
Cardiothoracic Institute
2 Beaumont Street
London W1N 2DX, United Kingdom

W. Rafflenbeul
Department of Medicine
Division of Cardiology
Hannover Medical School
Hannover, Federal Republic of Germany

H. Reuter
Department of Pharmacology
University of Berne
3010 Berne, Switzerland

V. Richard
Laboratoire de Physiologie Animale
Universite Scientifique et Medicale de
Grenoble
Grenoble, France

W. C. Roberts
Pathology Branch
National Heart, Lung & Blood Institute
National Institutes of Health
Bethesda, Maryland 20205

C. Rosendorff
MRC-University Circulation Research Unit
Departments of Physiology and Medicine
University of Witwatersrand Medical
School
Parktown 2193, Johannesburg, South
Africa

A. Schwartz
Department of Pharmacology and Cell
Biophysics
University of Cincinnati
231 Bethesda Avenue
Cincinnati, Ohio 45267

A. Scriabine
Miles Institute for Preclinical
Pharmacology
Box 1956
New Haven, Connecticut 06509

P. W. Serruys
Department of Cardiology
The Thoraxcenter
University Hospital
Rotterdam, The Netherlands

A. D. Sharma
Cardiovascular Division
Washington University
School of Medicine
St. Louis, Missouri 63110

N. Sperelakis
Physiology Department
University of Virginia School of Medicine
Charlottesville, Virginia 22908

D. G. Taylor
Miles Institute for Preclinical
Pharmacology
New Haven, Connecticut 06509

F. T. Thandroyen
MRC-UCT Ischaemic Heart Disease
Research Unit
Department of Medicine
Groote Schuur Hospital and University of
Cape Town
Cape Town, South Africa

J. Traber
Neurobiology Department
Troponwerke
D-5000 Cologne 80, Federal Republic of
Germany

P. D. Verdouw
Department of Cardiology
The Thoraxcenter
University Hospital
Rotterdam, The Netherlands

J. T. Willerson
*Department of Internal Medicine
  (Cardiovascular Division)
University of Texas Health Science Center
Dallas, Texas 75235*

H. Yasue
*Division of Cardiology
Shizuoka City Hospital
10-93 Ote-Cho
Shizuoka City, Japan 420*

Calcium Antagonists and Cardiovascular Disease, edited by L. H. Opie.
Raven Press, New York © 1984.

Chapter 1

Calcium, Calcium Ions, and Cardiovascular Disease

L. H. Opie

MRC-UCT Ischaemic Heart Disease Research Unit, Department of Medicine, Groote Schuur Hospital and University of Cape Town, Cape Town, South Africa

FUNDAMENTAL ROLE OF CALCIUM

Ca^{2+} ions play the most fundamental role in the regulation of the cardiovascular system. An influx of Ca^{2+} ions into the cytosol is required for myocardial contraction—a process which ejects blood from the heart against a peripheral resistance which, in turn, is determined by Ca^{2+}-regulated tone of vascular smooth muscle. Myocardial relaxation, induced by the uptake of Ca^{2+} ions by the sarcoplasmic reticulum, allows adequate diastolic filling for the next systole. Ca^{2+}-antagonist agents, by modifying these Ca^{2+}-induced effects, can exert most profound effects on the cardiovascular system. Fortunately, the therapeutic effects of Ca^{2+} antagonists are found in concentrations which inhibit vascular smooth muscle contraction (thereby causing coronary and peripheral vasodilation) or the atrioventricular node (in the case of verapamil and diltiazem) without exerting an undue negative inotropic effect.

Calcium Ion Fluxes

The major site of action of Ca^{2+} antagonists is the influx of Ca^{2+} across the sarcolemma (A. Fleckenstein, *Chapter 2;* E. Carafoli, *Chapter 3;* H. Reuter, *Chapter 4*). Ca^{2+} ions enter the heart cell through a voltage-controlled Ca^{2+} channel. The Ca^{2+} channel has a certain probability of opening in bursts which increases as the transsarcolemmal voltage becomes more positive than -40 mV, and then decreases with further depolarization as the driving force decreases (H. Reuter, *Chapter 4*). The density of the Ca^{2+} channels is about 0.1 Ca^{2+} channels per μm^2 of the surface of cardiac cells in culture, compared with a Na^+-channel density of 16 per μm^2; this difference explains the much greater amplitude of the "fast" Na^+ current.

Different Ca^{2+} channels in different tissues are proposed by Nayler et al. (*Chapter 17*) to explain different effects on myocardium (class I), vasculature (class II), and nodal tissue (class III); other explanations are also considered. An important practical point is that different Ca^{2+} antagonists act on different sites to produce clinically divergent effects—thus, verapamil and diltiazem can inhibit supraventricular tachycardias with circuits through the atrioventricular node, whereas nifedipine acts more powerfully on the peripheral vasculature.

Ca^{2+} ions leave the myocardial cells chiefly by a Na^+/Ca^{2+} exchange system which is designed to eject Ca^{2+} ions whenever the cytosolic Ca^{2+} ion concentration exceeds a certain value. The Ca^{2+} channel can be controlled by catecholamine stimulation, acting by a phosphorylation reaction dependent on cyclic AMP (the putative second messenger of β-stimulation), so that more channels are "opened." The Na^+/Ca^{2+} pump (E. Carafoli, *Chapter 3*) is also subject to phosphorylation which increases the affinity for Ca^{2+}; such phosphorylation occurs in response to Ca^{2+} and calmodulin, so that the intracellular surge of Ca^{2+} ions occurring in systole activates the exit processes. A back-up Ca^{2+} ejection system is that which uses ATP and pumps Ca^{2+} ions outwards (Ca^{2+}-pumping ATPase); this system may operate in diastole to help regulate intracellular Ca^{2+} (E. Carafoli, *Chapter 3*).

In the myocardium, a major mechanism controlling the pump function is the role of Ca^{2+} in governing contraction and relaxation, reflecting the rhythmical rise and fall of Ca^{2+} ion concentration in the cytosol (A. Katz, *Chapter 5*). The sarcoplasmic reticulum, which acts as an intracellular Ca^{2+} store, releases Ca^{2+} during depolarization either because the small amount of Ca^{2+} entering via the Ca^{2+} channel triggers the release of much more Ca^{2+}, or else depolarization itself releases Ca^{2+} ions. "This unresolved question represents the most important remaining mystery in excitation-contraction coupling" (A. Katz, *Chapter 5*).

Ca^{2+} uptake by the sarcoplasmic reticulum occurs by a Ca^{2+} pump which uses ATP. Phospholamban is a phosphoprotein found in the sarcoplasmic reticulum, whose activity can help regulate both the rates of Ca^{2+} uptake and release (A. Katz, *Chapter 5*). When phosphorylated by cyclic AMP (β-stimulation of cell), the Ca^{2+}-sensitivity of the sarcolemmal pump is enhanced so that Ca^{2+} uptake and release are accelerated. Interventions such as inotropic agents which ultimately act by an increase of intracellular Ca^{2+} (digitalis) theoretically can also activate the uptake process by enhanced activity of Ca^{2+}-calmodulin which, in turn, should accelerate Ca^{2+} uptake by the sarcoplasmic reticulum.

Contractile Mechanism

The contractile mechanism is Ca^{2+}-dependent, as outlined by Gevers (*Chapter 6*). In the heart, Ca^{2+} ions act as a reversible switch, binding to the troponin C subunit of troponin. According to the steric hindrance theory of Huxley, during diastole, tropomyosin obstructs the myosin-binding sites on actin subunits; systole starts when the arrival of Ca^{2+} and its binding to troponin C allows a local conformation twist to remove the obstruction and to allow contraction. Gevers proposes that troponin C phosphorylation (by cyclic AMP) lessens the size of the thin filament domain that can be activated (hence accelerating relaxation), and that phosphorylation of P light chains of myosin (by a myosin light chain kinase whose activation depends on Ca^{2+} and calmodulin) accelerates the rate of turnover of the ATPase site with faster cross-bridge cycling.

In vascular smooth muscle, actin does not interact with myosin at all if the P light chains are not phosphorylated by Ca^{2+}-calmodulin (W. Gevers, *Chapter 6;* R. Murphy and W. Gerthoffer, *Chapter 7*). Other potential mechanisms for smooth muscle contraction are: (a) the actin-linked protein, leiotonin, which is thought by Ebashi to have a role in vascular smooth muscle similar to troponin C in cardiac muscle; (b) caldesmon, which Sobue proposes as a large protein preventing myosin binding—when the Ca^{2+} concentration rises, then Ca^{2+}-calmodulin binds to caldesmon to free actins for attachment to myosin heads; and (c) the important "latch mechanism" proposed by Murphy. In vascular smooth muscle, Murphy and Gerthoffer (*Chapter 7*) propose two types of Ca^{2+}-dependent regulatory systems: First, there is a rapidly responding system somewhat similar to that of striated muscle, except that phosphorylation of myosin plays an important regulatory role; and second, there is a "latch" system whereby stress can be maintained tonically against a chronic load, such as the blood pressure, with little requirement for ATP. As both processes are ultimately Ca^{2+}-dependent, Ca^{2+} antagonists presumably will act on both.

CALCIUM ANTAGONISTS AND PATHOLOGY OF THE HEART

Calcium in Ischemic and Reperfusion Injury

The exact mechanism of irreversible injury to the myocyte is still under consideration (R. Jennings, *Chapter 8*). Early sarcolemmal damage is an important factor which is associated with depletion of high-energy phosphate compounds, but a cause-and-effect relationship is not proven. Willerson et al. (*Chapter 24*) provisionally link sarcolemmal damage with degradation of the phospholipids of the membrane and an associated increase in sarcolemmal permeability to Ca^{2+} ions. They propose that enhanced Ca^{2+} ion entry (as monitored indirectly by a lanthanum probe) precedes the development of irreversible ischemic injury. Next follows Ca^{2+} deposition in mitochondria, an irreversible process (R. Jennings, *Chapter 8*). Clinically, myocardial scantigrams with technetium 99m can detect accumulation of Ca^{2+} in the ischemic myocardium especially in cells with 10 to 40% of control blood flow. Cells damaged by severe ischemia undergo massive uptake of Ca^{2+} during reperfusion with contraction-band necrosis and mitochondrial overloading of Ca^{2+}. Whether accumulation of Ca^{2+} ions plays a role in the production of the original ischemic injury is still a matter of conjecture. An intriguing hypothesis (P. Poole-Wilson, *Chapter 9*) is that the entry of Ca^{2+} ions brings about some of the enzyme loss, possibly by activation of phospholipases and proteases. Small amounts of enzyme loss do not necessarily indicate small amounts of necrotic cells, but could be associated with reversible ischemic damage, according to Poole-Wilson (*Chapter 9*).

Calcium Antagonists in Experimental Ischemia and Infarction

There are many conflicting results about the use of Ca^{2+} antagonists in experimental ischemia or infarction. Many different preparations, doses, and varieties of Ca^{2+} antagonists have been used, as summarized by de Leiris et al. (*Chapter 10*). In the majority of cases, favorable effects are claimed (see also J. Willerson et al., *Chapter 24*) especially when the drug is given before the onset of ischemia. The proposed mechanisms of benefit are complex and may include an increased coronary blood flow or a decreased myocardial oxygen demand. Hugenholtz et al. (*Chapter 23*) proposed a "direct" antiischemic effect to maintain high-energy phosphate levels. The thoughtful chapter by Hearse (*Chapter 12*) points out that most interventions designed to decrease ischemic injury or the size of infarction may purely delay the whole process; quite possibly reperfusion by thrombolysis or other means is required to make a real difference to ultimate infarct size.

PHARMACOLOGY OF CALCIUM ANTAGONISTS

Sarcolemmal Binding Sites

Ca^{2+} antagonists, first developed by Fleckenstein, are a heterogeneous group of agents which potentially inhibit Ca^{2+}-dependent processes and regulatory mechanisms (A. Fleckenstein, *Chapter 2;* W. Nayler et al., *Chapter 17;* C. Cohen et al., *Chapter 14*). Theoretically, the Ca^{2+} channel inhibitors (slow-channel blockers) are specific subtypes of Ca^{2+} antagonists whose major site of action is to decrease Ca^{2+} influx through the slow Ca^{2+} channel; this inhibition of the Ca^{2+} channel has been recognized as the major site of action of Ca^{2+} antagonists for over 12 years (A. Fleckenstein, *Chapter 2*). Two types of sarcolemmal binding sites have been identified. First, the dihydropyridine site should bind nifedipine, but for technical reasons the related compound nitrendipine is usually used. Second, the other Ca^{2+} channel antagonists, such as verapamil and diltiazem, bind to another spatially separated ("allosteric") site to modify the dihydropyridine site. This dihydropyridine binding site may be near the Ca^{2+} channel or part of it. To explain different effects of different Ca^{2+} antagonists on various vascular beds and on nodal as opposed to myocardial contractile tissue, some investigators suggest that these drugs bind with different affinities to several populations of Ca^{2+} channels. Alternatively, the properties of one type of Ca^{2+} channel may be regulated differently by allosteric influences— the latter idea resembles the modulated receptor hypothesis proposed for the Na^+ channel.

Structural-Activity Relationships

The verapamil group of Ca^{2+} antagonists, structurally characterized by an aryl ring connected to an alkylamino or aralkylamino group, includes verapamil, diltiazem, cinnarizine, and tiapamil (H. Meyer, *Chapter 15*). This group probably binds to one type of site, sometimes identified by ^3H-cinnarizine. Both verapamil and diltiazem have stereoselectivity. A second ("nifedipine") group of Ca^{2+} antagonists includes the 1,4 dihydropyridines which probably bind to another site, identified by ^3H-nitrendipine. This second group, completely different in structure from the verapamil group, includes nicardipine, nitrendipine, nimodipine, nisoldipine, and felodipine. A third and very new type of Ca^{2+} antagonist, KB-944, resembles diltiazem from the pharmacological point of view, but has an aralkyl phosphonate group (H. Meyer, *Chapter 15*).

Calcium Antagonists Versus β-Blockade

At a cellular level, there are marked differences between the effects of β-adrenergic blockade and Ca^{2+} antagonists on the vascular smooth muscle, where β-blockade tends to vasoconstrict and Ca^{2+} antagonists to relax. In the case of the myocardium, however, a common property is shared—that of reducing Ca^{2+} influx by the slow channel (W. Nayler et al., *Chapter 17*). This the Ca^{2+} antagonists do directly by closing the number of slow channels (H. Reuter, *Chapter 4*), and the β-antagonists indirectly by decreasing the phosphorylation of a protein which is hypothetically involved with slow-channel control. In clinically relevant doses the chief Ca^{2+} antagonist drugs have their therapeutic effect without a negative inotropic effect, whereas in the case of β-blockade, the negative inotropic effect is an integrated part of the antianginal mechanism (L. Jee and L. Opie, *Chapter 32*).

α-Adrenoceptors and Calcium

The role of the β-adrenoceptor antagonists in the regulation of Ca^{2+} ion entry by the slow channel is well established (N. Sperelakis, *Chapter 26*). In contrast are the novel findings of Corr and Sharma (*Chapter 18*). They propose that myocardial α_1-receptors, which are increased in density in ischemia, act to enhance Ca^{2+} ion entry into ischemic cells and, thereby, help promote malignant arrhythmias. Experimentally, α_1 blockers, such as prazosin or labetalol (combined α_1-β-blockade), prevent such arrhythmias. Some Ca^{2+} antagonists, such as verapamil, have α-antagonist activity, which might explain in part their effect against ventricular arrhythmias found in some studies.

CALCIUM ANTAGONISTS FOR ISCHEMIC HEART DISEASE

The initial use of verapamil was for angina pectoris; thereafter, the powerful inhibitory effect on supraventricular tachycardias was ascribed to inhibition of

Ca^{2+}-dependent conduction through the atrioventricular node. Nifedipine, also originally introduced for angina pectoris, turned out to have powerful antihypertensive effects (see C. Rosendorff, *Chapter 30;* and L. Opie and L. Jee, *Chapter 31*). Diltiazem more closely resembles verapamil than nifedipine. In clinical practice, all three agents exert their pharmacological effects at dose ranges which do not depress the myocardium and may even improve myocardial infarction (in part through an unloading mechanism; in part from a "direct" myocardial mechanism). Very new experimental uses, proposed by Fleckenstein (*Chapter 2*) are in the prevention of (a) the calcinosis accompanying arterial disease, and (b) cataracts in the lens of the eye.

Coronary Artery Spasm

As originally described by Prinzmetal, typical variant angina may occur at the side of an atheromatous lesion of a large coronary artery. Yasue (*Chapter 11*) shows there is a marked circadian rhythm in the susceptibility to coronary artery spasm, with most attacks occurring at night or in the early morning— possibly as result of the high blood pH at night which, in turn, may induce an increase in the ionized serum Ca^{2+} to provoke attacks. Ca^{2+} antagonists (including diltiazem, nifedipine, verapamil) all inhibit these attacks, whereas β-blockade by propranolol is ineffective—and may be harmful (P. Hugenholtz et al., *Chapter 23*). At present, the best procedure for management of coronary artery spasm is the combination of nitrates and a Ca^{2+} antagonist. Thus, Conti et al. (*Chapter 25*) advise isosorbide dinitrate and nifedipine, each 10 to 30 mg 6-hourly.

Angina at Rest

Besides being more effective than β-adrenergic blockade in the therapy of variant angina, Ca^{2+} antagonists may also be better therapy in some patients with angina at rest (P. Hugenholtz et al., *Chapter 23*). Maseri (*Chapter 21*) has shown that β-blockade is ineffective and Ca^{2+} antagonism very effective when angina at rest is spasm-provoked. Spasm may contribute to the development of angina at rest, especially at night (H. Yasue, *Chapter 11*).

Because of the variable contribution of coronary spasm to unstable angina at rest, this potentially serious condition may not benefit from the "classic" therapy of nitrates and β-blockade. Hence Ca^{2+} antagonists are now increasingly added (P. Hugenholtz et al., *Chapter 23*) with apparently beneficial effects; large scale trials are, at present, comparing β-blockade with Ca^{2+} antagonists in unstable angina at rest.

A further extension of the concept of spasm is in the clarification of exercise-induced ST elevation (H. Yasue, *Chapter 11;* L. Jee and L. Opie, *Chapter 32*). Here, too, β-blockade is ineffective in contrast to Ca^{2+} antagonists. A novel proposal is that varying degrees of spasm play a role in determining the different and variable levels of exercise which provoke angina in some patients.

Stable Angina of Effort

Initially it was thought that Ca^{2+} antagonists aided angina of effort by unloading the heart, as a result of peripheral vasodilation. Lichtlen et al. (*Chapter 22*) show two further important effects: an increase of poststenotic coronary flow and actual relief of the previous coronary obstruction of the eccentric variety, where nifedipine has an effect similar to that of nitrates and where the effects of the two agents appear to be additive. Hence, Ca^{2+} antagonists are effective in most patients with stable angina of effort.

Calcium Antagonists and Atheroma: A Future Clinical Indication?

Recently, the logical proposition has been made that Ca^{2+} deposition is an important aspect of severe atherosclerosis; the Ca^{2+} antagonists can, therefore, be expected to be antiatherogenic agents. Experimentally, the data are convincing (A. Fleckenstein, *Chapter 2;* P. Henry, *Chapter 20*); clinically, the appropriate trials must be undertaken although such trials "have proved difficult in the past" (P. Henry, *Chapter 20*).

ARRHYTHMIAS

Slow-response action potentials are Ca^{2+}-dependent which may arise in ischemic tissue to initiate reentrant ventricular arrhythmias (N. Sperelakis, *Chapter 26*). Such action potentials are dependent on open slow channels, the number of which are, in turn, increased by agents elevating intracellular cyclic AMP such as β-agonists. According to the Sperelakis model (*Chapter 26*), cyclic AMP may phosphorylate a membrane protein constituent of the slow channel to make it available for voltage activation. This constituent is calciductin, according to Demaille's group. The voltage required for slow-channel activation is above -35 mV, compared with -55 mV for fast Na^+ channels. Slow responses also conduct slowly. Slow responses may be inhibited in severely ischemic cells by marked acidosis, rundown of ATP, and by a very high extracellular K^+. Hence, if slow responses play a role in ischemic ventricular fibrillation, then it may be expected that Ca^{2+} antagonists would not be active against ventricular arrhythmias arising in severely ischemic tissue (see also L. Opie et al. *Chapter 28*).

Another reason for ineffectiveness of Ca^{2+} antagonists in some models may be that the slow action potentials in ischemic tissue are not a "pure" slow action potential, but rather fast Na^+ channels whose activity is depressed. Clusin et al. (*Chapter 27*), however, propose that an ischemia-induced intracellular Ca^{2+} overload causes its arrhythmogenic effects by (a) shortening the action potential duration, and (b) ischemic depolarization.

Despite the encouraging data of Clusin et al. (*Chapter 27*), Ca^{2+} antagonists have not yet been recognized as agents effective against ventricular arrhythmias possibly because only some mechanisms of ventricular fibrillation are Ca^{2+}-dependent (L. Opie et al., *Chapter 28*). Rather, the prime antiarrhythmic qualities of the Ca^{2+} antagonists lie in the effectiveness of verapamil and diltiazem in supraventricular arrhythmias (acting by inhibition of excessively fast circus conduction through the atrioventricular node). In addition, all Ca^{2+} antagonists should relieve ventricular arrhythmias caused by severe coronary spasm.

HYPERTENSION

The marked effect of the Ca^{2+} antagonist, nifedipine, on arterial vascular smooth muscle, and the important role of Ca^{2+} ions in the contractile mechanism of vascular smooth muscle, makes nifedipine an important antihypertensive agent (C. Rosendorff, *Chapter 30*). Besides acute reduction of blood pressure, nifedipine has a sustained antihypertensive effect so that Opie and Jee (*Chapter 31*) use nifedipine as standard therapy for apparently refractory hypertension—with an almost uniformly satisfactory response. Part of the benefit of nifedipine may be a capacity to promote salt and water excretion while leaving K^+ excretion unchanged (R. Krebs, *Chapter 33*). Hence, Opie and Jee (*Chapter 31*) argue for "expanding indications in hypertension" suggesting that Ca^{2+} antagonists, such as nifedipine, are well on the way to becoming a standard vasodilator therapy, displacing hydralazine. Ca^{2+} antagonists have fewer contraindications that β-adrenergic blockade. Bühler et al. (*Chapter 29*) show a specific benefit of Ca^{2+} antagonism by verapamil (and nifedipine) in elderly patients, in whom there is a Ca^{2+} influx-dependent peripheral vasoconstriction. Bühler et al. find the best response to verapamil in elderly patients with a low plasma renin— the group which is less likely to respond to β-adrenergic blockade. Ca^{2+} antagonists normalize blood pressure in at least one-third of patients with essential hypertension.

FUTURE PERSPECTIVES

Ever-expanding indications for Ca^{2+} antagonists are prophesied by Krebs (*Chapter 33*) and Schwartz (*Chapter 34*). Cardiovascular indications currently under investigation include myocardial infarction, ventricular arrhythmias, congestive heart failure, pulmonary hypertension, cardioplegia, atherogenesis, hypertrophic cardiomyopathy, aortic insufficiency, cerebral stroke, and Raynaud's disease. In most cases, the results are sufficiently promising to warrant further clinical exploration. Krebs prophesizes not only new indications, but more tissue-specific Ca^{2+} antagonists—for example, nimodipine acts more specifically on the cerebral circulation, and nisoldipine resembles nifedipine, but also acts on venous smooth muscle. No wonder that Schwartz (*Chapter 34*) predicts that "calcium antagonists will dominate cerebrovascular pharmacology and perhaps other areas of pharmacology for years to come."

Calcium Antagonists and Cardiovascular Disease, edited by L. H. Opie.
Raven Press, New York © 1984.

Chapter 2

Calcium Antagonism: History and Prospects for a Multifaceted Pharmacodynamic Principle

A. Fleckenstein

*Physiologisches Institut, Albert-Ludwigs-Universität,
D-7800 Freiburg, Federal Republic of Germany*

PHYSIOLOGICAL AND BIOCHEMICAL BACKGROUND

The decisive role of Ca^{2+} in sustaining myocardial contractility was first appreciated 100 years ago by Sidney Ringer in 1882 (58). He found that Ca^{2+}-free saline leads to cardiac arrest of isolated frog hearts. As reported later by Mines (53) in 1913, Ca^{2+} withdrawal primarily impairs mechanical performance, whereas the bioelectric process of ventricular excitation may persist. Overwhelming evidence has accumulated in the past two decades, indicating that Ca^{2+} ions are required for the activation of the key-enzyme in contractile energy expenditure, i.e., myofibrillar ATPase. Excitation of the myocardial sarcolemma membrane produces a sudden influx of free Ca^{2+} ions from the extracellular space into the interior of the fibers. Simultaneously, further "activator Ca^{2+}" is released from intracellular stores. In this way, the Ca^{2+} ions act as mediators in excitation-contraction coupling between the Na^{+}-dependent bioelectric events at the fiber surface, and the Ca^{2+}-dependent intracellular processes that transform phosphate-bond energy into mechanical work. Therefore, contractility is reversibly lost upon withdrawal of extracellular Ca^{2+}.

As we have shown in studies on isolated rabbit auricles (59), the Ca^{2+}-deficient myocardium exhibits a striking insufficiency in utilizing its high-energy phosphate compounds during the state of excitation. But, after addition of Ca^{2+}, high-energy phosphate consumption is normalized. If, on the other hand, the extracellular Ca^{2+} concentration is increased above normal, more Ca^{2+} is taken up by the beating heart so that both splitting of high-energy phosphates and contractility are potentiated. In fact, Ca^{2+} ions not only trigger the contractile process, but also quantitatively control the output of mechanical tension by regulating the amount of ATP that is metabolized during activity.

The splitting of ATP will, in turn, give rise to intensified glycolytic and oxidative recovery processes which have to refill, thereafter, the high-energy phosphate stores. This explains why the whole chain of metabolic reactions following contraction is "Ca^{2+}-sensitive." Thus, alterations in transmembrane Ca^{2+} supply generally lead to parallel changes in the following three parameters: (a) the amount of ATP consumed by the contractile system, (b) the magnitude of mechanical tension developed, and (c) the extra-uptake of O_2 related to the contractile force generated (3,7,59). Moreover, it became clear in this context that many substances with a positive or negative inotropic effect on heart muscle are acting as promoters or inhibitors of the Ca^{2+} function in excitation-contraction coupling. For instance, β-receptor stimulation by sympathomimetic catecholamines, such as epinephrine, norepinephrine, or isoproterenol, facilitates the transmembrane Ca^{2+} influx during excitation. Therefore, Ca^{2+}-dependent splitting of ATP and contractile force are augmented. Also, under the influence of cardiac glycosides, more Ca^{2+} is made available for myofibrillar activation. Conversely, negative inotropism ensues from all drugs that restrict the access of Ca^{2+} to the contractile myofilaments by interference with transsarcolemmal Ca^{2+} uptake.

IDENTIFICATION OF CALCIUM-ANTAGONISTIC DRUGS ON HEART MUSCLE

Preliminary Investigations

Electrophysiological and biochemical evidence that a number of drugs can mimic the effects of simple Ca^{2+} withdrawal on isolated mammalian myocardium and intact hearts *in situ* was presented by Fleckenstein (8). That report was based on observations obtained with two new compounds, namely Isoptin (iproveratril, later given the generic name verapamil), and Segontin (prenylamine), as well as studies with high concentrations of certain adrenergic β-receptor blocking agents (propranolol, pronethalol, dichloroisoproterenol) or of barbituric acid derivatives. Under appropriate experimental conditions all these substances did the following: (a) they diminished contractile force without a major change in the action potential; (b) reduced the utilization of high-energy-phosphate compounds by the contractile system; (c) lowered extra O_2 consumption during contractile activity; and (d) lost their potency after administration of additional Ca^{2+}, β-adrenergic catecholamines, or cardiac glycosides, that is, following interventions that were designed to restore the Ca^{2+} supply to the contractile system.

These observations led us to suppose that the negative inotropic action of these drugs might predominantly consist of an interference with the mediator function of Ca^{2+} in excitation-contraction coupling of heart muscle.

To further clarify the pertinent problems, our investigations were primarily advanced in two directions (9,10,16,17,26,34). First, *it appeared necessary to distinguish the negative inotropic drug actions that were due to Ca^{2+} antagonism from those produced by β-receptor blockade.* Second, it seemed reasonable to search for more drugs that exert Ca^{2+} antagonism, not only as a side-effect, but also in a specific form. As to the differentiation of Ca^{2+} antagonism from β-blockade, it was, in fact, not difficult to show that the effective doses of propranolol, pronethalol, or dichloroisoproterenol (that directly inhibited Ca^{2+}-dependent excitation-contraction coupling of guinea pig hearts) were roughly 10 times greater than those needed for β-receptor blockade.

Accordingly, contractile function returned rapidly to normal upon administration of an extra dose of $CaCl_2$, whereas the β-blockade persisted. On the other hand, some highly potent β-receptor blocking agents, such as pindolol, oxprenolol, and sotalol, proved to be unable to produce cardiac contractile failure because they did not exert an appreciable Ca^{2+}-antagonistic action. Thus, the ability of directly interrupting Ca^{2+}-dependent excitation-contraction coupling of heart muscle certainly had nothing to do with β-receptor blockade.

Also, in our experiments with barbiturates, Ca^{2+} antagonism turned out to be a genuine pharmacodynamic principle. Earlier investigations of other researchers had already established that cardiac contractile incompetence produced by high doses of barbiturates exhibited criteria typical of Ca^{2+} antagonism, according to present knowledge. This applied particularly (a) to the selective depression of cardiac contractility by barbiturates without a loss of electric excitability (50), (b) to the high myocardial ATP and creatine phosphate contents at the climax of barbiturate-induced contractile failure (4,6,67), and (c) to the easy restitution of contractile force by cardiac glycosides (49,50,60) or epinephrine, even in the presence of high barbiturate concentrations. But these earlier researchers abstained from any explanation. Thus, the new concept of Ca^{2+} antagonism provided the first reasonable basis for the understanding of these scattered, old findings.

Discovery of Specific Calcium Antagonists

The decisive insight, however, into Ca^{2+} antagonism as a new pharmacodynamic principle resulted from the analysis of the mechanism of action of such compounds that, according to our observations, are capable of blocking excitation-contraction coupling specifically. "Specifically" means that in the scope of their actions the Ca^{2+}-antagonistic properties distinctly prevail. Prenylamine (Segontin) and verapamil (Isoptin) were the first drugs of this type that attracted our interest beginning in 1964. Prenylamine was still relatively weak and of modest specificity. Nevertheless, increasing doses of prenylamine inhibited Ca^{2+}-dependent excitation-contraction coupling of isolated papillary muscles from the hearts of rabbits, cats, guinea pigs, and rhesus monkeys by 50 to 70% before the Na^+-dependent excitatory process was also considerably affected (8,18,26). However, the Ca^{2+}-antagonistic action of verapamil, in comparison with that of prenylamine, proved to be of higher potency and selectivity. In fact, verapamil could completely suppress the contractile function of the isolated myocardium without a major alteration of action potential (9,10).

In 1968, Dr. Ferdinand Dengel, chief chemist of the Knoll Company, asked me to test a methoxy-derivative of verapamil. The new substance turned out to be much stronger than verapamil on both myocardium and smooth muscle, since myocardial contractility of guinea pig papillary muscles could totally be abolished by a concentration as low as 1×10^{-6} M. This methoxy-derivative of verapamil was the 600th compound Dr. Dengel had synthesized and so was named D 600. The more recent generic name is gallopamil. There is a powerful linear depression by D 600 of isometric tension development and extra O_2 consumption (due to mechanical activity).

One year later, in 1969, Professor Kroneberg, leading pharmacologist of the Bayer company at Elberfeld, handed me two other new compounds that carried only the labels "Bay a 1040" and "Bay a 7168." Both compounds were strong coronary vasodilators, according to pharmacological screening tests, and exerted significant negative inotropic effects on the myocardium. Kroneberg asked me to clarify the mechanism of action of these compounds which appeared to be similar to that of verapamil and D 600. This was, in fact, true (12,20,24,27,30). The drugs Bay a 1040 and Bay a 7168 are 1,4-dihydropyridine derivatives, and were later given the generic names nifedipine (Adalat) and niludipine, respectively. But the chemical formulas were kept secret for more than 3 years. Figure 1 shows an experiment with increasing concentrations of nifedipine. With 1 mg nifedipine/liter, Ca^{2+}-dependent contractility could totally be abolished. In the upper curve, the Na^+-dependent maximal upstroke velocity of action poten-

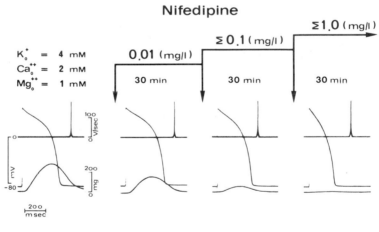

FIG. 1. Complete excitation-contraction uncoupling of a guinea pig papillary muscle by a stepwise increase of the nifedipine concentration in normal Tyrode's solution from 0.01 to 0.1 and, finally, 1 mg/liter: Whereas isometric tension development was totally suppressed, the upstroke velocity of the action potentials (dV/dt_{max} = 175 V/sec) indicating the fast Na^+ influx, did not change. The same was true of the height of the Na^+-dependent overshoot. Potentials were measured with an intracellular microelectrode of conventional type. Isometric tensions were recorded with a mechanoelectric transducer valve.

tial (dV/dt_{max}) was directly recorded. This Na^+-dependent parameter was obviously not affected by nifedipine, since the rate of upstroke remained at a steady level of about 190 V/sec. Eventually, in 1969, on the basis of these findings on heart muscle, we felt sufficiently entitled to emphasize the existence of a distinct pharmacological group of highly potent inhibitors of excitation-contraction coupling and to designate the members of this new family, with respect to their common mechanism of action, as *calcium antagonists* (14,15,26, 28). Simultaneously, it was shown that Ca^{2+} antagonists, as a further criterion, were also capable of affecting, in very low concentrations, Ca^{2+}-dependent excitation-contraction coupling of uterine and vascular smooth muscle (35,38). *Thus, we proposed, as a definition, that a specific Ca^{2+} antagonist is a substance which so predominantly exerts its inhibitory effects upon the Ca^{2+}-dependent functions in mammalian myocardium and smooth muscle that, in this dosage range, all other pharmacodynamic properties are more or less negligible.*

Although it was clear from these studies that the Ca^{2+} antagonists restrict the Ca^{2+} supply to the active myocardium, the exact site of action remained, until 1969, a matter of speculation. However, in this year, when methods became available that allowed the measurement of the transsarcolemmal Na^+ and Ca^{2+} currents independently of each other, the main problem to be examined was whether the Ca^{2+} antagonists specifically interfere with the slow transsarcolemmal inward Ca^{2+} current. The electrical device used in our experiments corresponded to the classical sucrose gap technique (39,62). The separation of the transmembrane Na^+ and Ca^{2+} currents was done by the voltage-clamp technique (57). The results of our studies are generally known: The slow transmembrane Ca^{2+} current was selectively suppressed by verapamil and D 600 (12,47), and the same was later shown also for nifedipine (48). On the other hand, there was no influence on the fast-channel-mediated transmembrane Na^+ influx that produces the action potential upstroke. With these findings, we delivered, in the years 1970 to 1972, the experimental basis for the term *slow-channel blocker* or *Ca^{2+} entry blocker*. It became clear from our electrophysiological data and from concomitant studies with labeled Ca^{2+} that the Ca^{2+} antagonists specifically restrict the influx of Ca^{2+} through the transmembrane Ca^{2+} channel. Our first comprehensive report on the basic principle of Ca^{2+} antagonism, as exemplified with prenylamine, verapamil, D 600, and nifedipine (Bay a 1040), was presented at a meeting of the European Section of the International Study Group for Research in Cardiac Metabolism in London in 1970. The proceedings appeared in 1971 in a volume entitled *Calcium and the Heart* (12). It was due to this publication that the Ca^{2+} antagonists aroused international interest for the first time. The fact that the Ca^{2+}-antagonistic action of these drugs is a consequence of inhibition of Ca^{2+} entry has been well known for over 12 years. Therefore, it is misleading to connect the impression of more recent scientific achievements with the synonym "Ca^{2+} entry blocker."

There has been a rapid numerical growth of the new drug family since 1970. We should like to divide these Ca^{2+} antagonists into two subgroups: Group A comprises the Ca^{2+} antagonists of outstanding efficacy and specificity such as verapamil, D 600, nifedipine, niludipine, nimodipine, and diltiazem. The substances of group A are capable of inhibiting Ca^{2+}-dependent excitation-contraction coupling of the mammalian ventricular myocardium by 90 to 100%, before the fast Na^+ influx during the rising phase of action potential is also affected (Fig. 1). Moreover, they do not interfere with electrogenic Mg^{2+} effects. Group B, on the other hand, includes prenylamine, fendiline, terodiline, perhexiline (and caroverine), which are somewhat less potent and specific. This means that under their influence a concomitant inhibition of the Na^+-dependent excitatory process can be seen when Ca^{2+}-dependent contractile tension development of isolated papillary muscles has been reduced by 50 to 70%. Interestingly enough, the substances of group B also interfere with Mg^{2+}-induced bioelectric phenomena in the myocardium.

Final evidence for the specific Ca^{2+}-antagonistic actions of the different compounds listed above was first presented in the following references: verapamil (9,10,12,26,28); D 600 (12,28); nifedipine (12,24,27,30,35); and niludipine (20).

CALCIUM-ANTAGONIST ACTIONS ON VASCULAR SMOOTH MUSCLE

In the period 1968 to 1969, it was also found that excitation-contraction coupling of intestinal and, particularly, of vascular smooth muscle cells was highly susceptible to the action of Ca^{2+} antagonists (23,25,36,37,40). Thus we proposed that, here again, the transmembrane Ca^{2+} conductivity is inhibited, since all Ca^{2+}-dependent contractile phenomena such as vascular tone and spastic vasoconstriction could be suppressed even with very small doses. Coronary smooth muscle exhibited the highest sensitivity to the spasmolytic action of Ca^{2+} antagonists (35), nifedipine being the most potent coronary relaxant. The fundamental coronary action of Ca^{2+} antagonists, namely excitation-contraction uncoupling, could be demonstrated most clearly on K^+-depolarized preparations (Fig. 2). Ca^{2+} antagonists also exerted outstanding vasodilator effects on peripheral resistance vessels as, for instance, in perfused isolated rabbit ears (35). Nifedipine was again the strongest Ca^{2+}-antagonistic vasodilator. However, addition of extra Ca^{2+} to the perfusion fluid in the presence of a Ca^{2+} antagonist restored, or even overcompensated, vascular tone immediately.

CELLULAR CARDIOPROTECTION BY CALCIUM ANTAGONISTS

According to the scheme of Fig. 3, heart muscle fibers undergo severe functional and structural alterations, finally resulting in necrotization, as soon as free Ca^{2+} ions penetrate excessively through the sarcolemma membrane into the myoplasm, so that the capacities of the Ca^{2+}-binding or extrusion processes are overpowered (11,12). The crucial event in the development of such lesions is high-energy phosphate deficiency, which results from (a) excessive activation

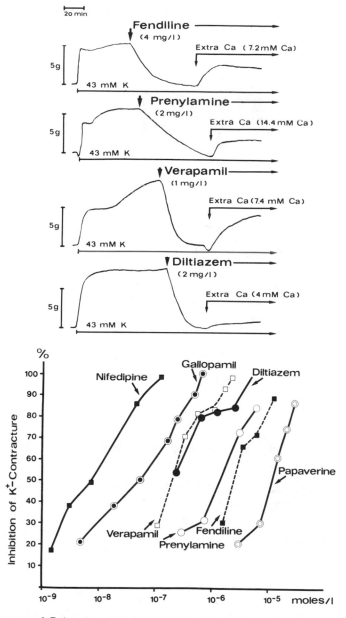

FIG. 2. Upper panel: Relaxation of K⁺-depolarized pig coronary strips by different Ca²⁺ antagonists. Partial restitution of contractile tension by additional Ca²⁺ at the end of the experiments. **Lower panel:** Comparison of the relaxing potencies of different Ca²⁺ antagonists, administered to K⁺-depolarized, contractured pig coronary strips. In these experiments, the time of exposure to the K⁺-rich (43 mM KCl) Tyrode's solution was kept constant (40 min). Then the Ca²⁺ antagonists were added and the maximum relaxation, reached within 1 hr, measured. In comparison with the coronary relaxing potency of papaverine, nifedipine is approximately 3,000 times, verapamil and diltiazem 50 to 100 times stronger. Each *point* represents the average relaxation calculated from at least 15 individual experiments for each concentration, SE not exceeding ± 2%. Ca²⁺ content always 1 mM; temperature: 35°C; pH: 7.4; oxygenation with a gas mixture of 97% O₂ and 3% CO₂. (From refs. 13, 14, 26a, and 35.)

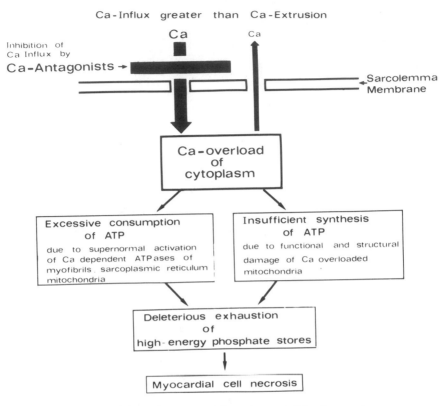

FIG. 3. Schematic representation of myocardial cell necrosis.

of Ca²⁺-dependent intracellular ATPases, and (b) Ca²⁺-induced impairment of the mitochondria that manifests itself as swelling, vacuolization, cristolysis, and loss of respiratory control and phosphorylation capacity.

Hence, we emphasized in 1968 the significance of myocardial Ca²⁺ overload as a new principle in cardiac pathophysiology and simultaneously demonstrated that development of necrosis could be totally prevented with the help of Ca²⁺ antagonists that counteracted the effects of excessive myocardial Ca²⁺ (Fig. 4). Sympathetic overstimulation, overdoses of vitamin D or dihydrotachysterol, as well as alimentary K⁺ and Mg²⁺ deficiency, also produced structural decay of myocardial tissue by this pathogenic mechanism. (For more details see refs. 12,15, and 22.) The same is true of cardiac ventricular lesions in hereditary cardiomyopathic hamsters. Here, too, an abundant incorporation of Ca²⁺ precedes the onset of myocardial necrosis (51,52). Therefore, in all these cases, Ca²⁺ antagonists minimized excessive Ca²⁺ uptake (Fig. 3) and high-energy phosphate breakdown, thereby preserving structural integrity. Ca²⁺ overload also proved to be responsible, to a significant extent, for the impairment of the mitochondria in anoxic or ischemic cardiac tissue, according to more recent

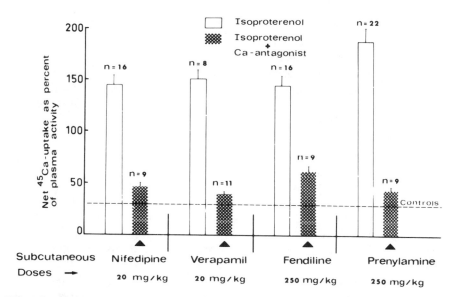

FIG. 4. Prevention of isoproterenol-induced right ventricular $^{45}Ca^{2+}$ overload in rats by different Ca^{2+} antagonists. All animals received a single subcutaneous dose of 30 mg isoproterenol/kg with or without the Ca^{2+} antagonists, applied at different injection sites. The radioactivity measurements were carried out 6 hr after i.p. administration of 10 μCi $^{45}Ca^{2+}$/kg body wt.

studies of other laboratories. Thus Ca^{2+} antagonists such as verapamil, nifedipine, or diltiazem could even protect hypoxic and ischemic hearts against additional Ca^{2+}-induced myocardial fiber damage that would otherwise precipitate structural disintegration (1,44,54,55,65).

CAN CALCIUM ANTAGONISTS PROVIDE PROTECTION AGAINST ARTERIAL CALCINOSIS IN VASCULAR SENESCENCE?

Admittedly, the present survey of Ca^{2+} antagonism is of limited scope and primarily concentrates on the physiological and pathophysiological roots. Thus, this report does not deal with the important implications of Ca^{2+} antagonism in clinical therapy. A comprehensive clinical review has recently been presented by Opie (56). Moreover, the present chapter omits a discussion of the interesting bioelectric effects of Ca^{2+} antagonists on normal and ectopic cardiac pacemakers. To be clarified in the future is the problem of vascular protection by Ca^{2+} antagonists against natural age-induced or premature arterial calcinosis.

Spontaneous Calcification of Aging Arteries

It is a well known fact that the arterial walls altered by sclerotic processes contain two main constituents, namely lipids, particularly cholesterol, and Ca^{2+}. However, it is rather puzzling that for many years only the lipid accumulation has been incriminated as a primary pathogenetic factor, whereas the concomitant calcinosis is generally considered a phenomenon of secondary importance. Thus, there is a striking numerical discrepancy between the nearly uncountable publications concerned with disturbances in arterial lipid content, and the scarce papers that refer to the pathophysiology of arterial Ca^{2+} metabolism. Calcinosis, whether symptomatic or not, appears to be an inevitable consequence of advanced age. This became particularly clear from our studies on age-dependent changes in Ca^{2+} and Mg^{2+} content of the human arterial walls. The investigation was carried out on *normal* tissue specimens that originated from 144 autopsies, mostly forensic, covering the whole life span from 1 to 90 years. The test arteries analyzed with atom absorption spectrometry were (a) the descending branch of the left coronary artery ($n = 86$), (b) the superior mesenteric artery ($n = 134$), and (c) the aorta ($n = 141$ autopsies). All artery segments with visible plaques were discarded.

The aging process of human arteries is reflected in a dramatic augmentation of their Ca^{2+} content (Fig. 5). Thus, in 81- to 90-year-old humans, the absolute amounts of arterial Ca^{2+} (mmoles Ca^{2+}/kg dry tissue) were about 7 times (coronary artery), 20 times (mesenteric artery), and nearly 100 times (aorta) higher than those in the corresponding infantile arteries, aged 0 to 10 years. In surprising contrast with the arterial walls, the myocardial fibers are exempt from any age-induced change in absolute Ca^{2+} content or Ca^{2+}/Mg^{2+} ratio: Thus 122 papillary muscles excised together with the arterial specimens from the same autopsies had a Mg^{2+} content which was always twice- to fourfold that of Ca^{2+}, regardless of whether at 10 or 90 years.

In a study on 35 dogs over an age-span of 16 years, we found a similar increase in Ca^{2+} content of the arterial walls as in humans; the Mg^{2+} concentra-

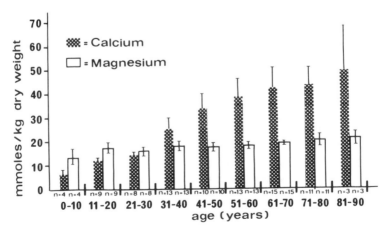

FIG. 5. Progressive arterial Ca^{2+} overload and increase in the ratio Ca^{2+}/Mg^+ with advanced age. Tissue samples were taken from the descending branch of the left human coronary artery ($n = 86$). The arteries mostly originated from autopsies on traffic victims. Only artery segments without visible plaques were analyzed using atom absorption spectrometry. (From refs. 21 and 31.)

tion remained again unchanged. Old dogs of an age of 13 to 16 years had about five times more Ca^{2+} in their coronary walls than the young animals did. In contrast to the ventricular myocardium of dogs, there was again no age-dependent change in the Ca^{2+} or Mg^{2+} contents. In all dog hearts, we found about 10 times more Mg^{2+} than Ca^{2+}.

Our results suggest that the steady rise in arterial Ca^{2+} content during lifetime is not only a most characteristic criterion of age, but also represents the decisive, inherent risk factor which predisposes senescent arteries to arteriosclerotic degeneration. Apart from augmentation of wall cholesterol, progressive Ca^{2+} overload appears to be the most important latent precursor of overt arteriosclerosis of aging arteries (21,22,31).

Prevention by Calcium Antagonists of Experimental Arterial Calcinosis Induced by Dihydrotachysterol or Vitamin D

Ca^{2+} antagonists have hitherto been used in vascular therapy for acute functional vasodilation and spasmolytic purposes. However, in the present context, it is a question of much greater medical significance whether these drugs are also capable of providing long-term protection of the arterial wall against Ca^{2+} overload and its severe consequences on structural integrity. This would mean that the Ca^{2+} antagonists do not only afford symptomatic improvement, but also interfere with the fundamental pathogenetic process of arterial calcinosis. To approach this problem experimentally, we have studied the influence of Ca^{2+} antagonists on vascular Ca^{2+} uptake in disease models in rats.

The easiest way of producing tremendous degrees of calcinosis of the arterial media within a few days consists of the administration of overdoses of dihydrotachysterol (AT 10) or vitamin D_3. These experimental vascular alterations are quite similar to Mönckeberg's type of calcifying arteriosclerosis in humans (5,42,45,61). As pointed out by Herzenberg (45), the process of media calcification particularly affects the smooth muscle cells and the elastic fibers. In Herzenberg's experiments on vitamin D-intoxicated rats, calcification of cardiac cells and arterial smooth muscle was always so intimately associated with degenerative processes that it appeared impossible to find out whether calcification or, alternatively, necrosis formation had to be considered the primary event. However, in the light of our present knowledge of Ca^{2+} overload as a causative factor in cellular disintegration, it was reasonable to assume that, also in experimental Mönckeberg sclerosis, histological damage ensues from abundant Ca^{2+}.

It was, in fact, not difficult to show that the background of experimental Mönckeberg sclerosis is an enormous intensification of Ca^{2+} uptake into the arterial walls (46).

The electron microscopic appearance of arteries from the vitamin D_3-treated animals was characterized by two morphological alterations, particularly of the media (5): cellular destruction, elastic fiber breakdown, and formation of extracellular and intracellular Ca^{2+} deposits of amorphous or crystalline structure.

The efficacy of certain Ca^{2+} antagonists, such as *prenylamine* and *verapamil*, in preventing experimental vascular Ca^{2+} overload was first shown on rats pre-treated with dihydrotachysterol and monosodium phosphate (46). However, the most impressive results were later obtained with *verapamil* in vitamin D_3-injected rats. Figure 6 (**top**) demonstrates the depression of the radiocalcium uptake rates by *verapamil,* whereas Fig. 6 (**bottom**) shows the prevention of the rise in absolute Ca^{2+} content of the aortic and mesenteric walls. The tremendous efficacy of *diltiazem* in inhibiting vitamin D_3-induced coronary calcinosis can be seen from Fig. 7**A.** Here, under the influence of vitamin D_3 alone, the Ca^{2+} content of the coronary wall tissue of rats rose from 12 to 220 mmoles/kg dry tissue wt. But with diltiazem, the effect of vitamin D_3 was completely neutralized. To visualize the prevention of experimental coronary calcinosis by Ca^{2+} antagonists, we also made use of histochemical techniques, particularly v. Kossa's stain for tissue calcium. In the presence of diltiazem, the coronary wall tissue is shielded from Ca^{2+} overload, and therefore remains completely intact. The anticalcinotic action of diltiazem is not restricted to the coronary vasculature. In fact, the coronary, cerebral, renal (Fig. 7**B**), mesenteric, and aortic arterial walls are similarly protected by the prophylactic diltiazem treatment. Previous investigations of other researchers (41–43,64) on rabbits and rhesus monkeys have shown that even small doses of vitamin D can produce progressive arteriosclerosis, arteritis, and thrombosis if combined with administration of nicotine and a cholesterol-rich diet. In the opinion of these authors, the uncontrolled intake of vitamin D_3 in men might even constitute one of the *"most important pathogenetic factors in human atherosclerosis."* Regardless of whether or not this hypothesis is true, the fact that certain Ca^{2+} antagonists interfere strongly with experimental vitamin D_3-induced calcinosis deserves more than purely academic interest.

Retardation by Calcium Antagonists of Arterial Calcium Accumulation in Aging, Hypertensive, and Alloxan-Diabetic Rats

As shown by us in previous studies on rats, increasing age, hypertension, and diabetes (experimentally produced with alloxan) favor Ca^{2+} accumulation in the arterial walls. Thus, the well-known ability of these factors to enhance the development of arteriosclerotic lesions in humans is paralleled by a distinct promoter effect on arterial Ca^{2+} incorporation in rats. Our studies have also shown that Ca^{2+} antagonists such as nifedipine and verapamil are not only capable of normalizing the elevated blood pressure in spontaneously hypertensive rats (19,32,66), but simultaneously prevent the abnormal accumulation of Ca^{2+} in the arterial vasculature of these animals (33). Figure 8 shows the regularization of blood pressure in spontaneously hypertensive rats by oral administration of nifedipine (50–150 mg/kg daily) for 5 months. Moreover, chronic treatment of the hypertensive rats with nifedipine, totally blocked the abnormal augmentation of Ca^{2+} in the aortic and mesenteric walls (Fig. 9). Thus, untreated 6-month-old hypertensive animals exhibited a Ca^{2+} content of 15.6 ($\pm$0.33) mmoles

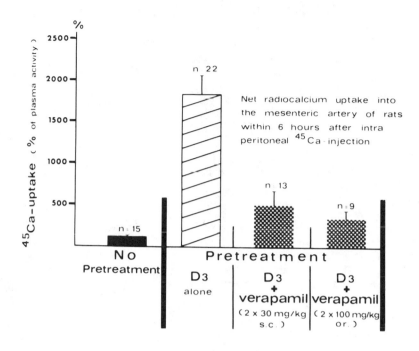

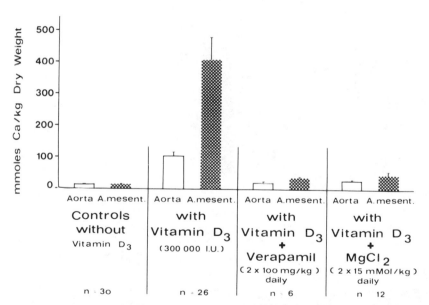

FIG. 6. Top: Inhibition of vitamin D₃-stimulated (300,000 IU/kg) net radiocalcium uptake into the wall of the mesenteric artery of rats by verapamil, administered subcutaneously or orally during 4 days. **Bottom:** Prevention of vitamin D₃-induced (300,000 IU/kg) rise in absolute Ca²⁺ content of the aortic and mesenteric walls by oral treatment with verapamil or MgCl₂ for 4 days. (From ref. 32a.)

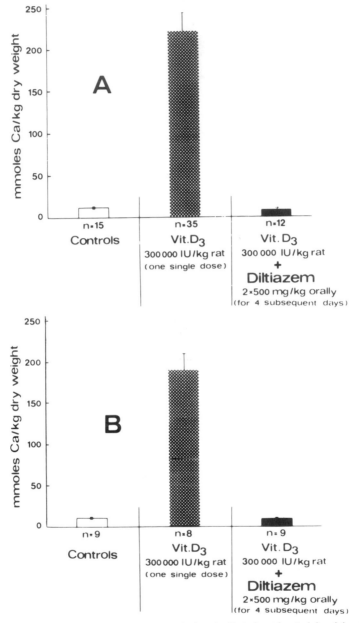

FIG. 7. Complete prevention by diltiazem of vitamin D_3-induced arterial calcinosis. **A:** Oral administration of 2×500 mg diltiazem/kg body wt to rats for 4 subsequent days completely neutralizes the tremendous stimulation of Ca^{2+} uptake into the coronary wall that otherwise would occur within 4 days following i.m. injection of vitamin D_3 (300,000 IU/kg). **B:** Same observations as in A made, however, on the rat renal arteries. Under the present experimental conditions, the relatively high oral doses of diltiazem were well tolerated during 4 days without any discernible negative side-effect.

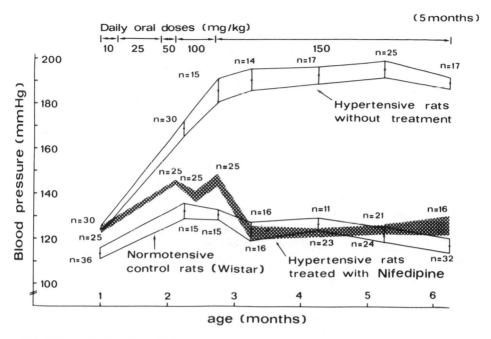

FIG. 8. Normalization of arterial blood pressure of rats suffering from spontaneous hypertension by chronic oral administration of nifedipine. The treatment lasted from the end of the first to the end of the sixth month of age. However, there was a rapid rise in tension to the level of untreated hypertensive rats as soon as the therapy was discontinued. (From refs. 19 and 66.)

(aorta), and 18.7 (±0.31) mmoles/kg dry tissue wt (mesenteric artery). Nifedipine lowered the corresponding values to 12.0 (±0.18) mmoles Ca^{2+}/kg for the aorta and 14.3 (±0.40) mmoles Ca^{2+}/kg for the mesenteric artery. These data, obtained in nifedipine-treated 6-month-old hypertensive rats, did not significantly differ from those found in normotensive 6-month-old Wistar rats. After cessation of the long-term treatment with nifedipine, blood pressure rose within 48 hr to the level of untreated hypertensive rats. However, it took 6 weeks before there was also a significant increase in arterial Ca^{2+} content up to 14.0 (±0.58) (aorta) and 15.96 (±0.95) mmoles/kg dry wt (mesenteric artery).

Our observations on hypertensive rats with nifedipine provide further evidence for a protective action of Ca^{2+} antagonists against vascular calcinosis. This conclusion is also backed by electron-optical studies on femoral, testicular, and tail arteries of spontaneously hypertensive rats (63). In the hypertensive rats without treatment, the excessive Ca^{2+} content of the arterial smooth muscle cells could be visualized in the form of multiple minute intracellular precipitates of Ca^{2+} antimonate, whereas the arterial vasculature of the nifedipine-protected animals was virtually free from such Ca^{2+} antimonate granules.

According to more recent investigations of our laboratory, the progressive arterial Ca^{2+} accumulation in *aging Sprague-Dawley* rats and in *alloxan-diabetic* rats also responds to certain Ca^{2+} antagonists. Thus, we were able to show that chronic administration of verapamil contained in the diet over 8 months (between the 2nd and the 10th month of age), prevented the natural age-dependent increase in the Ca^{2+} content of the arotic and mesenteric walls which otherwise would take place during this period (22). Similarly, long-term treatment of alloxan-diabetic rats with verapamil proved to be capable of keeping the mural Ca^{2+} contents of aorta and mesenteric artery within the normal range. More surprising was the fact that verapamil not only lowered arterial Ca^{2+} uptake, but also prevented the frequent development of diabetic eye cataracts (29). For instance, in a series of diabetic rats without verapamil, 70 lenses out of 113 (62%) became opaque within an observation period of 6.5 months. On the other hand, with verapamil (25 mg/kg daily given by means of a stomach tube), only 1 out of 26 lenses (3.9%) developed a cataract. Without verapamil, the Ca^{2+} content of the lenses of diabetic rats rose from 1.08 ($\pm$0.02) up to 10.89 ($\pm$0.85) mmoles/kg dry wt. With verapamil, the mean Ca^{2+} content remained in a low range of 3.46 ($\pm$0.61) mmoles/kg dry wt. There is a highly

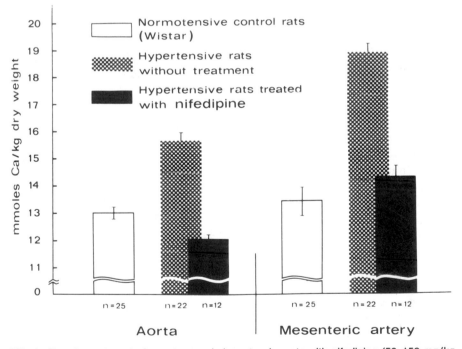

FIG. 9. Chronic treatment of spontaneously hypertensive rats with nifedipine (50–150 mg/kg daily) during 5 months (beginning at an age of one month) prevents the progressive rise in both arterial blood pressure and Ca^{2+} content of the arterial walls (aorta, mesenteric artery). All animals (normotensive controls, hypertensive rats without treatment, and nifedipine-treated hypertensive rats) were sacrificed at an age of exactly 6 months for the Ca^{2+} determination.

significant correlation between Ca^{2+} overload of the lenses and opacification, in that cataracts develop if the Ca^{2+} content of the lenses exceeds a threshold value of 7 to 8 mmoles/kg dry wt. Verapamil, by keeping the Ca^{2+} content of the lenses below this critical level, preserved transparency (Fig. 10).

In conclusion, verapamil and diltiazem provided excellent protection against vascular calcinosis in aging, vitamin D_3-treated and alloxan-diabetic rats, whereas nifedipine was most effective against excessive vascular Ca^{2+} uptake in hypertensive rats. Moreover, verapamil inhibited the development of alloxan-diabetic eye cataracts. Our results open new prospects with regard to the use of Ca^{2+} antagonists as anticalcinotic agents for long-term therapy. The most intriguing prospect is the possibility of an eventual control of the Ca^{2+}-dependent arterial aging process, and of the secondary circulatory complications. Apart from overt calcinosis, there are a number of other typical signs of vascular senescence

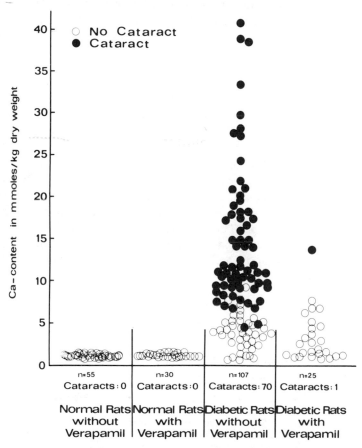

FIG. 10. Prevention of cataracts in alloxan-diabetic rats via inhibition of lenticular Ca^{2+} overload with verapamil (25 mg/kg daily given with a stomach tube over 6.5 months).

that are possibly attributable to the influence of progressive age-dependent arterial Ca^{2+} accumulation, namely:

1. The typical rarefaction of intact smooth muscle cells in the arterial media, possibly resulting from Ca^{2+}-induced mitochondrial destruction;

2. The typical loss of vascular elasticity that can fairly be related to Ca^{2+}-induced mineralization and degeneration of elastic fibers;

3. The typical inclination to a rise in systolic and diastolic blood pressure at an advanced age. This could also be a consequence of an elevated arterial Ca^{2+} content leading to increases in peripheral vascular tone. Accordingly, hypertension of elderly patients is most susceptible to a Ca^{2+}-antagonist treatment (2).

Regarding the fact that human life span is decisively determined by arterial senescence, any further progress in this field would be of utmost scientific and practical importance. It is now up to a joint effort of scientists and clinicians to clarify the important matter of a *possible geriatric significance of Ca²⁺ antagonists.*

CLOSING REMARKS

Ca^{2+} antagonism is a unifying concept that offers a common denominator for a multitude of pharmacological effects on myocardium, cardiac pacemakers, and smooth muscle cells. The term *calcium antagonist,* proposed by us in 1969 as a novel drug designation, represents more than a sophisticated scientific name, since it yields an explanation of the multifaceted practical consequences arising from the present worldwide application of these agents. The administration of Ca^{2+} antagonists as antianginal, antiarrhythmic, antihypertensive, or cardioprotective drugs makes use of the different manifestations of one and the same elementary membrane action. Thus, the elucidation of the involvement of Ca^{2+} into various physiological and pathophysiological processes has made the pharmacology of Ca^{2+} antagonists and the wide scope of their therapeutic actions easily understandable.

REFERENCES

1. Bing, R. J., Weishaar, R., Rackl, A., and Pawlik, G. (1978/79): *New Drug Therapy with a Calcium Antagonist, Diltiazem,* edited by R. J. Bing, pp. 27–37. Excerpta Medica, Amsterdam.
2. Bühler, F. R., and Hulthen, L. (1982): *Eur. J. Clin. Invest.,* 12:1–3.
3. Byon, Y. K., and Fleckenstein, A. (1969): *Pfluegers Arch.,* 312: R 8/9.
4. Döring, H. J., and Kammermeier, H. (1961): *Verh. Dtsch. Ges. Kreislaufforsch.,* 27:227–232.
5. Eisenstein, R., and Zeruolis, L. (1964): *Arch. Pathol.,* 77:27–35.
6. Fawaz, G., and Hawa, E. S. (1953): *Proc. Soc. Exp. Biol. Med.,* 84:277–280.
7. Fleckenstein, A. (1963): *The Cellular Functions of Membrane Transport,* edited by J. F. Hoffmann, pp. 71–93. Prentice-Hall, Englewood Cliffs, New Jersey.
8. Fleckenstein, A. (1964): *Verh. Dtsch. Ges. Inn. Med.,* 70:81–99.
9. Fleckenstein, A. (1968): *Verh. Dtsch. Ges. Kreislaufforsch.,* 34:15–34.
10. Fleckenstein, A. (1968): *Proceedings Vth European Congress of Cardiology,* Athens, pp. 255–269.

11. Fleckenstein, A. (1968): *Herzinfarkt und Schock,* edited by L. Heilmeyer and H. J. Holtmeier, pp. 94–109. Georg Thieme, Stuttgart.
12. Fleckenstein, A. (1970/71): *Calcium and the Heart,* edited by P. Harris and L. Opie, pp. 135–188. Academic Press, London.
13. Fleckenstein, A. (1970/71): *Vorträge der Erlanger Physiologentagung,* edited by W. D. Keidel and K. H. Plattig, pp. 13–52. Springer Verlag, Berlin.
14. Fleckenstein, A. (1977): *Annu. Rev. Pharmacol. Toxicol.,* 17:149–166.
15. Fleckenstein, A., Döring, H. J., Janke, J., and Byon, Y. K. (1975): *Handbook of Experimental Pharmacology,* New Series, Vol. XVI/3, edited by J. Schmier and O. Eichler, pp. 345–405. Springer Verlag, Berlin.
16. Fleckenstein, A., Döring, H. J., and Kammermeier, H. (1966/67): *Proceedings of International Symposium on the Coronary Circulation and Energetics of the Myocardium,* Milan, pp. 220–236. Karger, Basel.
17. Fleckenstein, A., Döring, H. J., and Kammermeier, H. (1968): *Klin. Wochenschr.,* 46:343–351.
18. Fleckenstein, A., Döring, H. J., Kammermeier, H., and Grün, G. (1968): *Biochim. Applic.,* 14 (Suppl. 1):323–344.
19. Fleckenstein, A., and Fleckenstein-Grün, G. (1980): *Eur. Heart J. 1,* (Suppl. B):15–21.
20. Fleckenstein, A., Fleckenstein-Grün, G., Byon, Y. K., Haastert, H. P., and Späh, F. (1979): *Arzneim. Forsch.,* 29:230–246.
21. Fleckenstein, A., Fleckenstein-Grün, G., Janke, J., and Frey, M. (1977): *Z. Praeklin. Klin. Geriatr.,* 7:269–284.
22. Fleckenstein, A., Frey, M., and Leder, O. (1983): *New Calcium Antagonists, Recent Developments and Prospects,* edited by A. Fleckenstein et al., pp. 15–31. Gustav Fischer Verlag, Stuttgart–New York.
23. Fleckenstein, A., and Grün, G. (1969): *Pfluegers Arch.,* 307:26.
24. Fleckenstein, A., Grün, G., Byon, Y. K., Döring, H. J., and Tritthart, H. (1973/75): *New Therapy of Ischemic Heart Disease,* edited by K. Hashimoto, E. Kimura, and T. Kobayashi, pp. 31–44. University of Tokyo Press, Tokyo.
25. Fleckenstein, A., Grün, G., Tritthart, H., and Byon, Y. K. (1971): *Klin. Wochenschr.,* 49:32–41.
26. Fleckenstein, A., Kammermeier, H., Döring, H. J., and Freund, H. J. (1967): *Z. Kreislaufforsch.,* 56:716–744; 839–853.
26a. Fleckenstein, A., Nakayama, K., Fleckenstein-Grün, G., and Byon, Y. K. (1976): *Ionic Actions on Vascular Smooth Muscle,* edited by E. Betz, pp. 117–123. Springer Verlag, Berlin.
27. Fleckenstein, A., Tritthart, H., Döring, H. J., and Byon, Y. K. (1972): *Arzneim. Forsch.,* 22:22–33.
28. Fleckenstein, A., Tritthart, H., Fleckenstein, B., Herbst, A., and Grün, G. (1969): *Pfluegers Arch.,* 307:R 25.
29. Fleckenstein, A., von Witzleben, H., Frey, M., and Milner, T. G. (1981): *Pfluegers Arch.,* 391 (Suppl.):R 12.
30. Fleckenstein-Grün, G., and Fleckenstein, A. (1975): *New Therapy of Ischemic Heart Disease,* edited by W. Lochner, W. Braasch, and G. Kroneberg, pp. 66–75. Springer Verlag, Berlin.
31. Fleckenstein-Grün, G., and Fleckenstein, A. (1978/80): *Calcium-Antagonismus,* edited by A. Fleckenstein and H. Roskamm, pp. 191–270. Springer Verlag, Berlin.
32. Fleckenstein-Grün, G., and Fleckenstein, A. (1980/81): *Calcium Antagonism in Cardiovascular Therapy—Experience with Verapamil,* edited by A. Zanchetti and D. M. Krikler, pp. 30–48. Excerpta Medica, Amsterdam.
32a. Frey, M., Keidel, J., and Fleckenstein, A. (1978/80): *Calcium-Antagonismus,* edited by A. Fleckenstein and H. Roskamm, pp. 258–264. Springer Verlag, Berlin.
33. Frey, M., von Witzleben, H., Keidel, J., and Fleckenstein, A. (1980): *Naunyn Schmiedebergs Arch. Pharmacol.,* (Suppl.)313:R 48.
34. Grün, G., Byon, Y. K., Kaufmann, R., and Fleckenstein, A. (1972): *Arztl. Forsch.,* 26:369–378.
35. Grün, G., and Fleckenstein, A. (1972): *Arzneim. Forsch.,* 22:334–344.
36. Grün, G., Fleckenstein, A., and Byon, Y. K. (1971): *Arzneim. Forsch.,* 21:1585–1590.
37. Grün, G., Fleckenstein, A., and Byon, Y. K. (1971): *Proceedings 25th Congress International Union Physiological Sciences,* Munich, Vol. 9, p. 221.
38. Grün, G., Fleckenstein, A., and Tritthart, H. (1969): *Pfluegers Arch.,* 264:239.

39. Haas, H. G., Kern, R., and Einwächter, H. M. (1970): *J. Membr. Biol.*, 3:180–209.
40. Haeusler, G. (1972): *J. Pharmacol. Exp. Ther.*, 180:672–682.
41. Hass, G. M., Landerholm, W., and Hemmens, A. (1966): *Am. J. Pathol.*, 49:739–771.
42. Hass, G. M., Trueheart, R. E., and Hemmens, A. (1960): *Am. J. Pathol.*, 37:521–539.
43. Hass, G. M., Trueheart, R. E., and Hemmens, A. (1961): *Am. J. Pathol.*, 38:289–312.
44. Henry, P. D., Shuchleib, R., Borda, L. J., Roberts, R., Williamson, J. R., and Sobel, B. E. (1978): *Circ. Res.*, 43:372–380.
45. Herzenberg, H. (1929): *Beitr. Pathol. Anat.*, 82:27–56.
46. Janke, J., Hein, B., Pachinger, O., Leder, O., and Fleckenstein, A. (1971/72): *Vascular Smooth Muscle*, edited by E. Betz, pp. 71–72. Springer Verlag, Berlin.
47. Kohlhardt, M., Bauer, B., Krause, H., and Fleckenstein, A. (1972): *Pfluegers Arch.*, 335:309–322.
48. Kohlhardt, M., and Fleckenstein, A. (1977): *Naunyn Schmiedebergs Arch. Pharmacol.*, 298:267–272.
49. Krayer, O. (1931): *Naunyn Schmiedebergs Arch. Pharmacol.*, 161:1–28.
50. Krayer, O., and Schütz, E. (1932): *Z. Biol.*, 92:453–461.
51. Lossnitzer, K., Janke, J., Hein, B., Stauch, M., and Fleckenstein, A. (1975): *Recent Advances in Studies on Cardiac Structure and Metabolism*, Vol. 6, edited by A. Fleckenstein and G. Rona, pp. 207–217. University Park Press, Baltimore.
52. Lossnitzer, K., and Mohr, W. (1973): *Int. Res. Commun. Sys.*, (73–10):1–5–9.
53. Mines, G. R. (1913): *J. Physiol. (Lond.)*, 46:188–235.
54. Nagao, T., Matlib, M. A., Franklin, D., Millard, R. W., and Schwartz, A. (1980): *J. Mol. Cell. Cardiol.*, 12:29–43.
55. Nayler, W. G., Grau, A., and Slade, A. (1976): *Cardiovasc. Res.*, 10:650–662.
56. Opie, L. H. (1980): *Lancet*, 1:806–810.
57. Reuter, H., and Beeler, G. W. (1969): *Science*, 162:399–401.
58. Ringer, S. (1882): *J. Physiol. (Lond.)*, 4:29–42.
59. Schildberg, F. W., and Fleckenstein, A. (1965): *Pfluegers Arch.*, 283:137–150.
60. Schwiegk, H. (1931): *Naunyn Schmiedebergs Arch. Pharmacol.*, 162:56–69.
61. Selye, H. (1958): *Am. Heart J.*, 55:805–809.
62. Stämpfli, R. (1954): *Experientia (Basel)*, 10:508–509.
63. Staubesand, J., and von Seydewitz, V. (1982): *Kalziumantagonisten zur Kardioplegie und Myocardprotektion in der offenen Herzchirurgie*, edited by H. Just, A. Tschirkov, and A. V. Schlosser, pp. 165–172. Georg Thieme Verlag, Stuttgart–New York.
64. Taylor, C. B., Hass, G. M., Liu, L. B., and Ho, K. J. (1972): *Ann. Clin. Lab. Sci.*, 2:239.
65. Weishaar, R., Ashikawa, K., and Bing, R. J. (1979): *Am. J. Cardiol.*, 43:1136–1143.
66. von Witzleben, H., Frey, M., Keidel, J., and Fleckenstein, A. (1980): *Pfluegers Arch.*, 384 (Suppl.):R 9.
67. Wollenberger, A. (1947): *Am. J. Physiol.*, 150:733–745.

Calcium Antagonists and Cardiovascular Disease, edited by L. H. Opie.
Raven Press, New York © 1984.

Chapter 3

How Calcium Crosses Plasma Membranes Including the Sarcolemma

Ernesto Carafoli

Laboratory of Biochemistry, Swiss Federal Institute of Technology (ETH), 8092 Zurich, Switzerland

Since the subject matter of this book is heart and heart diseases, this summary of ways and means by which Ca^{2+} crosses plasma cell membranes will concentrate on the cardiac sarcolemma. Considerable progress has now been made on the mechanisms by which Ca^{2+} is exchanged between heart sarcoplasm and the extracellular spaces, and it appears that some of the properties of the Ca^{2+} transporting systems may be peculiar to heart plasma membranes. However, the basic characteristics of the three systems involved—the Ca^{2+} channel, the Ca^{2+}-pumping ATPase, and the Na^+/Ca^{2+} exchanger—are probably similar in all plasma membranes. Thus, even if the data are eventually referred to the case of the heart, other plasma membranes will also be considered, depending on the cell type where the most important progresses have been made.

CALCIUM CHANNELS

Ca^{2+} action potentials, implying a Ca^{2+} component in plasma membrane conductance, were first recorded in 1958 for the crayfish muscle fiber membrane (30). In the years that followed, the observation was extended to a large variety of excitable plasma membranes, including heart sarcolemma (see refs. 42 and 69 for reviews). The Ca^{2+} component of the action potential current was attributed to the existence of a specific Ca^{2+} channel, which is different from the well-known Na^+ channel. The traditional method for the investigation of the Ca^{2+} channel has been the recording of electrical currents in intact, or near intact, tissue/cell preparations. Recently, the concept of a specific channel which allows the passage of Ca^{2+} has been extended to nonexcitable cells, for example, the erythrocytes (51,84). Here, the definition of a specific channel has been based on the conventional criteria for the characterization of carrier-

(channel)-mediated processes, among them saturation kinetics of the Ca^{2+} transport process, competitive inhibition by ions like Co^{2+}, and specific inhibition by the so-called Ca^{2+} antagonists or Ca^{2+} entry blockers (32).

In axonal membranes, the Ca^{2+} conductance has been calculated to be almost one order of magnitude lower than the Na^+ conductance (39), making the measurement of Ca^{2+} currents all but impossible. In the soma of nervous cells, by contrast, inward Ca^{2+} currents can be easily measured, and they are differentiated from the Na^+ current by their insensitivity to the well-known antagonist of the Na^+ channel, tetrodotoxin, by the specific sensitivity to Cd^{2+}, Co^{2+}, and other competing cations (see later), and by the inhibition by antagonists like verapamil and its derivatives (28,41). The measurement of Ca^{2+} currents in heart plasma membranes has been greatly facilitated by the introduction of the *voltage-patch technique* (37) which permits the study of single channels, and has allowed the definition of the kinetic parameters of the Ca^{2+} channel with adequate precision (71) (see later).

The selectivity of the Ca^{2+} channel has been tested by measuring the maximum values of current produced in media, when Ca^{2+} is replaced by other ions. For the somatic plasma membrane of neurons, the preference order is Ba^{2+}, Sr^{2+}, Ca^{2+}, and Mg^{2+} (2). Ba^{2+} is about twice as permeable through the channel as Ca^{2+}, a fact that is exploited in experiments where the conductance of single channels is studied. The cations mentioned above bind to the external opening of the channel prior to being transported across, explaining the saturation effect of the inward current at high cation concentrations. This also explains the channel-blocking effect of cations, such as Cd^{2+}, Ni^{2+}, La^{3+}, Co^{2+}, and Mn^{2+}, which bind to the external opening of the channel with high affinity. The K_d for the binding of the transported and blocking ions varies from about 5 mM (Ca^{2+}) to about 15 mM (Ba^{2+}) (3,85), and between 0.07 mM (Cd^{2+}) to about 0.7 mM (Ni^{2+} and Co^{2+}) (48,62).

Ca^{2+} action potentials in neuronal plasma membranes are eliminated when the pH of the medium decreases to 6.5, suggesting that protonation of a binding group plays a role (78). From a comparison of the pK values of the complexes formed by H^+, Ca^{2+}, and Ba^{2+} with the binding site of the Ca^{2+} channel and with different functional groups of proteins, it has been inferred that one carboxylic group is involved in the binding of penetrating cations at the outer opening of the channel (45). It has also been proposed that the Ca^{2+} channel possesses a selectivity filter responsible for the exclusion of monovalent cations in front of the site of binding of the carried ions. The *selectivity filter* may become damaged under certain experimental conditions, permitting as a consequence the transfer of Na^+ ions across the channel (as discussed in ref. 42).

Upon depolarization of the plasma membrane, the Ca^{2+} current rises at a slower rate than the Na^+ current: For this reason, the current carried by the Ca^{2+} channel is usually defined as "slow." During protracted depolarization of the plasma membrane, the Ca^{2+} current becomes spontaneously inactivated (43). This could either result from a voltage-dependent gating mechanism of inactivation (82), or from the inhibition of the channel by the increased intracellular Ca^{2+} (44), or from both.

The current produced by single Ca^{2+} channels has recently been evaluated indirectly from the fluctuation of Ca^{2+} currents in micropatches of plasma membranes of neuronal cells (1), or from the analysis of fluctuations in Ca^{2+} currents from large portions of neuronal plasma membranes: The Ca^{2+} components of the membrane noise were extracted from the difference between the total membrane noise and the noise in the presence of blockers of the Ca^{2+} channel like Ni^+ (1,85). Substitution of Ca^{2+} with the more readily permeable Ba^{2+} increases the current through the Ca^{2+} channel, thus facilitating the experiment.

The conductance for single channels extrapolated from experiments of this type is rather low: A single channel can pass up to 3.10^5 Ca^{2+} ions/sec, and the conductance of a unitary Ca^{2+} channel is of the order of 0.5 pS. The calculated density of Ca^{2+} channels (in the plasma membrane of molluscan neurons) is of the order of 250 to $330/\mu M^2$. Direct measurements of single channels in the sarcolemma of cultured heart myocytes with the voltage-patch technique (71) have yielded conductance values that are at least one order of magnitude higher, but, being based on direct measurements, are probably more realistic: 10 to 15 pS per unitary Ca^{2+} channel. The calculated density of the Ca^{2+} channel in heart is about 0.1 channel per 1 μM^2 (see H. Reuter, *this volume*).

NEUROTRANSMITTER EFFECTS

One important aspect of the Ca^{2+} channel is its sensitivity to adrenergic neurotransmitters. This was first shown by Grossmann and Furchgott (36) and Reuter (68) on the basis of experiments concerning the stimulation of Ca^{2+} influx during excitation of atrial cardiac preparations by catecholamines. Later, it was suggested by Tsien et al. (83) and Reuter (68), on the basis of experiments with butyrate derivatives of cyclic AMP, that this cyclic nucleotide is responsible for increased Ca^{2+} influx. Furthermore, Wollenberger et al. have observed that cyclic AMP promoted the phosphorylation of a 24,000 M_r in a sarcolemma-rich preparation of cardiac muscle (87). The phosphorylation increased the affinity of the binding sites for Ca^{2+} in the membrane.

The observations on catecholamines and cyclic AMP have recently been extended by Reuter et al. (71) to experiments with the voltage-patch technique on cultured heart myocytes, and by Veselovsky et al. and Fedulova et al. (31,86) to experiments on noise analysis on dialyzed dorsal root ganglion neurons of newborn rats. In both cases, potentiation of the influx of Ca^{2+} has been observed. Reuter et al. (71) have demonstrated that the treatment with catecholamines increases the probability of the opening of the Ca^{2+} channels.

CALCIUM CHANNELS IN ISOLATED VESICLES

One interesting recent development has been the possibility of studying the Ca^{2+} channel in vesicles isolated from heart sarcolemma. Opening of the channel is caused by the development of a diffusion potential produced by the exit of K^+ from the vesicle (10). Under these conditions, the activity of the Ca^{2+} channel can be followed directly by measuring the uptake of radioactive Ca^{2+} into the sarcolemmal vesicles. As expected, the uptake is inhibited by verapamil and La^{3+} (65,66). The experiments on isolated sarcolemmal vesicles have been extended to the effect of cyclic AMP, and have led to the biochemical characterization of the phosphorylation system responsible for the activation of the Ca^{2+} channel (i.e., the increase in the uptake of Ca^{2+}). Stimulation of the Ca^{2+} channel activity is induced by the addition of the catalytic subunit of the cyclic AMP-dependent protein kinase, and is paralleled by the phosphorylation of a membrane-bound acidic proteolipid which has been termed calciductin (66). This acidic proteolipid, which has a M_r of 23,000, resembles the acidic proteolipid phospholamban, which is active on the Ca^{2+}-transporting ATPase of heart sarcoplasmic reticulum.

THE CALCIUM-PUMPING ATPase

The involvement of a specific ATPase in the pumping of Ca^{2+} out of cells was first suggested by Dunham and Glynn in 1961 (27), and demonstrated by Schatzmann in 1970 (76). Originally, the system was considered specific to nonexcitable cells, but recent research (see ref. 59 for a review) has shown it to be present in excitable cells as well. The plasma membrane used in most of the studies of the Ca^{2+}-pumping ATPase has been the erythrocyte, for which the essential properties of the enzyme have been established, and from which the ATPase was first isolated and purified. Comprehensive reviews on the enzyme *in situ* (73,74,77) and on the purified enzyme (18) have recently appeared.

The Ca^{2+} ATPase can be essentially considered as a high-affinity, low-capacity enzyme: In heart sarcolemma, it interacts with Ca^{2+} with a K_m of about 0.5 μM, and pumps it out of the cell with a V_{max} of the order of 0.5 nmole/mg protein/sec. It belongs to the ATPases of the E_1–E_2 type, which form acyl phosphates during the enzyme cycle, and are sensitive to vanadate. Table 1 offers a summary of the most important properties of the Ca^{2+} ATPase.

The sensitivity to calmodulin, first reported by Jarrett and Penniston (53) and Gopinath and Vincenzi (34), is worth a special comment: While it may have some exceptions, notable among them the case of liver (46), it appears sufficiently general in distribution to be considered a characteristic property. In fact, the calmodulin-insensitive plasma membrane Ca^{2+}-pumping ATPases might be of different type. The interaction between calmodulin and the Ca^{2+} ATPase is direct (52,56), at variance with what is known for the case of the Ca^{2+} ATPase of heart sarcoplasmic reticulum (50), where it is mediated by the acidic proteolipid phospholamban. In an important new development, it has been exploited to isolate the Ca^{2+}-ATPase enzyme on calmodulin affinity chromatography columns (see later).

Following the demonstration of the existence of a *Ca^{2+}-pumping ATPase in*

TABLE 1. *The Ca²⁺-pumping ATPase of plasma membranes*

Affinity for Ca^{2+} (K_m)	0.4–0.5 μM
V_{max} of Ca^{2+} transport (nmoles/mg protein/sec)	0.5 nmoles/mg protein/sec
Ca^{2+}/ATP stoichiometry	1–2[a]
Inhibition	Vanadate, $I_{50} < 1$ μM
Calmodulin sensitivity	Present[b]
Enzyme cycle	E_1–E_2 type, formation of acyl phosphate
Membrane content	~0.1% of Total membrane protein
Effect of phospholipids	Acidic phospholipids activate
Limited proteolysis	Activates
Modulation by phosphorylation/ dephosphorylation	Present[c]

[a] Opinions on this point differ (see ref. 73 for discussion).
[b] In two cases, liver and luteal cells (see refs. 46 and 59), calmodulin has no effect.
[c] Only in heart sarcolemma.

heart sarcolemma (19) and its characterization as a high-affinity, low-capacity Ca²⁺-pumping system, efforts have been directed to the characterization of mechanisms for the regulation of its activity. One system, calmodulin, has already been mentioned. Other compounds that possess the ability to activate the ATPase (i.e., to induce the same K_m and V_{max} shifts which are induced by calmodulin) are acidic phospholipids and polyunsaturated fatty acids. They have been studied mostly in the case of the erythrocyte enzyme, both *in situ* (72) and in the purified state (see later), and their effects have recently been confirmed for the case of the heart sarcolemmal (purified) enzyme (24). The interest of the effects of acidic phospholipids resides in the fact that they are present in plasma membranes, and are concentrated in the inner layer of the bilayer leaflet, where the active site of the Ca²⁺ ATPase is presumably located. Assuming homogeneous distribution in the horizontal plane of the membrane, acidic phospholipids are present in sufficient amounts to produce about 50% activation of the Ca²⁺ ATPase (53). It is thus possible to think of them as modulators of the enzyme, operating in parallel with calmodulin. Changes in the phospholipid composition in the ambient surrounding the Ca²⁺ ATPase (lateral motion?) would determine its modulation. Of potential interest is also the activation of the Ca²⁺-transporting ATPase by the di- and triphosphoinositides (18,58), metabolites that are known to be produced in plasma membranes. In contrast, the activation of the enzyme by limited proteolysis, which has now been described for the erythrocyte (54, 75,79,80) and the heart sarcolemmal enzymes (24), is probably of no physiological interest. Controlled proteolysis, however, has now become an important tool for the molecular study of the purified ATPase.

Studies on heart sarcolemmal vesicles have shown that the Ca²⁺-pumping ATPase is modulated by a *phosphorylation/dephosphorylation cycle* (21). The demonstration of the phenomenon required the previous dephosphorylation of the sarcolemmal membranes by an exogenous protein phosphatase: Only after this treatment could the stimulatory effect of ATP be demonstrated. The activating effect of ATP is evidently mediated by a cyclic AMP-dependent, membrane-bound protein kinase, since it is inhibited by a protein-kinase inhibitor which is cyclic AMP-dependent. It is, however, apparently controlled also by Ca^{2+}, since the activation of the pumping of Ca^{2+} by ATP is considerably decreased by the absence of Ca^{2+}. The identity of the putative endogenous protein phosphatase that deactivates the ATP-activated Ca^{2+}-pumping ATPase is at the moment unknown. It is of interest that the target of the phosphorylation/dephosphorylation process is not the ATPase enzyme itself, but some other accessory protein of the sarcolemmal membrane. This conclusion is based on the finding that the purified Ca^{2+}-pumping ATPase of sarcolemma (24) is not influenced by the phosphorylation/dephosphorylation cycle described.

The Ca^{2+}-pumping ATPase has now been isolated using calmodulin-affinity chromatography columns. The procedure has so far been applied successfully to two plasma membranes: erythrocytes (55) and heart (20). The enzyme purifies as a single polypeptide of M_r 138,000, which forms an acyl phosphate when incubated in the presence of Ca^{2+} and ATP, and which can be reconstituted to optimal pumping efficiency in liposomal systems. The purified enzyme repeats the known properties of the enzyme *in situ*, except that the V_{max} of Ca^{2+} transport is up to 500 units. The Ca^{2+}/ATP stoichiometry of a reconstituted system is certainly $1:1$. It may be of interest here that controlled proteolysis studies (so far carried out almost exclusively on the purified erythrocyte enzyme) have permitted the mapping of different zones of functional interest in the ATPase molecule. The information so far collected from proteolysis experiments is summarized in the model of the molecular architecture of the enzyme molecule shown in Fig. 1.

THE SODIUM/CALCIUM EXCHANGE

Experiments carried out in the late 1960s by Reuter and Seitz (70) and Blaustein, Baker, Hodgkin, and their co-workers (15,16) on the effects of external Na^+ on the exit of Ca^{2+} from mammalian cardiac muscle and giant squid axons led to the discovery of an exchange diffusion carrier that is now recognized as the (quantitatively) most important system for the ejection of Ca^{2+} from excitable cells. Other experiments have established that the system may operate also in the "reverse" direction, i.e., mediate the influx of Ca^{2+} into cells (e.g., see refs. 4,5,7,15) and that it exists in nonexcitable plasma membranes as well. These include endocrine secretory tissues (38), epithelial cells in various organs (12, 29,33,35,49,81), and bone cells (47). In fact, the erythrocyte may be the only eucaryotic membrane where the Na^+/Ca^{2+} exchange diffusion carrier is absent (dog erythrocytes possess a Na^+-coupled Ca^{2+} transport system, but its properties are different from those of the Na^+/Ca^{2+} exchange system in the cells mentioned

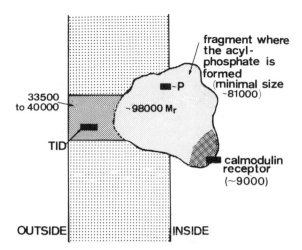

FIG. 1. A tentative scheme of the organization of the Ca^{2+} ATPase in the (erythrocyte) plasma membrane (from ref. 18). TID is the hydrophobic photoactivatable probe 3(trifluoromethyl)-3-[m(^{125}I)-iodophenyl] diazirine, which has been shown to bind preferentially to the proteolytic product of M_r about 35,000.

above) (see ref. 57). Anticipating a conclusion to be made at the end of this article, it seems that the two Ca^{2+} efflux systems, the Ca^{2+} ATPase and the Na^+/Ca^{2+} exchange system, are probably present in all plasma membrane species, their respective activity depending on the specific physiological demands of the different cells.

The basic observation made was that the rate of Ca^{2+} efflux from the cells studied depended in large part on the presence of Na^+ in the extracellular medium. Raising the intracellular Na^+ in squid axons, or lowering the extracellular Na^+ concentration, "reversed" the system, i.e., promoted inward Ca^{2+} transport (4,5,7,15). It was also shown that the efflux of Na^+ from squid axons was partially dependent on external Ca^{2+} (4,7). The exchange system was evidently separated from the Na^+/K^+ pump, since it was unaffected by ouabain (6).

One important problem connected with the discovery of the Na^+/Ca^{2+} exchange system, and with the suggestion that it is responsible for the maintenance of the Ca^{2+} gradient across the plasma membrane, is whether the energy content of the *electrochemical Na^+ gradient* is adequate. It was argued (see ref. 16) that an electroneutral exchange system, whereby 2 Na^+ are exchanged for 1 Ca^{2+}, could not account for the very low concentration of free Ca^{2+} existing within squid axons. An electrogenic exchange of 3 Na^+ for 1 Ca^{2+} was apparently necessary, and was indeed supported by several lines of evidence coming from experiments on squid axons and barnacle muscle fibers carried out in a number of laboratories (see ref. 14 for a recent review). In the case of the heart, clear-cut evidence for the electrogenicity of the exchanger has recently come from experiments on isolated heart plasma membrane vesicles. Pitts (61) has directly measured Na^+ influx and Ca^{2+} efflux, and has extrapolated a $3:1$ stoichiometry. Reeves and Sutko (64) and Caroni et al. (22) have used, as a tool, the movements of lipophilic cations during the operation of the exchanger, and have found that the interior of the vesicles becomes negative as Na^+ leaves them in exchange for Ca^{2+}. Philipson and Nishimoto (60) and Bers et al. (11) have shown that the operation of the exchanger, whereby Ca^{2+} uptake is driven by the exit of Na^+, is stimulated by establishing a positive potential inside the vesicles and inhibited by establishing a negative potential. It thus seems established, on the basis of a 3 Na^+ per 1 Ca^{2+} stoichiometry, that the energy content of the electrochemical Na^+ gradient is adequate for the maintenance of the low free Ca^{2+} concentrations measured in the cytosol. The electrogenicity of the exchange, however, will have as a consequence its sensitivity to the polarization level of the plasma membrane. In heart, one may expect that Ca^{2+} enters the cell by the Na^+/Ca^{2+} exchanger during the depolarization phase, and leaves it during repolarization of the plasma membrane.

The experiments on isolated heart sarcolemmal vesicles have permitted the definition of some important *kinetic parameters* of the exchange reaction. Reeves and Sutko (63) have measured a K_m for Ca^{2+} of the order of 20 μM and for Na^+ of the order of 15 mM. They have measured a V_{max} of approximately 0.4 nmoles Ca^{2+} transported per mg of sarcolemmal protein per sec. More recent experiments in which the constraint imposed on the reaction by its electrogenicity has been eliminated (22) have established that the affinity of the exchanger for Ca^{2+} is much higher (K_m about 2 μM) and its maximal velocity of Ca^{2+} pumping considerably faster (up to 30 nmoles per mg of sarcolemmal protein per sec). Thus, the exchanger appears to be a high capacity Ca^{2+} transporting system, which interacts with Ca^{2+} with a lower affinity than the Ca^{2+}-pumping ATPase.

One interesting aspect of the Na^+/Ca^{2+} exchange process is its *sensitivity to ATP*. A series of observations on squid axons have shown that ATP in the cytoplasm increases the affinity of the exchanger for internal Ca^{2+} and external Na^+ (8,9,13,25). The stimulatory effect of ATP evidently requires its hydrolysis, since only hydrolyzable ATP analogs are effective (26). This observation suggests the involvement of a phosphorylation reaction, which has now been demonstrated in isolated heart sarcolemmal vesicles (23). The affinity of the exchanger for Ca^{2+} is enhanced (to a K_m of about 0.8 μM) by a kinase-mediated phosphorylation step, and decreased by a phosphatase-mediated dephosphorylation reaction. Both the kinase and the phosphatase are membrane-bound, both are dependent on Ca^{2+} and calmodulin. The kinase is cyclic AMP-independent and has higher affinity for Ca^{2+} than the phosphatase.

INTEGRATED PICTURE OF CALCIUM HOMEOSTASIS

Naturally, an integrated picture of the overall Ca^{2+} homeostasis in cells must consider also the intracellular Ca^{2+} transporting membrane systems, i.e., the

TABLE 2. An integrated view of the transport of Ca^{2+} in heart cells

| Membrane system | Ca²⁺ transporting area of heart cells | | Ca²⁺ uptake | | | | | |
| | | | At 10 µM Ca²⁺ | | | At 1 µM Ca²⁺ + 1–3 mM Mg²⁺ | | |
	(m²/g)	[% Total area (a)]	Rate (b) (nmoles/mg protein/s)	"Total" uptake (a × b) (nmoles/mg proteins)	% Total uptake	Rate (b) (nmoles/mg protein/s)	"Total" uptake (a × b) (nmoles/mg proteins)	% Total uptake
Sarcolemma								
Ca²⁺–ATPase	0.10	0.8	1.5	1.2	0.4	1.5	1.2	0.7
Na⁺–Ca²⁺ exchange			20	16	3.1	10	8	4.9
Sarcoplasmic reticulum	1.5	12.1	20	242	46.5	12	145	88
Mitochondria	10.6	87	3	261	50	0.12	10.4	6.3

For mitochondria, only the inner membrane has been considered. Uptakes are given at 38°C. In the case of mitochondria, the rates have been doubled, on the assumption that the inner membrane represents 50% of the total protein of heart mitochondrial preparations. The following additional assumptions have been made: (a) the degree of contamination of all preparations with extraneous organelles is the same; (b) the protein content for the unit of membrane area is the same in all organelles.
From ref. 17.

(endo) sarcoplasmic reticulum and the mitochondria. In heart, the kinetic parameters of the four Ca^{2+} transporting systems (the two in the plasma membrane described here, plus mitochondria and the sarcoplasmic reticulum) have all been defined. Thus, a comprehensive picture of the respective importance of the four systems in the cellular homeostasis of Ca^{2+} can be attempted (Table 2). Under conditions approaching physiology, only minor fractions of the intracellular Ca^{2+} are handled by the plasma membrane and the mitochondria, the most active organelle being the sarcoplasmic reticulum. Under conditions of relative intracellular Ca^{2+} overload, however, the role of mitochondria becomes proportionately more important, and may equal or exceed that of sarcoplasmic reticulum. The picture that emerges is that of mitochondria as long-term Ca^{2+} buffers, which can handle very large amounts of Ca^{2+} whenever the need arises. In so doing, evidently, they serve an essential function, since they are responsible for maintaining the Ca^{2+} levels in the cell within limits compatible with the demands of the regulatory function of Ca^{2+}. The sarcoplasmic reticulum, by contrast, handles most of the Ca^{2+} which is responsible for the rapid and fine regulation of heart intracellular events, including the contraction and relaxation of myofibrils.

CONCLUSIONS

The picture that emerges from this overview can be summarized as follows:

1. A (proteinaceous) Ca^{2+} *channel,* responsible for the intake of Ca^{2+}, is ubiquitously distributed in eucaryotic cells. Its operation is voltage-controlled in excitable cells like heart or neurons. In cells where the transmembrane potential is insignificant and not modulated (e.g., the erythrocyte), the channel is not gated electrically, and presumably not gated at all. Whether the Ca^{2+} channel and/or all of its molecular components are the same in excitable and not-excitable tissues is an open problem. The effect of cyclic AMP on the channel represents a mechanism for the hormonal control of the amount of Ca^{2+} that enters the cell.

2. The Ca^{2+}*-pumping ATPase* is probably represented in the plasma membrane of all eucaryotic cells. It can be defined as a high-affinity, low-capacity system, designed to eject Ca^{2+} from the cells at rest. In heart, this would correspond to the diastolic period during which high Ca^{2+} affinity is required for efficient interaction with the low free Ca^{2+} concentration in the environment, but during which a low pumping rate is probably adequate. The cyclic AMP-dependent stimulation of the ATPase can be described as a control system additional to calmodulin for the translation of the hormonal message into the regulation of Ca^{2+} fluxes across the plasma membrane.

3. The Na^+/Ca^{2+} *exchange system* is probably also represented in all eucaryotic plasma membranes. It can be defined as a low-affinity, high-capacity pumping system, designed to eject Ca^{2+} whenever its concentration in the cytosol increases to a level which exceeds its K_m (Ca^{2+}). Under these conditions, its

low Ca^{2+} affinity is probably not a limiting factor, but its high pumping velocity is particularly useful. In heart, the recently discovered kinase/phosphatase system may be described as a control device, having the role of translating hormonal stimulation into modulation of the Ca^{2+} transport across the sarcolemma.

It may be proposed that the Na^+/Ca^{2+} exchanger predominates over the Ca^{2+}-pumping ATPase in cells where the concentration of Ca^{2+} in the cytosol undergoes cyclic fluctuations (heart, nervous tissue). In cells where this is not expected (e.g., liver), the Ca^{2+} ATPase predominates, and the exchanger can be visualized as an additional back-up system.

REFERENCES

1. Akaike, N., Fishman, H. N., Lee, K. S., Moore, L. E., and Brown, A. M. (1978): *Nature,* 274:379–382.
2. Akaike, N., Lee, K. S., and Brown, A. M. (1978): *J. Gen. Physiol.,* 71:509–531.
3. Akaike, N., Lee, K. S., Fishman, H. M., Moore, L. E., and Brown, A. M. (1978): *Biophys. J.,* 21:208a.
4. Baker, P. F., Blaustein, M. P., Hodgkin, A. L., and Steinhardt, R. A. (1967): *J. Physiol. (Lond.),* 192:43–44P.
5. Baker, P. F., Blaustein, M. P., Hodgkin, A. L., and Steinhardt, R. A. (1969): *J. Physiol. (Lond.),* 200:431–458.
6. Baker, P. F., Blaustein, M. P., Keynes, R. D., Manil, J., Shaw, T. I., and Steinhardt, R. A. (1969): *J. Physiol. (Lond.),* 200:459–496.
7. Baker, P. F., Blaustein, M. P., Manil, J., and Steinhardt, R. A. (1967): *J. Physiol. (Lond.),* 191:100–102P.
8. Baker, P. F., and Glitsch, H. G. (1973): *J. Physiol. (Lond.),* 233:44–46P.
9. Baker, P. F., and McNaughton, P. A. (1976): *J. Physiol. (Lond.),* 259:103–144.
10. Bartschat, D. K., Cyr, D. L., and Lindenmeyer, G. E. (1980): *J. Biol. Chem.,* 255:10044–10047.
11. Bers, D. M., Philipson, K. D., and Nishimoto, A. Y. (1980): *Biochim. Biophys. Acta,* 601:358–371.
12. Blaustein, M. P. (1974): *Rev. Physiol. Biochem. Pharmacol.,* 70:33–82.
13. Blaustein, M. P. (1977): *Biophys. J.,* 20:79–111.
14. Blaustein, M. P. (1982): *Membrane Transport of Calcium,* edited by E. Carafoli, pp. 217–236. Academic Press, London.
15. Blaustein, M. P., and Hodgkin, A. L. (1968): *J. Physiol. (Lond.),* 198:46–48P.
16. Blaustein, M. P., and Hodgkin, A. L. (1969): *J. Physiol. (Lond.),* 200:496–527.
17. Carafoli, E. (1982): *Membrane Transport of Calcium,* edited by E. Carafoli, pp. 109–139. Academic Press, London.
18. Carafoli, E., and Zurini, M. (1982): *Biochim. Biophys. Acta,* 683:279–301.
19. Caroni, P., and Carafoli, E. (1980): *Nature,* 283:765–767.
20. Caroni, P., and Carafoli, E. (1981): *J. Biol. Chem.,* 256:3263–3270.
21. Caroni, P., and Carafoli, E. (1981): *J. Biol. Chem.,* 256:9371–9373.
22. Caroni, P., Reinlib, L., and Carafoli, E. (1980): *Proc. Natl. Acad. Sci. (USA),* 77:6354–6358.
23. Caroni, P., Soldati, L., and Carafoli, E. (1982): *Electrogenic Transport,* edited by M. P. Blaustein and M. Lieberman. Raven Press, New York (*in press*).
24. Caroni, P., Zurini, M., and Clark, A. (1982): *Ann. NY Acad. Sci. (in press).*
25. Di Polo, R. (1974): *J. Gen. Physiol.,* 64:503–517.
26. Di Polo, R. (1977): *J. Gen. Physiol.,* 69:795–813.
27. Dunahm, E. T., and Glynn, L. M. (1961): *J. Physiol. (Lond.),* 156:274.
28. Fain, G. L., Gerschefeld, H. M., and Quandt, F. N. (1980): *J. Physiol. (Lond.),* 303:495–513.
29. Famulski, K., and Carafoli, E. (1982): *Cell Calcium,* 3:263–281.
30. Fatt, P., and Ginsborg, B. L. (1958): *J. Physiol. (Lond.),* 142:516–543.
31. Fedulova, S. A., Kostyuk, P. S., and Veselovsky, N. S. *Brain Res.,* 214:210–214.

32. Fleckenstein, A., Tritthart, H., Fleckenstein, B., Herbst, A., and Grün, G. (1969): *Pfluegers Arch. Ges. Physiol.*, 307:25.
33. Gmaj, P., Murer, H., and Kinne, R. (1979): *Biochem. J.*, 178:549–557.
34. Gopinath, R. M., and Vincenzi, F. F. (1977): *Biochem. Biophys. Res. Commun.*, 77:1203–1209.
35. Grinstein, S., and Erlij, D. (1978): *Proc. R. Soc. Lond. (Biol.)*, 202:353–360.
36. Grossmann, A., and Furchgott, R. F. (1964): *J. Pharmacol. Exp. Ther.*, 145:162–172.
37. Hamill, O. P., Marty, A., Neher, E., Sakmann, B., and Sigworth, J. F. (1981): *Pfluegers Arch. Ges. Physiol.*, 391:85–100.
38. Herchuelz, A., Sener, A., and Malaisse, W. J. (1980): *J. Membr. Biol.*, 57:1–12.
39. Hodgkin, A. L., and Keynes, R. D. (1957): *J. Physiol. (Lond.)*, 138:253–281.
40. Jarrett, H. W., and Penniston, J. T. (1977): *Biochem. Biophys. Res. Commun.*, 77:1210–1216.
41. Kawa, K. (1979): *J. Membr. Biol.*, 49:325–344.
42. Kostyuk, P. G. (1981): *Biochim. Biophys. Acta*, 650:128–150.
43. Kostyuk, P. G., and Kristhal, O. A. (1977): *J. Physiol. (Lond.)*, 270:545–568.
44. Kostyuk, P. G., and Kristhal, O. A. (1977): *J. Physiol. (Lond.)*, 27:569–580.
45. Kostyuk, P. G., Mironov, S. L., and Doroshenko, P. A. (1980): *Dokl. Akad. Nauk SSSR* 253:978–981.
46. Kraus-Friedman, N., Biber J., Murer, H., and Carafoli, E. (1982): *Eur. J. Biochem.*, 129:7–12.
47. Krieger, N. S., and Tashjian, A. H., Jr. (1980): *Nature*, 287:843–845.
48. Kristhal, O. A. (1976): *Dokl. Akad. Nauk SSSR*, 231:1003–1005.
49. Lee, C. O., Taylor, A., and Windhager, E. E. (1980): *Nature*, 287:859–861.
50. LePeuch, A. M., Le Peuch, C. J., and Demaille, J. G. (1980): *Biochemistry*, 19:3368–3373.
51. Lew, V. L., and Ferreira, H. G. (1978): *Curr. Top. Membr. Transp.*, 10:218–279.
52. Lynch, T. J., and Cheung, W. Y. (1979): *Arch. Biochem. Biophys.*, 194:165–170.
53. Niggli, V., Adunyah, E. S., and Carafoli, E. (1982): *J. Biol. Chem.*, 256:8588–8592.
54. Niggli, V., Adunyah, E. S., Penniston, J. T., and Carafoli, E. (1981): *J. Biol. Chem.*, 256:395–401.
55. Niggli, V., Penniston, J. T., and Carafoli, E. (1979): *J. Biol. Chem.*, 254:9955–9958.
56. Niggli, V., Ronner, P., Carafoli, E., and Penniston, J. T. (1979): *Arch. Biochem. Biophys.*, 198:124–130.
57. Parker, J. C. (1980): *J. Gen. Physiol.*, 71:1–17.
58. Penniston, J. T. (1982): *Ann. NY Acad. Sci.*, 402:296–303.
59. Penniston, J. T. (1983): *Calcium and Cell Function*, Vol. 4, edited by W. Y. Cheung (*in press*).
60. Philipson, K. D., and Nishimoto, A. Y. (1980): *J. Biol. Chem.*, 255:6880–6882.
61. Pitts, B. J. R. (1979): *J. Biol. Chem.*, 254:6232–6235.
62. Ponomarev, V. N., Narusevicius, E. V., and Chemeris, N. K. (1980): *Neurophysiology (Kiev)*, 12:221–223.
63. Reeves, J. P., and Sutko, J. L. (1979): *Proc. Natl. Acad. Sci. (USA)*, 76:590–594.
64. Reeves, J. P., and Sutko, J. L. (1980): *Science*, 208:1461–1464.
65. Rinaldi, M. L., Capony, J. P., and Demaille, J. G. (1982): *J. Molec. Cell. Cardiol.*, 14:279–289.
66. Rinaldi, M. L., Le Peuch, C. J., and Demaille, J. G. (1981): *FEBS Lett.*, 129:277–281.
67. Reuter, H. (1965): *Naunyn Schmiedebergs Arch. Pharmacol.*, 251:401–412.
68. Reuter, H. (1974): *J. Physiol. (Lond.)*, 242:429–451.
69. Reuter, H. (1975): *Calcium Movement in Excitable Cells*, edited by P. F. Baker and H. Reuter, pp. 55–97. Pergamon Press, New York.
70. Reuter, H., and Seitz, N. (1968): *J. Physiol. (Lond.)*, 195:451–470.
71. Reuter, A., Stevens, C. F., Tsien, R. W., and Yellen, G. (1982): *Nature*, 297:501–504.
72. Ronner, P., Gazzotti, P., and Carafoli, E. (1977): *Arch. Biochem. Biophys.*, 179:578–583.
73. Roufogalis, B. D. (1979): *Can. J. Physiol. Pharmacol.*, 57:1331–1339.
74. Sarkadi, B. (1980): *Biochim. Biophys. Acta*, 604:159–190.
75. Sarkadi, B., Enyedi, A., and Gardos, G. (1980): *Cell Calcium*, 1:287–297.
76. Schatzmann, H. J. (1970): *Experientia*, 26:687.
77. Schatzmann, H. J. (1982): *Membrane Transport of Calcium*, edited by E. Carafoli, pp. 41–108. Academic Press, New York.
78. Spitzer, N. C. (1979): *Brain Res.*, 161:555–559.

79. Stieger, J., and Schatzmann, H. G. (1981): *Cell Calcium,* 2:601–616.
80. Taverna, R. D., and Hanahan, D. J. (1980): *Biochem. Biophys. Res. Commun.,* 94:652–659.
81. Taylor, A., and Windhager, E. E. (1979): *Annu. J. Physiol.,* 236:F505–F512.
82. Tillotson, D. (1979): *Proc. Nat. Acad. Sci. (USA),* 76:1497–1500.
83. Tsien, R. W., Giles, W., and Greengard, P. (1972): *Nature (New Biol.),* 240:120–122.
84. Varecka, L., and Carafoli, E. (1982): *J. Biol. Chem.,* 257:7414–7421.
85. Veleyev, A. E. (1979): *Neurophysiology (Kiev),* 11:371–374.
86. Veselovsky, N. S., and Fedulova, S. A. (1980): *Dokl. Akad. Nauk SSSR,* 253:1493–1495.
87. Wollenberger, A., Will, H., and Krause, E. G. (1975): *Recent Advances in Studies on Cardiac Structure and Metabolism,* edited by A. Fleckenstein and N. S. Dhalla, pp. 81–93. University Park Press, Baltimore.

Calcium Antagonists and Cardiovascular Disease, edited by L. H. Opie.
Raven Press, New York © 1984.

Chapter 4

Electrophysiology of Calcium Channels in the Heart

Harald Reuter

Department of Pharmacology, University of Berne, 3010 Berne, Switzerland

More than 15 years ago, it was suggested by three independent reports (8, 17,19) that an influx of Ca^{2+} ions could contribute considerably to the total ionic membrane current that determines the shape of the cardiac action potential. However, the main evidence for a Ca^{2+} inward current in various cardiac preparations and its importance for the plateau phase of the action potential came from voltage-clamp experiments (see ref. 22). Since the kinetics of the Ca^{2+}-dependent inward current were much slower than those of the excitatory Na^+ inward current, it has been called the *slow inward current* (i_{si}) (20,23,26). Although there has been much debate and confusion about the ionic nature of the i_{si}, it is now generally accepted that the predominant charge carriers of this current component are indeed Ca^{2+} ions. Several recent reviews have dealt with specific properties of the slow inward Ca^{2+} current in cardiac muscle preparations (e.g., refs. 14,22,29). It is the aim of the present chapter to discuss various methods and their reliability in measuring i_{si} and properties of Ca^{2+} channels in the heart.

SLOW INWARD CALCIUM CURRENT AND THE CARDIAC ACTION POTENTIAL

Figure 1 shows the importance of the Ca^{2+} current in relation to the *cardiac action potential*. The *upper part* of Fig. 1 illustrates a cardiac action potential, and the *center part* shows, schematically, the main ionic current components as they can be recorded during a voltage-clamp step from −80 mV to 0 mV (*lower part*). These main current components that determine the shape of an action potential of a ventricular muscle fiber consist of a rapidly activating and inactivating Na^+ inward current, i_{Na}, of a more slowly activating and inactivating secondary inward current, predominantly carried by Ca^{2+} (i_{si} or i_{Ca}),

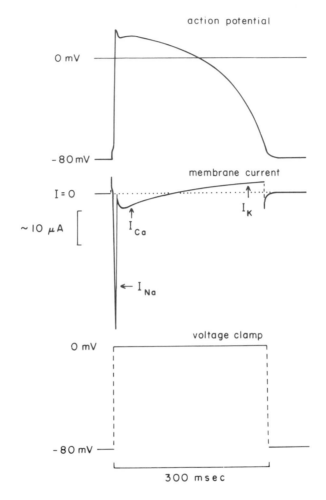

FIG. 1. Schematic drawing of a ventricular cardiac action potential (*top*), of total membrane current flowing at 0 mV (*middle*), and of a voltage-clamp step from a holding potential of −80 mV to 0 mV (*bottom*). Such a voltage step applied to a ventricular fiber bundle typically induces a pattern of ionic current flow (*middle*), where I_{Na} is the Na⁺ current responsible for the upstroke of the action potential, I_{Ca} is the slow inward Ca²⁺ current flowing predominantly during the plateau phase, and I_K is the K⁺ outward current that induces repolarization of the action potential.

and time-independent, and probably also time-dependent, outward currents, both of which are mainly carried by K⁺ (i_K). The shape of the typical plateau phase of the action potential is the result of various factors, the decrease of one of the K⁺ current components during depolarization of the membrane potential (inward rectification of i_{K_1}), a small noninactivating fraction of i_{Na} and, as the main factor, the contribution of i_{si}. The fast transient i_{Na}, of course, is essential for the rapid depolarization phase of the action potential.

Since i_{Na} can be specifically blocked by the poison of the buffer fish, tetrodo-toxin, one can study i_K and i_{si} unpolluted by i_{Na}. For example, one can plot the peak inward current that flows at the beginning of the step and the outward current at the end when the inward current has largely decayed (see Fig. 1) over a wide voltage range. Such a *current-voltage relationship* for peak inward (*open circles*) and late outward current (*closed circles*) is shown in Fig. 2. As indicated above, the total outward current has an N-shaped appearance over the voltage range of a normal action potential, that is, the K⁺ conductance falls, or rectifies in the inward direction, during depolarization in the voltage range −50 to −10 mV. Peak inward current becomes apparent at voltages more positive than −40 mV, reaches a maximum at about 0 mV, and decreases as the driving force for this current component becomes smaller. These current-voltage relationships for i_K and i_{si} cross over at about +45 mV. This corresponds

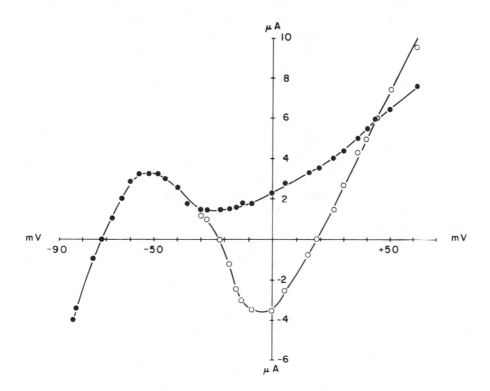

FIG. 2. Current voltage relationships of peak slow Ca²⁺ inward current (*open circles*) and of outward current at the end of a voltage pulse (*closed circles*) (c.f., Fig. 1 for an illustration of a current record, where the slow inward current has been labeled as I_{Ca} and outward current as I_K). Data were obtained from a thin (∼ 0.3 mm) ventricular trabeculum of a sheep heart by means of the single sucrose gap voltage-clamp method. The Na current (I_{Na} in Fig. 1) has been eliminated by the application of tetrodotoxin (20 μM). The *abscissa* indicates the membrane potential during voltage steps (resting potential −72 mV) and the *ordinate* the membrane currents. For further description see text. (H. Reuter, *unpublished results*.)

to the reversal potential of i_{si} (13,24). The fact that the reversal potential does not coincide with the Ca²⁺-equilibrium potential which, according to the Nernst equation, should be 50 to 70 mV more positive, is due to a small outward K⁺ current flowing through the Ca²⁺ channels (13,24). It should be kept in mind that none of the ion channels in biological membranes is exclusively selective for one single ion species. Ca²⁺ channels are among the most selective ones, although they also pass other divalent (Ba²⁺ and Sr²⁺) and monovalent (Na⁺ and K⁺) cations.

Another important feature that can be noticed from a current-voltage plot like that in Fig. 2 is the fact that the maximal net inward current resulting from the flow of i_{si} is usually only 3 to 4 times larger than the net outward K⁺ current at the same potential (about 0 mV). For comparison, peak i_{Na} is about 50 to 100 times larger than the corresponding outward current. This accounts for the fact that the upstroke of a "slow-response" action potential is sluggish (2–8 V/sec) in comparison to that of a normal action potential (150–500 V/sec). This means that any small change in i_{si} or i_{out} will have a major effect on the upstroke velocity and configuration of a slow-response action potential, that is, action potentials where i_{Na} has been inactivated, for example, by depolarization of the membrane with 20 to 30 mM KCl, while the normal action potential may only be slightly affected. I emphasize this fact *because slow-response action potentials are not a reliable measure of* i_{si}.

Three slow-response action potentials that were graphically superimposed after recording from a guinea pig papillary muscle are depicted in Fig. 3. The papillary muscle had been depolarized by 22 mM KCl in the Tyrode's solution in order to inactivate i_{Na}. A strong electrical stimulus elicited the slow-response action potential under control conditions (Fig. 3, trace 1). When isoproterenol (5×10^{-7} M) was added to the bathing solution, amplitude and duration of the slow response were markedly increased (Fig. 3, trace 2). After the addition of verapamil (2×10^{-6} M), however, the action potential was largely inhibited (Fig. 3, trace 3). Similar results have been described many times by various

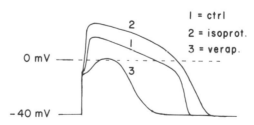

FIG. 3. "Slow-response" action potentials recorded from a guinea pig papillary muscle; drawings from original superimposed oscilloscope tracings. The membrane potential has been depolarized to −40 mV by 22 mM KCl in the bathing solution, in order to inactivate I_{Na} which normally causes the rapid depolarization phase of the action potential (c.f., Fig. 1). The control slow-response action potential is trace 1; the slow response in the presence of isoproterenol (0.5 μM) is trace 2, and that in the presence of verapamil (2 μM) is trace 3. (H. Reuter, *unpublished result.*)

investigators in the literature (for review see ref. 4). The interpretation of these effects is that β_1-adrenoceptor agonists, like isoproterenol, increase i_{si}, and thereby produce the indicated change in action potential. This has indeed been substantiated by voltage-clamp experiments (e.g., refs. 20,21,30). However, the same phenomenon could, in principle, arise just as well from a *decrease* in the K^+ conductance which may well be the reason for a similar effect of certain α-adrenoceptor agonists on the action potential (3,6,15). In other words, the shape change of the action potential alone does not provide clear evidence as to the underlying mechanism. For the very same reason, the initial evidence for Ca^{2+} influx contributing to the plateau phase of the action potential was ambiguous and the authors were well aware of this fact (17,19). Similarly, the inhibition of the slow-response action potential could arise from an increase in outward current by a drug, or a decrease of i_{si}, or both. In the case of verapamil and related drugs, voltage-clamp experiments revealed a strong inhibitory effect on i_{si} (10–12) which accounts for much of the effect illustrated in Fig. 3. However, most drugs are not entirely specific in their action. This applies also to verapamil-like substances which have been shown to have effects on Na^+ channels (1,7) and K^+ channels (11) as well. This further complicates the interpretation of drug effects on slow-response action potentials.

The question then arises: Are measurements of slow-response action potentials useless in the investigation of drug actions? The answer is "no." These measurements are simple and have their place in routine pharmacological studies which are aimed at obtaining first information about possible mechanisms of the action of a drug on cardiac cell membranes. However, they do not provide decisive evidence on the mechanism of drug actions and should be interpreted with great caution. On the other hand, voltage-clamp measurements and single-channel recordings (see ref. 9) are suitable tools for obtaining this kind of evidence.

RECORDING OF SINGLE CALCIUM CHANNELS

One of the most exciting new developments in electrophysiology is the possibility of recording properties of single ion channels in cell membranes directly. The first recordings were performed on the nicotinic ion channels in skeletal muscle activated by acetylcholine (16). Meanwhile, the method has been improved and extended to many biological cells (for a review of the method and its applications see ref. 9). The method allows, for the first time, the characterization of single membrane proteins that function as ion channels in terms of their molecular electrophysiological properties, that is, their responses to changes in membrane potential, to intracellular and extracellular ionic constituents, to enzyme activities, and to hormones, neurotransmitters, and drugs.

Ionic currents flowing through single Ca^{2+} channels have been recorded in cultured cardiac cells (25), chromaffin cells (5), snail neurons, vertebrate neurons, and vertebrate secretory cells (2). As pointed out by Brown et al. (2), the basic properties of Ca^{2+} channels seem to be very similar in all these tissues from

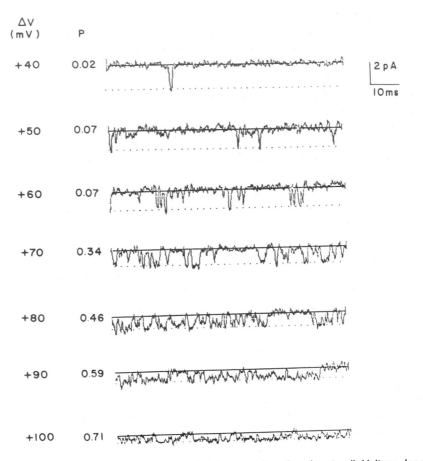

FIG. 4. Single Ca²⁺-channel currents recorded from a cultured rat heart cell. Voltage-dependence of single-channel currents, with Ba²⁺ as charge carriers. Membrane potential was stepped by the indicated step size (ΔV) from a holding potential of about −70 mV. The *solid lines* indicate the baseline after leak subtraction, the *dotted lines* indicate the measured open-channel current, *i.* Beside each record is the average probability (*p*) that the channel was open during the voltage step, ΔV. Single-channel current, *i,* becomes smaller during depolarization because of the reduction in driving force. (From ref. 25.)

widely different species. Some of those properties are illustrated in Fig. 4. These recordings were obtained from cultured myocytes of neonatal rat hearts by Reuter et al. (25). The potential of a small patch of membrane in a single cardiac cell was depolarized by voltage-clamp steps (ΔV). Small depolarizations from the holding potential, which was about −70 mV in this cell, did not cause any openings of the channels. If the membrane potential was depolarized by 40 mV, occasional openings occurred, and voltage-clamp steps of larger sizes greatly increased the probability of the single Ca²⁺ channel entering an "open" state. With a probability $p = 1.0$, the channel would be open all the time throughout the clamp pulse. The probability, p, can be calculated from $I = Npi$, where I is the time-averaged mean current flowing through an open channel during a depolarizing pulse, i is the magnitude of the single-channel current, and N is the number of channels functioning in the patch of membrane ($N = 1$ in Fig. 4). The single-channel current, i, decreases with depolarization because the driving force for current flow decreases. An interesting feature of Ca^{2+} channels is that their openings frequently occur in bursts (see, for example, $\Delta V = 60$ and 70 mV in Fig. 4). This burst behavior of single Ca^{2+} channels determines the relatively slow time course of Ca^{2+} currents measured by conventional voltage-clamp methods. With long depolarizing clamp steps (1 sec), the frequency of openings decreases during the pulse, indicating inactivation of the channels. Inactivation is partially voltage-dependent and results from a decreased probability of Ca^{2+} channels opening when the holding potential is made more positive (25). By knowing the total membrane Ca^{2+}-current density, single-channel current, and membrane capacity, one can calculate a density of about 0.5 Ca^{2+} channel per μm^2 membrane surface area in the cultured cardiac cells. For comparison, the Na^+-channel density is approximately 16 per μm^2 in these cells. Na^+ channels do not show bursting behavior and with increasing depolarization virtually all channel openings occur during the first 10 to 20 msec of a clamp step (ref. 27; A. Cachelin, J. de Peyer, and H. Reuter, *unpublished*). The much smaller density of Ca^{2+} channels than that of Na^+ channels in the membrane accounts for the large difference in amplitude of the two inward currents, as illustrated in Fig. 1. The current flowing through single Ca^{2+} channels is only slightly smaller than that flowing through single Na^+ channels.

Another interesting feature of cardiac Ca^{2+} channels, in contrast to Na^+ channels, is that they do not survive in isolated inside/out membrane patches. It seems that these channels need some input from cell metabolism for their proper function. It has long been known that the Ca^{2+} current in the heart is greatly increased by β-adrenergic catecholamines (see previous section). As has been suggested by various authors (see refs. 22 and 28 for reviews) phosphorylation of Ca^{2+} channels by cyclic AMP-dependent protein kinase may be the ultimate reaction step in the whole cascade of events following β-adrenoceptor occupancy by the respective agonists. This hypothesis has gained considerable support by the injection of the catalytic subunit of cyclic AMP-dependent protein kinase into single myocardial cells which caused an effect on the slow inward Ca^{2+} current identical to that obtained after application of epinephrine (18). It is quite possible then that phosphorylation of the Ca^{2+} channel, or of a protein closely associated with the channel, is an important metabolic step that regulates the probability of the channel to enter an open state during membrane depolarization.

The method of single-channel recording is one of the most powerful tools in elucidating mechanisms of drug actions on cell membranes. In the near future considerable new insight will probably be gained about molecular reactions involved in ion channel regulation by hormones and drugs.

CONCLUSIONS

The various electrophysiological methods currently used to measure Ca^{2+} currents in the heart are of different quality and reliability. So-called slow-response action potentials, which partly depend on inward Ca^{2+} current through the membrane, are technically easy to record. Although drug-induced changes in the shape of such action potentials may give useful hints concerning possible mechanisms of actions of the drugs, the interpretation of the results can be very difficult and even misleading. Voltage-clamp techniques are much better suited to evaluate drug effects on the individual membrane current components underlying the cardiac action potential. Voltage-clamp experiments, however, are relatively difficult, not without problems in cardiac muscle, and therefore will probably remain in the hands of a few experts. The most advanced and reliable method of recording ion channels is the "patch-clamp" technique which permits direct recordings of the electrophysiological properties of individual channels. Ca^{2+} channels in cardiac cells have already been measured with this technique. It will be most interesting to analyze effects of hormones, neurotransmitters, and drugs at the molecular level of individual ion channels. A clearer and deeper understanding of mechanisms of drug actions, like those of Ca^{2+} antagonists, will help guide their therapeutic use.

ACKNOWLEDGMENT

Support by the Swiss National Science Foundation (Grant 3.154–0.81) is gratefully acknowledged.

REFERENCES

1. Bayer, R., Hennekes, R., Kaufmann, R., and Mannhold, R. (1975): *Naunyn Schmiedebergs Arch. Pharmacol.*, 290:49–68.
2. Brown, A. M., Camerer, H., Kunze, D. L., and Lux, H. D. (1982): *Nature*, 299:156–158.
3. Brückner, R., and Scholz, H. (1980): *Naunyn Schmiedebergs Arch. Pharmacol.*, 311:R37.
4. Cranefield, P. F. (1975): *The Conduction of the Cardiac Impulse.* Futura, Mount Kisco, New York.
5. Fenwick, E. M., Marty, A., and Neher, E. (1982): *J. Physiol. (Lond.)*, 331:599–635.
6. Gadsby, D. C., and Glitsch, H. G. (1982): *J. Physiol. (Lond.)*, 332:51 P.
7. Galper, J. B., and Catterall, W. A. (1978): *Dev. Biol.*, 65:216–227.
8. Hagiwara, S., and Nakajima, S. (1966): *J. Gen. Physiol.*, 43:793–806.
9. Hamill, O. P., Marty, A., Neher, E., Sakmann, B., and Sigworth, F. J. (1981): *Pfluegers Arch.*, 391:85–100.
10. Hescheler, J., Pelzer, D., Trube, G., and Trautwein, W. (1982): *Pfluegers Arch.*, 393:287–291.
11. Kass, R. S., and Tsien, R. W. (1975): *J. Gen. Physiol.*, 66:169–192.
12. Kohlhardt, M., Bauer, B., Krause, H., and Fleckenstein, A. (1972): *Pfluegers Arch.*, 335:309–322.
13. Lee, K. S., and Tsien R. W. (1982): *Nature*, 297:498–501.
14. McDonald, T. F. (1982): *Ann. Rev. Physiol.*, 44:425–434.
15. Miura, Y., Iuni, J., and Imamura, H. (1978): *Naunyn Schmiedebergs Arch. Pharmacol.*, 301:201–205.
16. Neher, E., and Sakmann, B. (1976): *Nature*, 260:799–802.

17. Niedergerke, R., and Orkand, R. K. (1966): *J. Physiol.* (*Lond.*), 184:291–311.
18. Osterrieder, W., Brum, G., Hescheler, J., Trautwein, W., Flockerzi, V., and Hofmann, F. (1982): *Nature,* 298:576–578.
19. Reuter, H. (1966): *Pfluegers Arch.,* 287:357–367.
20. Reuter, H. (1967): *J. Physiol.* (*Lond.*), 192:479–492.
21. Reuter, H. (1974): *J. Physiol.* (*Lond.*), 242:429–451.
22. Reuter, H. (1979): *Ann. Rev. Physiol.,* 41:413–424.
23. Reuter, H., and Beeler, G. W., Jr. (1969): *Science,* 163:399–401.
24. Reuter, H., and Scholz, H. (1977): *J. Physiol.* (*Lond.*), 264:17–47.
25. Reuter, H., Stevens, C. F., Tsien, R. W., and Yellen, G. (1982): *Nature,* 297:501–504.
26. Rougier, O., Vassort, G., Garnier, D., Gargouïl, Y. M., and Coraboeuf, E. (1969): *Pfluegers Arch.,* 308:91–110.
27. Sigworth, F. J., and Neher, E. (1980): *Nature,* 287:447–449.
28. Tsien, R. W. (1977): *Adv. Cyclic Nucleotide Res.,* 8:363–420.
29. Tsien, R. W., and Siegelbaum, S. (1978): *Physiology of Membrane Disorders,* edited by T. E. Andreoli, J. F. Hoffman, and D. D. Fanestil. Plenum, New York.
30. Vassort, G., Rougier, O., Garnier, D., Sauviat, M. P., Coraboeuf, E., and Gargouïl, Y. M. (1969): *Pfluegers Arch.,* 309:70–81.

Calcium Antagonists and Cardiovascular Disease, edited by L. H. Opie.
Raven Press, New York © 1984.

Chapter 5

Calcium Fluxes Across the Sarcoplasmic Reticulum

Arnold M. Katz

Cardiology Division, Department of Medicine, The University of Connecticut Health Center, Farmington, Connecticut 06032

The pumping action of the heart is regulated both by the changing requirements of the arterial and venous circulation, which define the load on the pump, and by the properties of the myocardium itself, which define the characteristics of the heart as a pump. The latter, like those of any pump, are defined by the frequency of cycling (heart rate) and the size of each stroke (stroke volume), which represents the difference between end-diastolic and end-systolic volumes. This simple analysis allows us to define a number of important mechanisms by which the pumping action of the heart can be controlled. Furthermore, it provides the basis for understanding the interplay between the multiple and interrelated effects of important physiological, pharmacological, and pathophysiological interventions that modify cardiovascular function.

In considering *the heart as a pump,* the dependence of the size of each stroke on both end-diastolic and end-systolic volumes allows this important parameter of cardiac function to be characterized in terms of two independent, though interrelated, properties of the myocardium: contraction and relaxation. Obviously, an intervention that altered end-diastolic and end-systolic volumes in the same direction and to the same degree would have no effect on stroke volume (although the geometry of the heart would undergo important changes). Conversely, a change in stroke volume would become maximal during interventions that exert opposing effects on end-diastolic and end-systolic volumes. Stated another way, a positive inotropic drug would exert its maximal effect on stroke volume, and thus the pumping action of the heart, if it promoted *both* contraction and relaxation so as to decrease end-systolic volume and increase end-diastolic volume. The hemodynamic manifestations of these considerations have long been recognized by cardiovascular physiologists, who have noted that most inotropic interventions do not significantly impair relaxation (16). Indeed, there is often a parallel effect of elevation of extracellular Ca^{2+} concentration in stimulating both contraction and relaxation (15), while catecholamines actually accelerate the relaxation phase of the cardiac cycle (34,44). It is only recently, however, that the biochemical basis for these effects has become clarified.

CALCIUM FLUXES AND THE CONTRACTION-RELAXATION CYCLE

The mechanisms responsible for myocardial contraction and relaxation are now understood in terms of the central role of Ca^{2+} as an activator of the contractile process. Cytosolic Ca^{2+} concentration is approximately 0.1 μM during diastole, rising more than 10-fold in systole. This increase in cytosolic Ca^{2+} concentration allows Ca^{2+} to bind to troponin, the Ca^{2+}-receptor protein of the contractile apparatus, and thereby to initiate the contractile process (5,17). As the amount of Ca^{2+} bound to the high-affinity Ca^{2+} binding site of troponin determines the number of active actin-myosin interactions, the intensity of contraction, and thus the ability of the heart to empty, will be determined by the amount of activator Ca^{2+} available in the cytosol for binding to troponin.

Relaxation occurs when lowering of cytosolic Ca^{2+} concentration causes Ca^{2+} to become dissociated from troponin, restoring the contractile proteins to their relaxed state. The rate of Ca^{2+} removal from the cytosol will thus determine the rate at which wall tension falls during isovolumic contraction; while the extent to which cytosolic Ca^{2+} concentration falls during diastole represents a major determinant of diastolic compliance, and thus of filling and end-diastolic volume. In this way, the transitions of the heart from rest to activity, and back to rest, can be viewed as reflections of the rise and fall of cytosolic Ca^{2+} concentration during each cardiac cycle that determine, respectively, end-systolic and end-diastolic volumes.

The changes in cytosolic Ca^{2+} concentration that occur during each cardiac cycle are the result of regulated Ca^{2+} fluxes into and out of the cytosol. There are two sources of activator Ca^{2+}, and thus two sinks into which Ca^{2+} is transported during diastole; these are the extracellular fluid and the lumen of the sarcoplasmic reticulum. These important Ca^{2+} fluxes take place across the membrane barriers of the sarcolemma and sarcoplasmic reticulum (SR), which separate the cytosol from the extracellular space and interior of the SR, respectively.

As the Ca^{2+} concentrations in the extracellular space and within the SR are much higher than those in the cytosol, activation is readily seen to depend on passive ion fluxes in which increases in the Ca^{2+} permeability of the sarcolemma and SR membranes allow this cation to flow down its electrochemical gradient into the area of the cell occupied by the contractile proteins. Conversely, the Ca^{2+} fluxes responsible for relaxation are active, in that energy must be expended to transport Ca^{2+} out of the cytosol, both into the extracellular space and the lumen of the SR.

CALCIUM FLUXES ACROSS THE SARCOLEMMA

As discussed in other chapters, the major pathway by which Ca^{2+} enters the cardiac cytosol is via voltage-dependent Ca^{2+} channels; the resulting electrogenic Ca^{2+} flux gives rise to the slow inward current. Ca^{2+} efflux across the sarcolemma occurs mainly in exchange for Na^+, which enters the cytosol down an electrochemical gradient that provides the energy needed to move Ca^{2+} into the extracellular space. There is also evidence for an ATP-dependent Ca^{2+} pump in the sarcolemma, which couples the energy derived from hydrolysis of this nucleotide to the active transport of Ca^{2+} out of the cytosol (2,41). Although the physiological characteristics of these active Ca^{2+} fluxes have been studied extensively, the complexity of the sarcolemma has, so far, prevented detailed studies of the molecular characteristics of the membrane pumps and channels by which they are effected.

SARCOPLASMIC RETICULUM

The SR is a relatively simple membrane, as its primary, if not exclusive, function is to regulate cytosolic Ca^{2+} concentration. In mammalian fast skeletal muscle, in which contraction of an individual muscle cell is essentially an all-or-none process, Ca^{2+} fluxes across the SR appear not to be extensively regulated. This fact probably accounts for the ease with which active membrane vesicles of rabbit white skeletal SR can be prepared, and the finding that even with little purification, approximately 90% of the protein in these vesicles is of a single molecular species: the Ca^{2+} pump ATPase protein. It is, therefore, not surprising that the membranes of the skeletal SR have been studied extensively. Myocardial contractile function depends to a significant extent on the amount of Ca^{2+} stored within, and released from the cardiac SR (7). As Ca^{2+} fluxes across this membrane are much more extensively regulated than in skeletal muscle, cardiac SR preparations are more complex. Because of its simplicity, the skeletal SR membrane has come to represent the "gold standard" in this field, much as the frog sartorius has been for muscle mechanics, and the squid axon for electrophysiology. For this reason, the following descriptions focus on the properties of rabbit skeletal muscle SR, which allows our discussion of the special properties of cardiac SR to be presented in terms of the more precisely defined skeletal SR membranes.

Structure

Both skeletal and cardiac SR represent intracellular membrane structures that enclose a space within, but distinct from the cytosol that contains a store of Ca^{2+} that can be released during excitation. The state of the Ca^{2+} within these membrane structures is not clear; whereas it is generally assumed that some of this Ca^{2+} is free and at an activity considerably higher than that in the cytosol, it is possible that under normal or pathological conditions at least a portion of this Ca^{2+} is bound to an anion, such as phosphate (28), to the anionic phospholipid head groups of the SR membrane, or to Ca^{2+}-binding proteins within the SR (33). Recent evidence suggests that palmitic acid, thought to be formed in large quantities in the ischemic myocardium, can trap Ca^{2+} in the SR as a Ca^{2+}-palmitate complex (32).

The structure of the SR membrane in skeletal muscle has been studied extensively, and the location of the Ca^{2+} pump ATPase protein within these membranes has been defined by a combination of electron microscopy, and X-ray and neutron diffraction (1,12) (Fig. 1). The Ca^{2+} pump proteins appear to be imbedded in the phospholipid bilayer as dimers (3) which are arranged in a weak lattice structure (36). A large portion (approximately half) of the protein molecule extends from the cytosolic (outer) surface of the phospholipid bilayer into the aqueous space of the cytosol (Fig. 1B) (1). This cytosolic portion of the Ca^{2+} pump ATPase protein probably contains the high-affinity Ca^{2+}- and ATP-binding sites that participate in active Ca^{2+} transport (see later). The other half of this protein is imbedded in the bilayer, contacting the aqueous space within the SR (Fig. 1B). In this way, the Ca^{2+} pump ATPase protein spans the membrane in a manner that allows it to function as a "channel" through which Ca^{2+} can move between the aqueous spaces on the two sides of the membrane.

The SR forms special, and functionally important, junctions with the sarcolemma and with the transverse tubular system (t-tubules), an extension of the sarcolemma that appears to play a key role in excitation-contraction coupling. These junctions are believed to provide a functional link between the membranes of the sarcolemma and the SR, and may serve as the site at which the changing electrical potential across the sarcolemma initiates the release of Ca^{2+} by the SR in response to an action potential. Studies of the t-tubule-SR junction of skeletal muscle have shown structures linking these two membrane systems (Fig. 2) (6,9,39). There is evidence that these structures represent potential connections between the extracellular space and the interior of the SR (Fig. 2), and that this structure changes during excitation (9). A "fanciful" reconstruction of one of these structures is shown in the inset to Fig. 2. It should be emphasized that the composition of the fluid within the SR differs significantly from that of the extracellular fluid (40). For this reason, the appearance of a channel between the extracellular space and the interior of the SR (which probably involves permeability changes in both the t-tubule and the SR) would be expected to have important functional consequences. Such a mechanism could, for example, explain the as yet poorly understood, nature of the signal by which the action potential that spreads along the sarcolemma and down the t-tubule initiates release of the Ca^{2+} stored within the SR (8).

At least three mechanisms have been postulated to explain this key step in excitation-contraction coupling. An *electrical coupling* may allow the change in charge distribution across the t-tubule caused by depolarization to influence

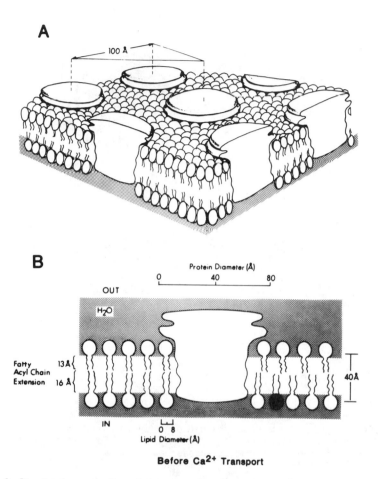

FIG. 1. A: Structural organization of the sarcoplasmic reticulum (SR) membrane depicting the random configuration of the Ca^{2+} pump protein in the membrane bilayer. Each structure probably represents a dimer of the Ca^{2+} pump protein. The nearest distance between these structures is approximately 100 Å. **B:** Cross-section of the SR membrane showing in detail the resting conformation of the Ca^{2+} pump protein, which is seen to span the membrane bilayer with a substantial portion protruding to the outside. Water (*shaded*) penetrates the layer of phospholipid head groups so that both ends of the protein are in contact with these water layers. The phospholipid head groups are separated by 40 Å with different fatty acyl extensions for the outer and inner monolayers. In addition, there are 6 to 10% more phospholipid molecules in the inner than in the outer monolayer (see *shaded* phospholipid). (From ref. 25a.)

the structure of a channel in the SR so as to cause the latter to open. Alternatively, a *structural rearrangement* of a protein or proteins within the t-tubule may open a Ca^{2+} channel in the SR by removing a "plug-like" mechanism that, at resting potential, occludes this channel. Finally, the transfer of a small amount of Ca^{2+} from the extracellular space to the interior of the cell immediately "below" the t-tubule membrane may increase Ca^{2+} concentration outside the

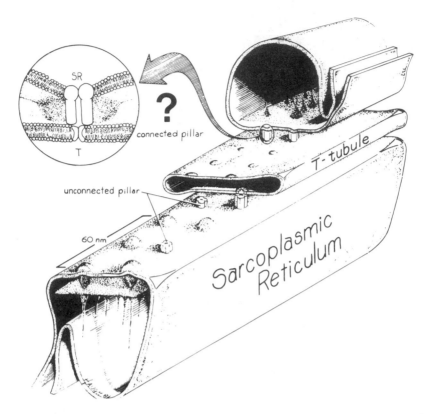

FIG. 2. Hypothetical model of the junction between the t-tubule and SR showing "pillars" as connections between the lumens of the t-tubules and SR. The *inset* shows one possible mechanism for the formation of channels across these membranes. (From ref. 6.)

SR in a manner that provides a stimulus to the opening of a Ca^{2+} channel in the SR by a *"Ca^{2+}-induced Ca^{2+} release"* (8). This unresolved question represents the most important remaining mystery in excitation-contraction coupling.

Calcium Uptake

As has already been pointed out, the process by which Ca^{2+} is transported into the SR is an active one, in which Ca^{2+} is moved against its electrochemical gradient by an ion pump that involves expenditure of the chemical energy derived from the hydrolysis of the terminal phosphate of ATP. This energy transduction is effected by the Ca^{2+} pump ATPase, a 100,000 dalton protein that, through a sequence of steps involving the formation and subsequent breakdown of phosphorylated enzyme intermediates (EPs), allows the terminal high-energy phosphate of ATP to be transferred to this protein (10,14,42). These changes are accompanied by the binding of Ca^{2+} to the external (cytosolic) portion of the

Ca^{2+} pump ATPase and the subsequent transport of the cation to the interior of the SR, an active process that requires the expenditure of energy. The nature of the bond linking the phosphate group that is derived from ATP to the Ca^{2+} pump changes during the Ca^{2+} transport reaction: Initially, when the Ca^{2+} pump is energized and the Ca^{2+} is at the low-energy level of the cytosol, this is a high-energy acyl phosphate bond ($\sim$P), while in the later steps of this reaction sequence—when the energy has been used to "raise" the Ca^{2+} to the higher activity found within the SR—the bond is transformed into a low-energy acyl phosphate ($-$P) (35,38). [Both bonds differ chemically from the phosphoester formed by protein kinase-catalyzed phosphorylation (see later).]

The reaction steps in the Ca^{2+} transport reaction can be simplified according to the scheme shown in Fig. 3, in which E represents the Ca^{2+} pump ATPase protein, E$_1$ $\cdot$ P is the high-energy acyl phosphate and E$_2$ $\cdot$ P is the low-energy acyl phosphate. Ca$_i$ and Ca$_o$ refer, respectively, to the low and high Ca^{2+} concentrations inside and outside the SR. The forward reaction of the Ca^{2+} pump begins when ATP and Ca^{2+} bind to the cytosolic portion of the enzyme (Fig. 3, step 1), forming a short-lived Ca$_o$ E-ATP complex that is rapidly converted to the high-energy acyl phosphoenzyme, Ca$_o$E$_1$ $\cdot$ P (Fig. 3, step 2). This step captures the energy of the terminal phosphate bond of ATP in the high-energy phosphoenzyme E$_1$ $\cdot$ P to which two Ca^{2+} ions are also bound in their low-energy state, i.e., at or near their activity in the cytosol. The key step in Ca^{2+} transport occurs in the next step (Fig. 3, step 3), where E$_1$ $\cdot$ P, the high-energy acyl phosphate, is converted to E$_2$ $\cdot$ P, the low-energy intermediate. In this step, the energy previously present in the acyl phosphate bond of E$_1$ $\cdot$ P is utilized to move the 2 Ca^{2+} ions from the region of low activity outside the SR (Ca$_o$) to the interior of the SR, where Ca^{2+} activity is high (Ca$_i$). The nature of the conformational change that occurs at this step remains poorly understood, but a large entropy change may play a role in this active transport process (27).

Release of Ca^{2+} from the low-energy acyl phosphoprotein, E$_2$ $\cdot$ P, into the region of high Ca^{2+} concentration inside the SR may require replacement of the bound Ca^{2+} by Mg^{2+}, resulting in the formation of MgE$_2$ $\cdot$ P (Fig. 3, step 3). The low-energy phosphorylated intermediate then breaks down with release of inorganic phosphate outside the SR to form free E (Fig. 4, step 4). There is evidence that the state of the nonphosphorylated Ca^{2+} pump ATPase

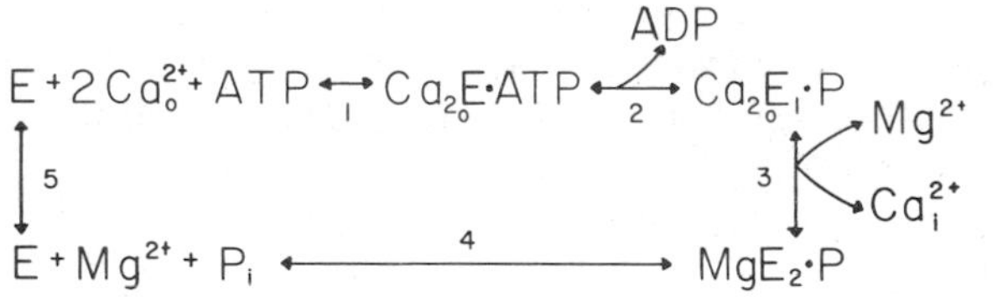

FIG. 3. Schematic representation of the reactions of the Ca^{2+} pump ATPase of the SR. See text for explanation.

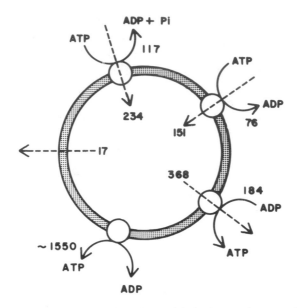

FIG. 4. Schematic representation of Ca²⁺ fluxes (*dashed arrows*) across the sarcoplasmic reticulum membrane (*shaded*), and their relationship to reactions involving ATP and ADP (*solid arrows*). Reading clockwise from top: a rapid Ca²⁺ influx (234 nmoles/mg/min) coupled to ATP hydrolysis by the Ca²⁺ pump; a somewhat less rapid Ca²⁺ influx (151 nmoles/ min) accompanied by EP formation; a rapid Ca²⁺ efflux (368 nmoles/mg/min) that occurs when ATP is formed from ADP; ATP hydrolysis not coupled to a Ca²⁺ flux; and (*dashed line*) a slow (17 nmoles/mg/min) passive Ca²⁺ "leak." Although each of these fluxes is depicted in the figure as occurring via a separate process, it is probable that, with the exception of the passive leak, they involve the Ca²⁺ pump ATPase protein. Data from ref. 43 assume a ratio of 2 moles Ca²⁺ transported by the Ca²⁺ pump for each mole of ATP hydrolyzed or regenerated.

protein immediately after $E_2 \cdot P$ is degraded differs from that to which Ca²⁺ is bound initially, so that completion of the Ca²⁺ pump cycle requires the conversion of this E to that originally present at the start of the reaction (Fig. 3, step 5). Overall, the rate-limiting step in the Ca²⁺ pump reaction is generally agreed to occur at one of the steps of EP degradation.

It should be noted that all of the steps in the Ca²⁺ pump reaction are reversible. Thus, under conditions favorable for the back reaction (i.e., when Ca_i and ADP are high, Ca_o and ATP are low, and in the presence of high concentrations of Mg²⁺ and phosphate), the downhill Ca²⁺ efflux from the SR can be coupled to the resynthesis of ATP from ADP and inorganic phosphate that is accompanied by the formation of phosphorylated enzyme from inorganic phosphate.

Calcium Release

Unlike the mechanism for active Ca²⁺ uptake by the SR, the nature of the process by which Ca²⁺ is released from this structure in the intact muscle remains poorly understood. While there is general agreement that Ca^{2+} release from the SR is a passive, downhill process, little is known of the nature of the "channel" that mediates the permeability change that allows Ca^{2+} to flow out of the SR (8). As already mentioned, the backward reaction of the Ca^{2+} pump ATPase can mediate a Ca^{2+} efflux that is coupled to ATP synthesis from P_i; however, the conditions needed to produce this complete reversal of the Ca^{2+} pump reaction (notably, low ATP, high ADP, and low Ca_o) are not normally found in the cytosol of living muscles.

Several years ago, we observed a slow Ca^{2+} efflux from Ca^{2+}-loaded SR vesicles that was increased by elevation of Ca_o (23,24), and found that elevation of Ca_o could promote a slow Ca^{2+}-induced Ca^{2+} release when ATP levels outside the vesicles were high and ADP concentrations were low (20). More recently, analysis of more rapid Ca^{2+} fluxes across the SR membrane in terms of their relationship to various partial reactions of the Ca^{2+} pump ATPase protein demonstrated a rapid Ca^{2+} efflux, probably mediated by the Ca^{2+} pump, that occurs when external Ca^{2+} concentrations are well above those found in resting muscle (43) (Fig. 4). These findings are consistent with the view that some of the partial reaction steps of the backward reaction of the Ca^{2+} pump ATPase can mediate the release of Ca^{2+} from the SR, although whether this process is responsible for the Ca^{2+}-induced Ca^{2+} release seen in more intact preparations (8) remains unsettled.

Pharmacologic Regulation

It is now generally agreed that neither the cardiac glycosides nor catecholamines have *direct* effects on the cardiac SR (22). However, the β-adrenergic agonists are recognized to have important *indirect* effects on the cardiac SR. These are mediated by cyclic AMP-dependent protein kinases that catalyze the phosphorylation of *phospholamban,* a 22,000 dalton protein within the SR membrane that regulates the rates of both Ca^{2+} uptake and Ca^{2+} release by these membranes (see refs. 18 and 41 for review). It should be emphasized that the phosphate bond formed in phospholamban by the protein kinase is a phosphoester, which differs from both the high- and low-energy acyl phosphate bonds found in the Ca^{2+} pump ATPase protein.

The effects of phospholamban phosphorylation on the cardiac SR are complex, but the overall result is acceleration of both Ca^{2+} uptake and Ca^{2+} release by these membrane vesicles. The stimulation of Ca^{2+} uptake, which has been studied most extensively, is due to several effects (41). The rate of EP formation is accelerated, due mainly to an increase in the rate of the transition between the two nonphosphorylated states of the enzyme (Fig. 3, step 5). More important is the acceleration of the rate-limiting steps of EP degradation (especially step 3 in Fig. 3) which allows phosphorylation of phospholamban to increase the overall rate of the forward reaction. A quite different effect has also been observed to accompany phospholamban phosphorylation: This is an increase in the Ca^{2+}

sensitivity of the Ca^{2+}-uptake reaction that enhances the ability of low cytosolic Ca^{2+} concentrations to promote and participate in Ca^{2+} transport (13). This increased Ca^{2+} sensitivity of the Ca^{2+} pump is accompanied by a loss of a positive cooperativity observed for the Ca^{2+}-dependence of Ca^{2+} transport by cardiac SR when phospholamban is in its dephospho-form. Together, these effects allow β-adrenergic agonists and other agents that increase cellular cyclic AMP levels to accelerate both Ca^{2+} uptake and Ca^{2+} release by the SR (Fig. 5).

The physiological importance of these effects of β-adrenergic agonists on Ca^{2+} uptake by the SR can be understood in view of the ability of these agents to accelerate heart rate. Indeed, if systole were not shortened by these agents, then the catecholamine-stimulated heart would, at the high heart rates produced by these agents, fail to relax sufficiently rapidly to allow for filling. It is, therefore, not surprising that β-adrenergic stimulation increases the rate of Ca^{2+} transport by the cardiac SR, an effect that both shortens the duration of systole and accelerates the rate of relaxation. The increased Ca^{2+} sensitivity of the Ca^{2+} pump associated with phospholamban phosphorylation (13) is also important in allowing the heart to relax completely, in view of the ability of positive inotropic effects of the β-adrenergic agonists to increase the amount of Ca^{2+} released during excitation-contraction coupling.

There is evidence that phosphorylation of phospholamban by the cyclic AMP-dependent protein kinases increases the rate of Ca^{2+} efflux from cardiac SR vesicles (18). This effect of phospholamban phosphorylation may play a role in the acceleration of contraction associated with the response of the heart to β-adrenergic agonists.

Regulation by Calcium

Cytosolic Ca^{2+} concentration has a dual effect on the rate of Ca^{2+} transport by the SR. Simplest is its role as substrate for the forward reaction of the Ca^{2+} pump (Fig. 3, step 1), which allows increasing Ca^{2+} concentration in the micromolar range to accelerate directly the rate of Ca^{2+} uptake by the SR. More recently, a second, indirect, effect of Ca^{2+} has been observed that is mediated by phospholamban. It is now clear that this regulatory protein can also be phosphorylated by a Ca^{2+} (calmodulin)-dependent protein kinase; and that, like cyclic AMP-dependent protein kinase-catalyzed phosphorylation, the Ca^{2+}-dependent phosphorylation stimulates the rate of Ca^{2+} uptake (26,41).

The physiological implications of the indirect effects of the Ca^{2+} (calmodulin)-dependent phosphorylation of phospholamban are related to the resulting stimulation of Ca^{2+} uptake by the SR, which allows an increase in the level of cytosolic Ca^{2+} during systole to accelerate the mechanism responsible for Ca^{2+} removal from the cytosol during diastole. In other words, this mechanism makes it possible for interventions that increase cytosolic Ca^{2+} and thereby promote ventricular emptying to activate the mechanisms responsible for ventricular filling.

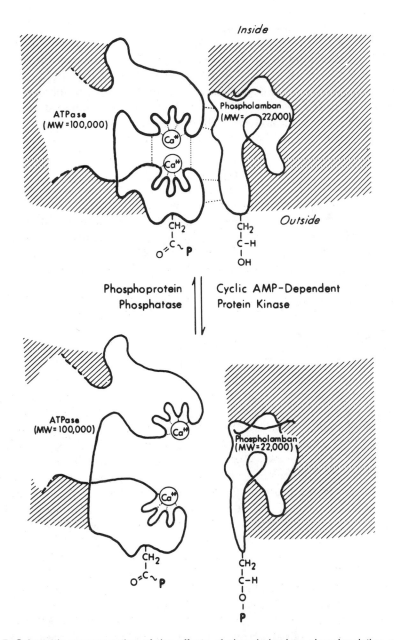

FIG. 5. Schematic representation of the effects of phospholamban phosphorylation on the Ca²⁺ pump of the cardiac sarcoplasmic reticulum. **Top:** Phospholamban in the dephospho-form interacts with the Ca²⁺ pump ATPase protein so as to confer positive cooperativity between its 2 Ca²⁺ binding sites and to slow pump turnover rate. **Bottom:** Phosphorylation of phospholamban reduces its interactions with the Ca²⁺ pump ATPase protein, allowing each Ca²⁺ binding site to act independently with Ca²⁺, thereby increasing both Ca²⁺ sensitivity and turnover of the Ca²⁺ pump. (From ref. 13.)

As has already been discussed, inotropic agents, which by definition enhance the ability of the heart to empty, would fail to increase the ability of the heart to function as a pump unless there was a concomitant increase in the ability of the more fully emptied heart to fill. This latter effect appears to be due, at least in part, to the Ca^{2+}-dependent phosphorylation of phospholamban that allows the increased cytosolic Ca^{2+} in the inotropically stimulated heart to enhance cardiac filling through its ability to accelerate Ca^{2+} transport into the SR.

Nonspecific "Membrane Stabilizing" Effects

For many years, investigators who examined the response of the SR to a variety of membrane-active drugs, including local anesthetics, antiarrhythmic agents, and β-adrenergic receptor antagonists, have generally found that these agents inhibit the Ca^{2+}-uptake reaction (4,11,19,21,30,31,37). These drugs commonly have an amphiphilic structure; that is, they contain both hydrophobic and hydrophilic regions in their molecular structure and so can insert into the membrane bilayer of the SR.

A general observation regarding the effects of a wide variety of amphiphiles on Ca^{2+} fluxes across the SR is that their potency to inhibit Ca^{2+} efflux from Ca^{2+}-filled SR vesicles is much greater than their effects on active Ca^{2+} influx. This effect explains the ability of low concentrations of these amphiphiles, which slightly inhibit the Ca^{2+} pump, to increase Ca^{2+} content when added to Ca^{2+}-filled vesicles that are rapidly exchanging this cation (4,21,25,29,30,37). The much greater sensitivity of Ca^{2+} efflux than Ca^{2+} influx to the inhibitory effects of these amphiphiles allows them, in low concentrations, to increase both Ca^{2+} filling and Ca^{2+} retention by the SR. The significance of these observations in terms of the function of the intact heart remains uncertain. However, high doses of many of these amphiphilic substances when administered to intact animals, or to whole heart preparations, generally have a negative inotropic effect that may be related in part to the ability of these amphiphiles to promote calcium retention within these membranes in the intact heart.

CONCLUSIONS

Ca^{2+} fluxes across the SR play a central role in both the initiation and termination of cardiac systole. The rate and extent of contraction are determined by the passive efflux of Ca^{2+} from the SR through a "channel" that may be related to the Ca^{2+} pump ATPase protein in these membranes. Ca^{2+} uptake by the SR, which is an active process by which the Ca^{2+} pump ATPase protein utilizes the chemical energy of ATP to transport Ca^{2+} against its electrochemical gradient, determines the rate and extent of relaxation. Agents that promote Ca^{2+} efflux from the SR would be expected to increase myocardial contractility, produce rigor, or both. Conversely, agents that inhibit Ca^{2+} efflux probably have a negative inotropic action. Interventions that activate the Ca^{2+} pump would increase the rate of relaxation, while those that increase its Ca^{2+} sensitivity might also increase diastolic compliance. Those interventions that inhibit the SR Ca^{2+} pump, or desensitize it to Ca^{2+}, would be expected to have an opposite effect. Studies of the effects of the β-adrenergic agonists and a variety of drugs that can be shown to modify these Ca^{2+} fluxes across the SR *in vitro* can explain at least some of their actions on myocardial function in the intact heart.

ACKNOWLEDGMENTS

These studies have been supported by Grants HL-22135, HL-21812, and HL-26903 from The National Institutes of Health.

REFERENCES

1. Blasie, J. K., Pachence, J. M., and Herbette L. G. (1983): *Brookhaven Symposia: Neurons in Biology,* edited by B. P. Schoenborn (*in press*).
2. Caroni, P., and Carafoli, E. (1981): *J. Biol. Chem.,* 256:3263–3270.
3. Coan, C., and Keating, S. (1982): *Biochemistry,* 21:3214–3220.
4. Colvin, R., Pearson, N., Messineo, F. C., and Katz, A. M. (1982): *J. Cardiovasc. Pharmacol.,* 4:935–941.
5. Ebashi, S. (1980): *Proc. R. Soc. Lond. (Biol.)* 207:259–286.
6. Eisenberg, B. R., and Eisenberg, R. S. (1982): *J. Gen. Physiol.,* 79:1–19.
7. Fabiato, A. (1981): *J. Gen. Physiol.,* 78:457–497.
8. Fabiato, A., and Fabiato, F. (1977): *Circ. Res.,* 40:119–129.
9. Franzini-Armstrong, C. (1980): *Fed. Proc.,* 39:2403–2409.
10. Hasselbach, W. (1981): *Membrane Transport,* edited by S. J. Bonting and J. J. H. H. M. de Pont, pp. 183–208. Elsevier/North-Holland, Amsterdam.
11. Herbette, L., Messineo, F. C., and Katz, A. M. (1982): *Ann. Rev. Pharmacol. Toxicol.,* 22:413–430.
12. Herbette, L., Scrapa, A., Blasie, J. K., Wang, C. T., Saito, A., and Fleischer, S. (1981): *Biophys. J.,* 36:47–72.
13. Hicks, M., Shigekawa, M., and Katz, A. M. (1979): *Circ. Res.,* 44:384–391.
14. Inesi, G. (1979): *Membrane Transport in Biology,* edited by G. Giebisch, D. C. Tosteson, and H. H. Ussing, pp. 357–393. Springer-Verlag, Berlin.
15. Kapelko, V. I., Gorina, M. S., and Novikova, N. A. (1982): *J. Mol. Cell. Cardiol.,* 14(Suppl. 3):21–29.
16. Karliner, J. S., Lewinter, M. M., Mahler, F., Engler, R., and O'Rourke, R. A. (1977): *J. Clin. Invest.,* 60:511–521.
17. Katz, A. M. (1970): *Physiol. Rev.,* 50:63–158.
18. Katz, A. M. (1979): *Adv. Cyclic Nucleotide Res.,* 11:303–343.
19. Katz, A. M. (1982): *Fed. Proc.,* 41:2456–2459.
20. Katz, A. M., Louis, C. F., Repke, D. I., Fudyma, G., Nash-Adler, P., Kupsaw, R., and Shigekawa, M. (1980): *Biochim. Biophys. Acta,* 596:94–107.
21. Katz, A. M., Nash-Adler, P., Watras, J., Messineo, F. C., Takenaka, H., and Louis, C. F. (1982): *Biochim. Biophys. Acta,* 687:17–26.
22. Katz, A. M., and Repke, D. I. (1973): *Am. J. Cardiol.,* 31:193–201.
23. Katz, A. M., Repke, D. I., Dunnett, J., and Hasselbach, W. (1977): *J. Biol. Chem.,* 252:1950–1956.
24. Katz, A. M., Repke, D. I., Fudyma, G., and Shigekawa, M. (1977): *J. Biol. Chem.,* 252:4210–4214.
25. Katz, A. M., Repke, D. I., and Hasselbach, W. (1977): *J. Biol. Chem.,* 252:1938–1956.
25a. Katz, A. M., Messinco, F. C., and Herbette, L. (1982): *Circulation,* 65(Suppl. I):I-2-I-10.

26. Kirchberger, M. A., and Antonatz, T. (1982): *J. Biol. Chem.*, 257:5685–5691.
27. Kodama, T., Kurebayashi, N., Harafuji, H., and Ogawa, Y. (1982): *J. Biol. Chem.*, 257:4238–4241.
28. Kübler, W., and Katz, A. M. (1977): *Am. J. Cardiol.*, 40:467–471.
29. Louis, C. F., Nash-Adler, P., Fudyma, G., Shigekawa, M., and Katz, A. M. (1980): *Biochim. Biophys. Acta,* 599:610–622.
30. Messineo, F. C., and Katz, A. M. (1979): *Cardiovasc. Pharmacol.,* 1:449–459.
31. Messineo, F. C., Pinto, P. B., and Katz, A. M. (1982): *Adv. Myocardiol.,* 3:407–415.
32. Messineo, F., Rathier, M., Favreau, C., Pinto, P., and Katz, A. M. (1982): *Circulation,* 66(Suppl. II):II-200.
33. Michalak, M., Campbell, K. P., and MacLennan, D. H. (1980): *J. Biol. Chem.*, 255:1317–1326.
34. Morad, M., and Rolett, E. (1972): *J. Physiol. (Lond.),* 224:537–558.
35. Nakamura, Y., and Tonomura, Y. (1982): *J. Biochem. (Tokyo),* 91:449–461.
36. Napolitano, C. A., Cooke, P., Segalman, K., and Herbette, L. (1983): *Biophys. J.,* 42:119–125.
37. Nash-Adler, P., Louis, C. F., Fudyma, G., and Katz, A. M. (1980): *Mol. Pharmacol.,* 17:61–65.
38. Shigekawa, M., and Dougherty, J. P. (1978): *J. Biol. Chem.*, 253:1458–1464.
39. Somlyo, A. V. (1979): *J. Cell Biol.,* 80:743–750.
40. Somlyo, A. V., Gonzalez-Serratos, H., Shuman, H., McClellan, G., and Somlyo, A. P. (1981): *J. Cell Biol.,* 90:577–594.
41. Tada, M., and Katz, A. M. (1982): *Ann. Rev. Physiol.,* 44:401–423.
42. Tada, M., Yamamoto, T., and Tonomura, Y. (1978): *Physiol. Rev.,* 58:1–79.
43. Takenaka, H., Adler, P. N., and Katz, A. M. (1982): *J. Biol. Chem.*, 257:12649–12656.
44. Wiggers, C. J., and Katz, L. N. (1920): *Am. J. Physiol.,* 53:49–64.

Calcium Antagonists and Cardiovascular Disease, edited by L. H. Opie.
Raven Press, New York © 1984.

Chapter 6

Calcium and the Contractile Mechanism in Heart and Smooth Muscle

Wieland Gevers

Muscle Research Unit of the South African Medical Research Council and the University of Cape Town Medical School, Department of Medical Biochemistry, Observatory 7925, Cape Town, South Africa

The fact is beyond dispute that contraction in all types of muscles is decisively influenced by the Ca^{2+} concentration in the vicinity of filamentous contractile proteins (see refs. 1 and 12 for general reviews). We have also learned to accept that the site of control by Ca^{2+} differs in various kinds of muscles, and may even be multiple in a single type of cell.

In *striated muscles,* including the heart, Ca^{2+}-binding "sensors/transducers," in the form of troponin complexes, are bound at regular intervals to the thin filaments made up of actin and tropomyosin (25). In addition, one of the light chains (often called the P light chain) present in each head of the thick filament-based myosin molecules, binds Ca^{2+} at roughly the same sensitivity as does troponin (15), and the same chain can be reversibly phosphorylated by an enzyme system (myosin light chain kinase) which is also controlled by Ca^{2+}, through calmodulin, again in the critical range of concentrations found in contracting striated muscles (6).

Of these *three separate Ca^{2+}-sensitive sites,* the first-mentioned is generally accepted to be the key element which permits cross-bridges (tension-generating actin-myosin interactions) to occur in localized, subjacent regions of each sarcomere. This affords a mechanism for a graduated tension development in the whole muscle dependent on the particular Ca^{2+} concentration in the myoplasm bathing the sarcomeres. The significance of the two other sites for Ca^{2+} action is not yet clear, but there are strong indications that, in the heart, the phosphorylated state of the myosin P light chains is associated with an improved catalytic performance of the myosin as an ATPase (7,27). This is a modulatory influence of Ca^{2+} that is exerted over a series of beats, to enhance the speed of shortening according to the well-established positive "Barany relationship" between the quality of a given myosin in respect of its actin-activated Mg^{2+}-ATPase activity on the one hand, and the *in situ* shortening velocity at zero load, on the other (5). It is possible that this "second" role of Ca^{2+} is only played at the unusually high myoplasmic Ca^{2+} concentrations encountered in hearts subjected to marked adrenergic stimulation, especially in trained subjects (28), but the mechanism may be more general (20).

Another problem awaiting resolution is the precise mechanism by which the binding of Ca^{2+} by troponin (specifically by troponin C) switches on a region of the adjacent thin filament so that myosin heads can interact with actins and carry out the tension-generating cross-bridge cycles. The popular *steric hindrance theory of Huxley* and co-workers supposes that tropomyosin obstructs the myosin-binding sites on actin subunits in the "relaxed" or Ca^{2+}-free state, and that the thin filament undergoes a local conformational twist, after Ca^{2+} is bound to troponin, to remove the obstruction (16). Perry (25) believes that there is a direct "actin-to-actin" transmission of the Ca^{2+}-initiated impulse. Whichever view is right, there is some evidence that phosphorylation of troponin I, another subunit of troponin, diminishes the size of the thin filament domain that can be switched on by Ca^{2+} binding to troponin C, and thus diminishes the potential number of tension-generating sites in the sarcomeres (27,34). In addition, the binding of Ca^{2+} to troponin C is strongly diminished when troponin I is phosphorylated (which occurs in adrenergic responses because the protein kinase concerned is the one activated by cyclic AMP) (29). This protein phosphorylation thus represents a doubly negative modulatory influence on the Ca^{2+} sensitivity of contraction (4,11,15,25,27).

In summary, then, the control of contraction in cardiac cells by Ca^{2+} fluctuations is largely centered on the binding of Ca^{2+} to troponin C in the thin filaments (diminished when troponin I is phosphorylated) which switches on a number of adjacent actin units (fewer when troponin I is phosphorylated) for interaction with myosin heads, and thus for tension development, accompanied by ATP hydrolysis. The cycling rate of individual cross-bridges is increased when Ca^{2+}-dependent phosphorylation of the P light chains of myosin heads has occurred. These phenomena may be expected to lead to increased $+dT/dt_{max}$ and $-dT/dt_{max}$ values for individual beats, together with increased peak tensions, in any situation where both Ca^{2+} and cyclic AMP accumulate in the myoplasm of heart cells, which typically occurs during acute β-adrenergic responses (27). It should be mentioned, however, that there are a number of reports in which the positive inotropism following β-adrenergic stimulation has not been found to be accompanied by enhanced phosphorylation of the myosin P light chains (13,14,17,33).

Although we are dealing in this chapter mainly with Ca^{2+} and its influence on the contractile apparatus, reference must be made to the effects of the *two second messengers, Ca^{2+} and cyclic AMP,* on the promotion of separate and specific phosphorylations of the Ca^{2+} pump-associated protein phospholamban in the sarcoplasmic reticulum, which both enhance the rate of Ca^{2+} sequestration by this system, and are supportive of the above myofibril-based mechanisms in shortening the duration of each beat (31). The main determinants of peak Ca^{2+} concentrations are known to be the amounts of "trigger" Ca^{2+} entering the heart cells during the plateau phase of each action potential (22), influenced by certain subtle effects exerted by resting length on the release rates of Ca^{2+} from the sarcoplasmic reticulum (18), plus the "loading" with Ca^{2+} of the junctional sarcoplasmic reticulum. This results, on the one hand, from the enhanced sequestration rates arising from phospholamban phosphorylation, and, on the other, from increased net entry of Ca^{2+} into the heart cells at fast beating rates (Bowditch staircase) (19).

Figure 1 represents a general contemporary view of the regulation of Ca^{2+}-controlled cardiac contraction. *Smooth muscles provide a striking contrast to striated muscles in the regulatory sites controlled by Ca^{2+}.* Whereas the absence of a sarcomeric structure and a preponderance of actin over myosin points to a different basic contraction mechanism, there is no reason to doubt that actin-myosin cross-bridges also generate the tension that can be exerted by smooth muscles (24). In principle, one is thus also dealing with separate thin filament- and thick filament-based regulatory possibilities, and there is, at present, no agreement on the relative importance of a number of proposed mechanisms, some of which are not mutually exclusive (see later).

Much support has been given to the concept of regulation of actin-myosin

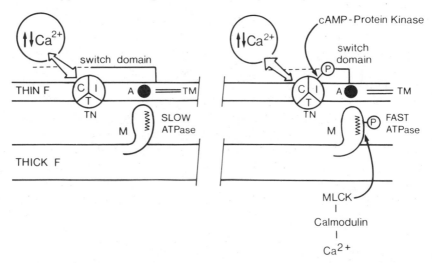

FIG. 1. Control of cardiac contractility by Ca^{2+}, acting as a reversible switch, by binding to troponin C subunit (TnC) of troponin (TN), for activation of local domain of thin filaments. Modulation occurs when TnI subunit of TN is phosphorylated by cyclic AMP-dependent protein kinase; this lessens the thin filament domain which can be activated and diminishes the ability of TnC to bind Ca^{2+}. Phosphorylation of the P light chains of myosin (M) by Ca^{2+} and calmodulin-dependent myosin light chain kinase (MLCK) may increase the catalytic efficiency of the ATPase site (faster cross-bridge cycles) which consist of cyclical, tension-generating interactions between myosin heads and actin (A) units bound to tropomyosin (TM) in the thin filaments.

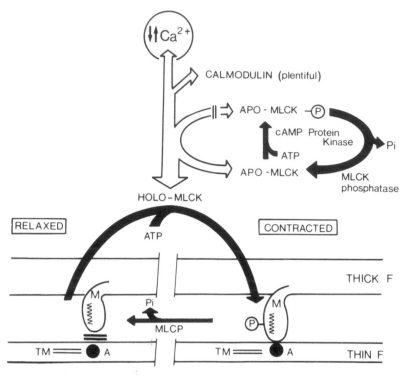

FIG. 2. Two-way control of cross-bridge activity in smooth muscle, with Ca²⁺-dependent phosphorylation of P light chains in myosin heads permitting actin-myosin interactions which do not occur when the P light chains are not phosphorylated (see text for details). MLCK: myosin light chain kinase; Pᵢ: inorganic phosphate; PLC: P light chain; —P (*encircled*): phosphorylated protein; MLCP: myosin light chain phosphatase; A: actin; M: myosin; TM: tropomyosin.

interactions in various kinds of smooth muscles, including those derived from blood vessel walls, by Ca²⁺- and calmodulin-dependent phosphorylation of the P light chains of myosin by *myosin light chain kinase* (MLCK) (See ref. 1) (Fig. 2). In its simplest form, the signal for contraction is believed to be a rise in the myoplasmic Ca²⁺ concentration; Ca²⁺-calmodulin complexes form and then bind to and activate apo-MLCK molecules, which phosphorylate the P light chains of myosin. Only in this form can the myosin heads readily interact with actin units. Termination of contraction occurs when Ca²⁺ is removed from the vicinity of the myofilaments, bringing about disaggregation and inactivation of the Ca²⁺-calmodulin-apo-MLCK complexes. Myosin light chain phosphatase(s) now act unopposed to produce unreactive myosin heads and relaxed smooth muscle cells (23,32). Grading of the tension generation at various Ca²⁺ levels is brought about by the varying degree of recruitment of MLCK and the consequent varying proportion of myosin heads which are phosphorylated and able to form cross-bridges.

Adelstein and Hathaway (2) have provided evidence that phosphorylation of the apo-MLCK protein by cyclic AMP-dependent protein kinase severely depresses its affinity for Ca^{2+}-calmodulin complexes, promoting relaxation, or more correctly, lessening the contractile response to elevated Ca^{2+} concentrations (Fig. 2).

Because of increasing evidence that the above scheme is not adequate to explain the contractile behavior of smooth muscles, attention has been given to *alternative or additional sites for Ca²⁺ regulation in smooth muscles.* Ebashi and co-workers have characterized an actin-linked (thin filament) protein called *leiotonin,* in which a larger subunit cofunctions with a Ca^{2+}-binding, troponin-C-like subunit and with tropomyosin to provide an "on-off" switch for cross-bridge formation (9). Marston et al. (21) have isolated a smooth muscle "troponin" which resembles its striated muscle counterpart and differs from leiotonin. Both of these Ca^{2+}-sensitive systems may, perhaps almost certainly do, coexist with the above-described P light chain phosphorylation cycle, but bear the sort of relationship to it which troponin C bears to the P light chain in heart muscle (Fig. 3). Yet another site of Ca^{2+}-binding in smooth muscle is the P light chain itself, and it has been suggested that this may be where the direct regulation of contraction occurs (8,26), always strongly and additionally modulated by the phosphorylation status of the light chain (Fig. 3).

A finding of great interest in the context of vascular smooth muscle is the apparent existence of a *"latch" mechanism* by which tension can be maintained after Ca^{2+} concentrations, rates of ATP hydrolysis at cross-bridge cycles, and extents of P light chain phosphorylation have all fallen (3). This is believed to occur when dephosphorylation of the P light chains coincides with attachment

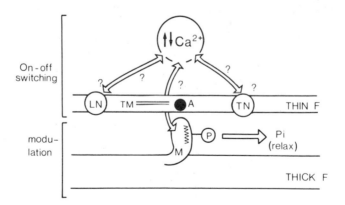

FIG. 3. Potential Ca^{2+} binding sites of regulatory importance for smooth muscle. Leiotonin (LN) and troponin (TN) are linked to tropomyosin (TM) and actin (A) in thin filaments. The P light chain of myosin (M) heads can be reversibly phosphorylated (see Fig. 2) but can serve as a third potential Ca^{2+} sensitivity site, this time on the thick filaments. The relative merits of these not necessarily contradictory postulates are currently not clear (see text).

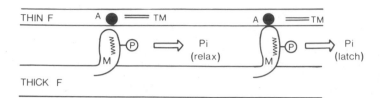

FIG. 4. "Latch" hypothesis (Murphy) for the maintenance of tension in smooth muscles, requiring no ATP hydrolysis and independent of Ca^{2+} changes (see text for details).

of myosin heads to actin-containing filaments, thus removing the stimulus that phosphorylation normally provides for the slow steps of the ATPase cycle. The cross-bridges accordingly remain attached for considerable lengths of time, maintaining tension at low energy cost (Fig. 4). This proposed latch mechanism illustrates clearly how kinetic aspects of the biochemical steps of cross-bridge cycles are relevant to physiological parameters of function (10).

Yet another proposal for the reversible control by Ca^{2+} of smooth muscle contraction emanates from Sobue et al. (30). A large protein called *caldesmon* interacts with tropomyosin-bound actin units under resting conditions to prevent myosin-binding; when Ca^{2+} concentrations rise in stimulated smooth muscle cells, Ca^{2+}-calmodulin complexes form and bind to caldesmon, freeing actins for attachment to myosin heads and for the completion of tension-producing cross-bridge cycles (Fig. 5).

Clearly, there is a great need to define in detail the precise mechanisms by which the contractile apparatus in smooth muscles is activated, in a graded fashion and subject to modulating influences. The sources of activating Ca^{2+} and the mechanisms for its removal or sequestration need also to be clarified, so that the actions of many hormones and drugs, now beginning to be understood with reasonable clarity in the case of heart muscle, can also be elucidated in

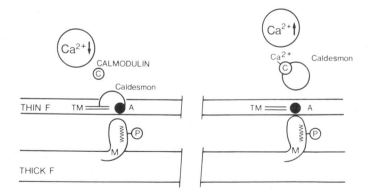

FIG. 5. Proposed roles of caldesmon and calmodulin in sensitizing thin filaments to interaction of actin units with myosin heads (see text).

blood vessels and other organs containing smooth muscle. This will have profound implications for the therapy of a wide range of important diseases.

SUMMARY

Fluctuations in Ca^{2+} concentrations in the vicinity of contractile proteins are probably the most important, perhaps the only "on-off" switches for the tension-producing interactions of myosin and actin molecules in all kinds of muscles. Differences in the organization of the aggregated proteins, the existence of a number of alternative Ca^{2+}-binding sites, and the operation of modulatory influences provide different muscles with physiologically appropriate locomotory apparatuses of great complexity and medical importance.

ACKNOWLEDGMENTS

The South African Medical Research Council and Atomic Energy Board, as well as the Research Committee of the University of Cape Town, have generously supported research by the author and colleagues mentioned in this article.

REFERENCES

1. Adelstein, R. S., and Eisenberg, E. (1980): *Annu. Rev. Biochem.*, 49:921–956.
2. Adelstein, R. S., and Hathaway, D. R. (1979): *Am. J. Cardiol.*, 44:783–787.
3. Aksoy, M. O., Murphy, R. A., and Kamm, R. E. (1982): *Am. J. Physiol.*, 242:C109–116.
4. Bailin, G. (1979): *Am. J. Physiol.*, 236:C41–46.
5. Barany, M. (1967): *J. Gen. Physiol.*, 50:197–218.
6. Barany, M., and Barany, K. (1981): *Am. J. Physiol.*, 241:H117–128.
7. Bhan, A., Malhotra, A., Scheuer, J., Conti, M. A., and Adelstein, R. S. (1981): *J. Biol. Chem.*, 256:7741–7743.
8. Chacko, S., Conti, M. A., and Adelstein, R. S. (1977): *Proc. Natl. Acad. Sci. USA*, 74:129–133.
9. Ebashi, S., Mikawa, T., Hirata, M., Toyo-Oka, T., and Nonomura, Y. (1977): *Excitation-Contraction Coupling in Smooth Muscle*, edited by R. Casteels, pp. 325–334. Elsevier/North-Holland, Amsterdam.
10. Eisenberg, E., and Greene, L. E. (1980): *Annu. Rev. Physiol.*, 42:293–309.
11. England, P. J. (1975): *FEBS Lett.*, 50:57–60.
12. Franzini-Armstrong, C., and Peachey, L. D. (1981): *J. Cell. Biol.*, 91:166s–186s.
13. High, C. W., and Stull, J. T. (1979): *Am. J. Physiol.*, 239:H756–764.
14. Holroyde, M. J., Potter, J. D., and Solaro, R. J. (1979): *J. Biol. Chem.*, 254:6478–6482.
15. Holroyde, M. J., Small, D. A. P., Howe, E., and Solaro, R. J. (1979): *Biochim. Biophys. Acta*, 587:628–637.
16. Huxley, H. (1964): *Science*, 164:1356–1366.
17. Jeacocke, S. A., and England, P. J. (1980): *Biochem. J.*, 128:763–768.
18. Jewell, B. R. (1977): *Circ. Res.*, 40:225–230.
19. Katz, A. M. (1976): *The Physiology of the Heart*, pp. 182–184. Raven Press, New York.
20. Kopp, S. J., and Barany, M. (1979): *J. Biol. Chem.*, 254:12007–12012.
21. Marston, S. B., Trevett, R. M., and Walters, M. (1980): *Biochem. J.*, 185:315–365.
22. McDonald, T. F. (1982): *Annu. Rev. Physiol.*, 44:425–434.
23. Morgan, M., Perry, S. V., and Ottaway, J. (1976): *Biochem. J.*, 157:687–697.
24. Murphy, R. A. (1979): *Annu. Rev. Physiol.*, 41:737–748.
25. Perry, S. V. (1979): *Biochem. Soc. Trans.*, 7:593–617.

26. Rees, D. D., and Frederikson, D. W. (1981): *J. Biol. Chem.*, 256:357–364.
27. Resink, T. J., and Gevers, W. (1981): *Cell Calcium*, 2:105–123.
28. Resink, T. J., Gevers, W., Noakes, T. D., and Opie, L. H. (1981): *J. Mol. Cell Cardiol.*, 13:679–654.
29. Robertson, S. R., Johnson, J. D., Holroyde, M. J., Kranias, E. G., Potter, T. D., and Solaro, R. J. (1982): *J. Biol. Chem.*, 257:260–263.
30. Sobue, K., Morimoto, K., Inui, M., Kanda, K., and Kakiuchi, S. (1982): *Biomed. Res.*, 3:188–196.
31. Tada, M., and Katz, A. M. (1982): *Annu. Rev. Physiol.*, 44:401–423.
32. Werth, D. K., Haeberle, J. R., and Hathaway, D. R. (1982): *J. Biol. Chem.*, 257:7306–7309.
33. Westwood, S. A., and Perry, S. V. (1981): *Biochem. J.*, 197:185–193.
34. Yamamoto, K., and Ohtsuki, I. (1982): *J. Biochem.* (*Tokyo*), 91:1669–1677.

Calcium Antagonists and Cardiovascular Disease, edited by L. H. Opie.
Raven Press, New York © 1984.

Chapter 7

Cell Calcium and Contractile System Regulation in Arterial Smooth Muscle

Richard A. Murphy and William T. Gerthoffer

Department of Physiology, School of Medicine, University of Virginia,
Charlottesville, Virginia 22908

The overall activation process in vascular smooth muscle is depicted in Fig. 1. The mechanisms involved in steps 1 and 2 (Fig. 1) are extensively characterized, as shown in other chapters in this volume. An implicit assumption underlying studies of vascular smooth muscle contraction is that Ca^{2+} binds to a myofilament regulatory site to "turn on" cross-bridges (Fig. 1, steps 3 and 4). This assumption is based upon the well-known Ca^{2+}-dependent regulatory process in skeletal and cardiac muscle (Fig. 1, *dashed arrows*), where Ca^{2+} binding to troponin regulates force by allowing cross-bridge attachment and cycling. If the same type of mechanism applies to vascular smooth muscle, then changes in tissue force, wall stress, or vascular resistance provide an adequate estimate of the effects of a drug on activation and cell Ca^{2+}.

Recent studies show that contractile system regulation by Ca^{2+} is more complicated than was assumed. This chapter summarizes our current understanding of the Ca^{2+}-dependent molecular mechanisms regulating the contractile system in vascular smooth muscle. Ca^{2+} does regulate the number of activated cross-bridges and active stress generation. However, Ca^{2+} also regulates cross-bridge cycling rates and, thereby, the velocity and energetics of contraction.

BIOCHEMICAL EVIDENCE FOR CALCIUM-DEPENDENT REGULATORY MECHANISMS

The importance of Ca^{2+} in regulating the function of vascular smooth muscle was first demonstrated in studies which showed that the dependence of force on $[Ca^{2+}]$ was the same in skinned smooth and skeletal muscles (cf. ref. 6, Fig. 2). The molecular basis for activation by Ca^{2+} was not clear because vertebrate smooth muscles appear to lack troponin, the thin filament regulatory

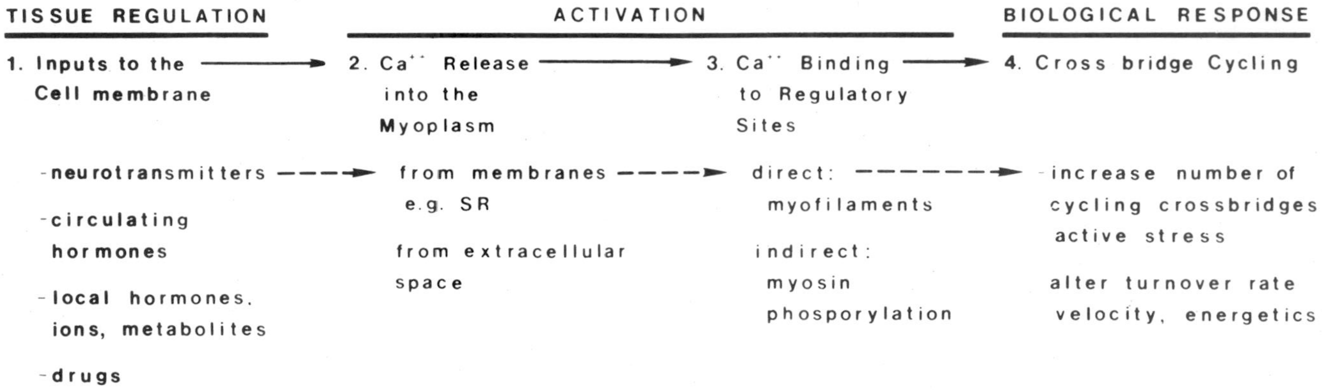

TISSUE REGULATION   ACTIVATION   BIOLOGICAL RESPONSE

1. Inputs to the → 2. Ca^{++} Release → 3. Ca^{++} Binding → 4. Cross bridge Cycling
Cell membrane   into the   to Regulatory
   Myoplasm   Sites

- neurotransmitters - - -→ from membranes - - -→ direct: - - - -→ - increase number of
               e.g. SR   myofilaments   cycling crossbridges

- circulating   active stress
hormones   from extracellular   indirect:

- local hormones.   space   myosin   alter turnover rate
ions, metabolites   phosporylation   velocity, energetics

- drugs

FIG. 1. Regulation of contraction in vascular smooth muscle. Our discussion is keyed to the four steps or processes depicted here. The *dashed arrows* indicate the primary mechanisms operating in skeletal muscle. Additional listed mechanisms are also involved in activation of vascular smooth muscle.

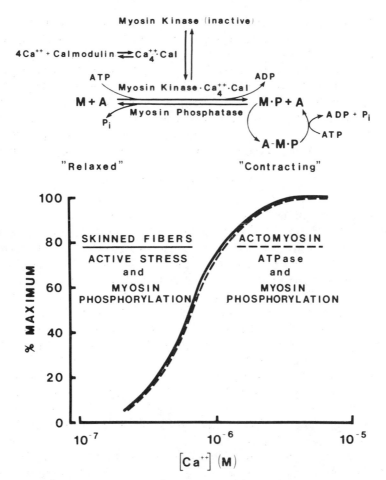

FIG. 2. Biochemical evidence showing that Ca^{2+}-stimulated phosphorylation can regulate cross-bridge cycling in smooth muscle. Cross-bridges (myosin, M) only show significant interaction with actin in the thin filament (A) when they are phosphorylated (M-P). Myosin is phosphorylated after a rise in [Ca^{2+}] leads to formation of the active myosin kinase·calmodulin·Ca_4^{2+} complex. The schematic Ca^{2+}-dependence curves summarize the results of many studies.

protein in striated muscle. However, several partially characterized proteins isolated from smooth muscle can increase the (Ca^{2+}-dependent) ATPase activity of pure actin and myosin (8,15).

The best characterized regulatory system in smooth muscle does not involve a direct allosteric action of Ca^{2+} binding to a myofilament site. Perry and his colleagues discovered that all muscles contain highly specific enzymes which can reversibly phosphorylate myosin: myosin kinase and myosin phosphatase (17). Increasing [Ca^{2+}] produces myosin phosphorylation (Fig. 2) by activating myosin kinase. Phosphorylation is not a primary regulatory mechanism in striated muscle and induces only small effects on the interaction between myosin and actin. In contrast, the actin-activated ATPase activity of smooth muscle myosin is highly dependent on Ca^{2+}-stimulated phosphorylation (8,15), as is force development by skinned smooth muscles (11). Such results (Fig. 2) suggest that *myosin phosphorylation is an important regulatory mechanism in smooth muscle.* According to the phosphorylation hypothesis, the increase in myoplasmic $[Ca^{2+}]$ following stimulation of smooth muscle leads to the formation of calmodulin · Ca_4^{2+} and then the active myosin kinase · calmodulin · Ca^{2+} complex. The cross-bridges are turned on by phosphorylation (i.e., enabled to interact with the thin filament), and contraction follows. Relaxation is postulated to reflect a lowering of myoplasmic $[Ca^{2+}]$, dissociation of the active myosin kinase · calmodulin · Ca_4^{2+} complex, and myosin dephosphorylation by the myosin phosphatase (Fig. 2). Myosin phosphatase activity is not Ca^{2+}-dependent, and no evidence has yet been obtained for cellular regulation of this enzyme.

Figure 2 summarizes the evidence from several laboratories supporting this hypothesis (3,8,11). Such evidence, obtained with isolated proteins or skinned tissues, meets two important criteria required to establish a significant physiological role for myosin phosphorylation in smooth muscle contraction (12): (a) pure smooth muscle myosin can be phosphorylated at a significant rate by an endogenous kinase and dephosphorylated by an endogenous phosphatase; and (b) phosphorylation of myosin increases actomyosin ATPase activity and force in skinned vascular smooth muscle.

REGULATION IN INTACT CELLS

A third criterion must also be met if the scheme depicted in Fig. 2 is true: the time course and the magnitude of phosphorylation must be proportional to force development, and dephosphorylation must be correlated with relaxation in intact vascular smooth muscle. We tested this criterion using a preparation dissected from the media of swine carotid arteries in which tissue mechanical measurements were shown to provide estimates of *cellular* contractile output (5). With the reasonable assumption that the sliding filament/cross-bridge model is valid for smooth muscle (9,14), measurements of the steady-state stress (S_o, force/cross-sectional area) obtained at the optimal tissue length for force development (L_o) is proportional to the number of cross-bridges generating force additively (1,4). Shortening velocities measured after a quick-release to constant loads allow the construction of stress-velocity curves. V_o, the maximum isotonic shortening velocity at zero external load, can be estimated from such curves (4). [V_o is the same as V_{max} as defined by Katz (10).] V_o is the most direct physiological estimate of cross-bridge cycling rates with the effect of the external load removed. V_o is not generally believed to be regulated by Ca^{2+} in skeletal muscle, and "Indeed, it has become an axiom that [V_o] of a muscle is controlled by the rate of turnover of ATP by its constituent myosin isoenzyme" (19).

This is the basis for the assumption that stress provides an adequate estimate of the level of activation. Thus, rigorous mechanical measurements in a suitable tissue preparation, with results expressed in absolute units (Newtons/m² for stress, and L_v/sec for velocity) provide quantitative estimates of the number of attached cross-bridges and their average turnover rate, respectively (14).

Myosin phosphorylation is a covalent modification and can be measured quantitatively in tissues quick-frozen during contractions. There is one regulatory light chain for each head of the myosin molecule or two per cross-bridge. Stoichiometric phosphorylation is one mole P_i/mole light chain or two moles P_i/mole myosin or per cross-bridge.

We cannot measure myoplasmic $[Ca^{2+}]$ in intact vascular smooth muscle cells, but can reasonably assume that it increases with stress in response to higher agonist concentrations during steady-state contractions. From studies of skinned tissues, we can relate levels of phosphorylation obtained with agonists to specific Ca^{2+} values. The results of our studies on intact and skinned tissues support the scheme shown in Fig. 3 (1,3,7): (a) Steady-state levels of S_o increase with the agonist concentration and, presumably, with cell $[Ca^{2+}]$ to a maximum value of 6×10^5 N/m² *cell* cross-section. This is most clearly shown in K^+-depolarized tissues where extracellular Ca^{2+} is the agonist. (b) Steady-state S_o values up to about 3.3×10^5 N/m² can be maintained with no significant increases in myosin phosphorylation or in V_o. (c) At higher agonist concentrations (and higher cell $[Ca^{2+}]$), phosphorylation and V_o are increased in parallel. None of the agonists studied produced steady-state levels of phosphorylation above 0.4 or 0.5 moles P_i/mole light chain although high $[Ca^{2+}]$ produces up to 0.8 moles P_i/mole light chain in skinned carotid tissues (3). Consequently, the curve for phosphorylation and V_o is extrapolated from other results (next section). (d) Finally, it was V_o and not S_o which was directly proportional to myosin phosphorylation under all experimental conditions (2).

The type of experiments illustrated in Fig. 2 shows that myosin phosphorylation can act as a switch allowing attachment and rapid cycling of cross-bridges. However, the results in intact tissues (Fig. 3) provide strong evidence that a second Ca^{2+}-dependent regulatory mechanism is operating to permit force maintenance. Furthermore, this system must be more sensitive to the cell $[Ca^{2+}]$ (3). From these steady-state results and other results (next section) we postulate that there are two populations of cross-bridges contributing to active stress in vascular smooth muscle. Phosphorylated cross-bridges cycle rapidly and are associated with high rates of energy consumption and high shortening velocities. However, Ca^{2+}-dependent stress can be maintained by dephosphorylated cross-bridges. We have termed these "latchbridges" because they are slowly cycling or perhaps remain attached without cycling. We interpret the dependence of V_o on phosphorylation in living tissues as a consequence of the internal load imposed by latchbridges on the phosphorylated, rapidly cycling cross-bridges (2,4).

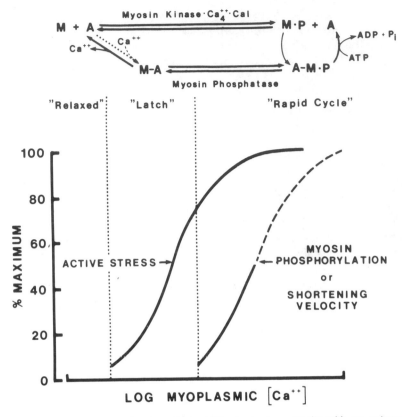

FIG. 3. Dependence of steady-state stress (S_o), shortening velocity with no external load (V_o), and myosin phosphorylation on the cell [Ca²⁺]. Contractions were induced by varying the agonist concentration (histamine or CaCl₂ in high K⁺-depolarizing solutions) (1) or the free [Ca²⁺] in skinned preparations (3). See text for details of how these curves were estimated. The model depicts our interpretation of the data. At very low myoplasmic [Ca²⁺], which does not support tone, the cross-bridge (M) cannot interact with the thin filament (A). Stimulation of tissues always results in an initial high level of cell Ca²⁺ (13) required to activate myosin kinase. Myosin phosphorylation results in rapidly cycling cross-bridges. A subsequent fall in cell [Ca²⁺] to intermediate levels is associated with stress maintenance by dephosphorylated non- or slowly cycling "latch-bridges" (1,3,7).

ACTIVATION-CONTRACTION COUPLING IN LIVING VASCULAR SMOOTH MUSCLE

The fourth and final criterion (12) which must be met to prove that Ca²⁺-dependent phosphorylation of myosin is a key regulatory mechanism is to correlate the time course of changes in phosphorylation with the time course of changes in cell [Ca²⁺] on stimulation. Figure 4 attempts to illustrate this correlation as accurately as possible for the swine carotid media responding to depolari-

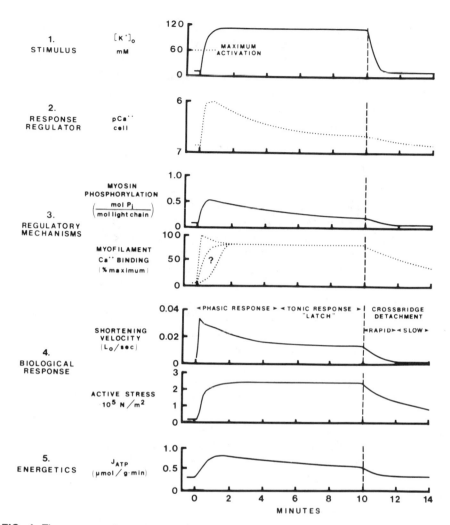

FIG. 4. Time course of events involved in activation and inactivation in the swine carotid media in response to K^+-depolarization in normal $CaCl_2$ (1.6 mM). *Solid lines* are measured values and *dashed lines* are indirect estimates (see text for details).

zation by 110 mM K^+ in normal $CaCl_2$ (1.6 mM). The numbered panels are keyed to the steps outlined for activation in Fig. 1.

1. The input to the cell membrane is the change in extracellular $[K^+]$. The kinetics of the increase in K^+ can be calculated from the K^+ dose-response curve, the tissue thickness (250 μm plus an estimated 70 μm diffusion boundary layer), and the diffusion coefficient for K^+ in carotid arteries, assuming plane sheet geometry. Other studies with electrically stimulated tissues suggest that

the diffusion of K^+ is slow, relative to the cellular events, and appears to limit the rates of many of the cellular responses when these events are averaged in the whole tissue.

2. The second step, represented by the time course of changes in myoplasmic $[Ca^{2+}]$, is unknown. The postulated curve is estimated from the time-dependent changes in phosphorylation and the $[Ca^{2+}]$-dependence for phosphorylation in skinned carotid tissues (3). However, the transient nature and time course of changes in cell $[Ca^{2+}]$ following addition of several agonists, including K^+, have been demonstrated directly by light emission from aequorin-loaded smooth muscles (13; and K. Morgan, *personal communication*).

3. Ca^{2+} binding to two regulatory systems must be involved in the third step. One, leading to formation of the active myosin kinase complex, can be directly followed by measuring myosin phosphorylation. The second, involving an unknown site which must be occupied for latchbridge formation, can be indirectly estimated in the steady state from mechanical measurements. Ca^{2+} occupancy of this site may follow cell $[Ca^{2+}]$ during the initial transients, may be a relatively slow process (18) or may require prior phosphorylation of the cross-bridge as suggested by studies of skinned tissues (3).

4. The final event is the biological response. This can be directly measured and consists of both the number of active cross-bridges contributing to stress, as in striated muscle, and the average cross-bridge turnover rates. The latter are estimated from shortening velocity at a constant load of 0.1 S_o. Velocity shows a transient response reflecting changes in $[Ca^{2+}]$ and phosphorylation (1,2,4). Measured velocities peak more rapidly than other parameters (Fig. 4). Most of the measurements are tissue averages and their rates of change are slowed by agonist diffusion. However, the initial shortening velocity of the tissue is determined by the velocities of superficial cells in the preparation, which are rapidly activated (1). The two curves depicted in *panel 4* (Fig. 4) define the latch state: force maintenance with reduced cross-bridge cycling rates (in this example, after 5 min).

Panel 5 (Fig. 4) shows data on a secondary biological response, i.e., energy consumption. It is calculated from measurements of O_2 consumption associated with cross-bridge cycling in the swine carotid media by Paul et al. (16) and is expressed as ATP utilization. O_2 consumption measurements have a low time resolution, but the results are consistent with an important prediction of the hypothesis that myosin phosphorylation and a second regulatory system can modulate cross-bridge cycling rates and, thereby, ATP consumption.

Figure 4 also illustrates the kinetics of relaxation of K^+ washout. Our studies indicate that relaxation is determined by the rate of Ca^{2+} extrusion or sequestration. Ca^{2+} removal is slow in the swine carotid, and two phases of relaxation can be identified (7): (a) A rapid exponential phase (rate constant of 1.2–1.8 min^{-1}) is correlated with dephosphorylation and inactivation of the rapidly cycling cross-bridge population, and (b) a slow exponential phase (rate constant,

0.10–0.14 min^{-1}) was found to reflect latchbridge inactivation as cell $[Ca^{2+}]$ gradually approaches resting levels.

FUNCTIONAL IMPLICATIONS

The complex mechanisms involved in steps 1 and 2 of activation (Fig. 1) have been explored in detail in efforts to explain the diversity of vascular smooth muscle responses. However, the role and relative importance of the mechanisms involved in steps 1 and 2 (Fig. 1) may be better understood after considering the molecular regulatory systems involved in steps 3 and 4 (Fig. 1).

An important contribution of the molecular regulatory mechanisms described above is that vascular smooth muscle can maintain stress tonically against an opposing load (e.g., blood pressure) with a greatly reduced energy expenditure. This is a property that is largely unnecessary in skeletal muscles. ATP consumption at a given stress is 300-fold less in the swine carotid than in the frog sartorius. However, Ca^{2+} transients in vascular smooth muscle allow a rapid initial vasoconstriction on stimulation.

The combination of two regulatory mechanisms with different Ca^{2+} sensitivities producing fast or slow cross-bridge turnover rates may also contribute to smooth muscle diversity. Depending on the nature of the Ca^{2+} transients elicited, the responses could be phasic, tonic, or biphasic, as illustrated by contractions of rat portal vein, swine carotid artery, and rabbit ear artery. There is little reason to believe that the Ca^{2+}-dependence curves for the two regulatory systems (cf. Fig. 3) are the same in all tissues, and such differences would also contribute to functional specialization.

Optimum operation of our hypothesized regulatory scheme requires fine control of myoplasmic $[Ca^{2+}]$. This is much more demanding than the situation in striated muscle, where Ca^{2+} release in response to an action potential is quantal and rises from below threshold to supramaximal levels. The many inputs to the smooth muscle cell membrane and various Ca^{2+} pools involved in activation presumably contribute to the necessary fine control of cell $[Ca^{2+}]$.

ACKNOWLEDGMENTS

This summary of our research (supported by NIH Grant 2 PO1 HL19242) incorporates the contributions of our colleagues and we acknowledge a considerable debt to Drs. M. O. Aksoy, M. Chatterjee, P. F. Dillon, S. P. Driska, K. E. Kamm, and S. Mras.

W. T. Gerthoffer was a recipient of a NIH Research Service Award (F32 HL05991).

REFERENCES

1. Aksoy, M. O., Mras, S., Kamm, K. E., and Murphy, R. A. (1983): *Am. J. Physiol.*, 245 (*in press*).

2. Aksoy, M. O., Murphy, R. A., and Kamm, K. E. (1982): *Am. J. Physiol.*, 242:C109–C116.
3. Chatterjee, M., and Murphy, R. A. (1983): *Science*, 221:464–466.
4. Dillon, P. F., Murphy, R. A., and Claes, V. A. (1982): *Am. J. Physiol.*, 242:C102–C108.
5. Driska, S. P., Damon, D. N., and Murphy, R. A. (1978): *Biophys. J.*, 24:525–540.
6. Filo, R. S., Bohr, D. F., and Ruegg, J. C. (1965): *Science*, 147:1581–1583.
7. Gerthoffer, W. T., and Murphy, R. A. (1983): *Am. J. Physiol.*, 245 (*in press*).
8. Hartshorne, D. J., and Siemankowski, R. F. (1981): *Annu. Rev. Physiol.*, 43:519–530.
9. Johansson, B. (1978): *Circ. Res.*, 43 (Suppl. I):14–20.
10. Katz, A. (1977): *Physiology of the Heart.* Raven Press, New York.
11. Kerrick, W. G. L., Hoar, P. E. and Cassidy, P. S. (1980): *Fed. Proc.*, 39:1558–1563.
12. Krebs, E. G., and Beavo, J. A. (1979): *Annu. Rev. Biochem.*, 48:923–959.
13. Morgan, J. P., and Morgan, K. G. (1982): *Pfluegers Arch.*, 395:75–77.
14. Murphy, R. A. (1980): *Handbook of Physiology*, Section 2, Vol. II, edited by D. F. Bohr, A. P. Somlyo, and H. V. Sparks, Jr., pp. 325–351. American Physiological Society, Bethesda.
15. Marston, S. B. (1982): *Prog. Biophys. Molec. Biol.*, 41:1–41.
16. Paul, R. J. (1983): *Fed. Proc.*, 42:62–66.
17. Perry, S. V. (1979): *Biochem. Soc. Trans.*, 7:593–617.
18. Robertson, S. P., Johnson, J. D., and Potter, J. D. (1981): *Biophys. J.*, 34:559–569.
19. Weeds, A. (1978): *Nature*, 274:417.

Calcium Antagonists and Cardiovascular
Disease, edited by L. H. Opie.
Raven Press, New York © 1984.

Chapter 8

Calcium Ions in Ischemia

Robert B. Jennings

Department of Pathology, Duke University Medical Center, Durham, North Carolina 27710

Calcium ions are involved in multiple processes in normal myocytes, including contraction, excitation, and the response of the heart to stress via the adenyl cyclase mechanism. These functions all require that the level of intracellular Ca^{2+} be maintained with precision by modulation of its rate of entry and efflux and of the function of the sarcoplasmic reticulum and mitochondria. If intracellular Ca^{2+} rises to an abnormally high level, it may cause lethal injury or, in ischemia, it may accelerate the rate at which cells become irreversibly injured. This chapter will review the biology of ischemic injury in terms of the role Ca^{2+} may play in causing lethal injury.

Sudden proximal occlusion of a major coronary artery in the dog heart is followed by variable degrees of reduction of arterial flow to the myocardium supplied by the occluded vessel. A transmural gradient of ischemia results with the subendocardial myocardium receiving the least and the subepicardial myocardium the greatest collateral flow (21). Flows to the subendocardial myocardium are usually between 0 and 14% of control and are defined as severe or low-flow ischemia. Most of our studies of the metabolic and structural changes occurring as a consequence of ischemic injury have been done on zones of low-flow ischemia identified by the use of thioflavine S to establish the location of the severely ischemic tissue (10).

METABOLIC AND STRUCTURAL CHANGES IN ISCHEMIA

The metabolic and structural changes found in zones of severe or total ischemia have been reviewed in detail elsewhere (12) and are summarized here to serve as a background for understanding alterations in Ca^{2+} ion in ischemia.

The depressed arterial flow in the ischemic tissue provides inadequate O_2 to maintain aerobic metabolism and to support the diffusion of various end products of metabolism to the circulation. Since aerobic (mitochondrial) metabolism is required to produce sufficient high-energy phosphates to support contraction, macromolecular synthesis, the resynthesis of adenine nucleotides, and a number of other reactions, the ischemic cell loses these functions but survives for a period of time on energy produced by anaerobic glycolysis (20). However, this source is limited by the relatively small quantity of glycogen present in the myocytes and by the fact that the glycolytic rate is much slower in zones of low-flow ischemia than it is in control myocardium. Moreover, the low collateral flow provides little or no exogenous glucose for entry into the glycolytic pathway. Lactate, the end product of glycolysis, accumulates in the tissue because arterial flow is reduced and because no O_2 is available to support its further metabolism to CO_2 and H_2O.

Because the demand of the acutely ischemic tissue for high-energy phosphates exceeds the reserve supply of high-energy phosphates and the capacity of anaerobic glycolysis to produce it, sarcoplasmic ADP rises. Myokinase is activated to salvage the high-energy phosphate of ADP. The ATP produced in this reaction is utilized, but the AMP produced is dephosphorylated to adenosine; adenosine is lost from the cell and further degraded (13). As a consequence, the adenine nucleotide pool of the severely ischemic myocytes quickly is destroyed. Products of continued metabolism such as protons, inosine, hypoxanthine, xanthine, P_i, etc. accumulate. These changes are progressive until the supply of high-energy phosphates is exhausted and the cells disintegrate (12).

These metabolic changes of ischemia are accompanied by modest reversible changes in ultrastructure including relaxation of the myofibrils and glycogen depletion. However, as the period of ischemia is extended, the ischemic injury becomes biologically irreversible, a transition associated with new ultrastructural changes. These include mitochondrial swelling with the amorphous matrix densities, the virtual absence of glycogen, peripheral aggregation of nuclear chromatin, and the appearance of discontinuities in the plasmalemma of the sarcolemma (see Figs. 3 and 4 in ref. 12). The mitochondrial and sarcolemmal changes appear to be pathognomonic of irreversibility in this model. It seems likely that the sarcolemmal changes are lethal; however, insufficient work has been completed to establish either the mechanism through which they develop or whether this change is the first change which dictates that ischemic injury is irreversible (12).

In summary, the early stage of lethal ischemic injury is associated with a series of metabolic changes including very low contents of high-energy phosphate (creatine phosphate $= 0$, ATP $< 10\%$ of control), a low adenine nucleotide pool, proton excess, cessation of anaerobic glycolysis, high lactate, low glycogen, high inosine, and numerous other changes. From the ultrastructural point of view, mitochondrial damage and membrane damage are prominent. From the functional point of view, slices of such tissue demonstrate signs of membrane damage and cannot maintain volume and ion gradients. The best evidence available indicates that significant membrane damage is a lethal event (12).

ELECTROLYTE CHANGES IN SEVERE OR TOTAL ISCHEMIA

Studies of ischemic tissue *in vivo* (4,5) with ion selective electrodes have shown redistribution of ions within the tissue during the first few minutes of ischemia; moreover, ultrastructural analysis indicates that when these changes are marked, they are associated with cell swelling. The swelling probably occurs because of osmotic changes. For example, an increase in intracellular particles such as lactate, creatine, inorganic phosphate, etc., should have osmotic consequences as should the net influx of Cl^- which follows the loss of membrane potential (17). Later, when the concentration of sarcoplasmic ATP becomes very low, depressed activity of the Na^+,K^+-ATPase of the cell membrane and the presence of small holes in the plasmalemma should contribute to volume changes (10,13).

On the other hand, direct study of severely ischemic tissue reveals little change in either electrolytes or water. For example, only a small decrease in total tissue K^+ (14) is found after 240 min of *in vivo* low-flow ischemia. Eventually, however, the tissue K^+ falls close to the extracellular levels (8). Tissue H_2O, Na^+, Cl^-, Mg^{2+}, and Ca^{2+} also exhibit similar modest changes from control at 240 min (14). Since there is abundant biologic evidence that the myocytes were irreversibly injured at least 3 hr earlier, the explanation for the small rate of change in total electrolytes and water is considered to be the low rate of coronary collateral arterial flow.

CALCIUM IN ISCHEMIC INJURY

The concentration of sarcoplasmic Ca^{2+} ion $[Ca^{2+}]_i$ in healthy myocytes is controlled primarily by the rate of entry of extracellular Ca^{2+}, the rate of exit of intracellular Ca^{2+}, and by the activity of the sarcoplasmic reticulum and the mitochondria (19). The latter organelles both require ATP for cation transport, cease functioning in the absence of ATP, and should exhibit depressed function when the ATP concentration falls below the effective K_m of the enzyme systems involved (9,26). In addition, due to the absence of O_2, mitochondria of ischemic cells with low intracellular ATP should be essentially nonfunctional in terms of cation transport. Thus, increases in $[Ca^{2+}]_i$ in ischemia could occur as a consequence of release of Ca^{2+} ion from the sarcoplasmic reticulum, mitochondria and, perhaps, troponin, as well as from failure of ischemic cells to extrude Ca^{2+} entering from the extracellular space.

The extent of any redistribution of Ca^{2+} ion during the early phases of severe ischemia *in vivo* is unknown because there is no method currently available to estimate the sarcoplasmic concentration of Ca^{2+} versus the stores of Ca^{2+} in the sarcoplasmic reticulum or mitochondria. The maximum concentration achievable, taking into account the fact that free Ca^{2+} ion is bound strongly by membrane phospholipid or protein, is in the micromolar range, and any deleterious effects of Ca^{2+} in severe ischemia must be mediated by this or an even more dilute concentration. On the other hand, much higher Ca^{2+} may accumulate in zones of moderate ischemia where coronary arterial collateral flow can supply significant quantities of Ca^{2+} ion to the ischemic cells.

An increased $[Ca^{2+}]_i$ could have a variety of detrimental consequences. It could accelerate the depletion of ATP from the ischemic myocyte by stimulating Ca^{2+}-activated ATPases or by inhibiting glycolysis. In addition, Ca^{2+} ion may activate endogenous phospholipases (12), and thereby lead to the disruption of the cell membrane. The latter enzymes can be activated by intracellular Ca^{2+} levels of 100 μM, i.e., levels achievable without the entry of extracellular Ca^{2+} (7). Either of these potential effects of Ca^{2+} may contribute to lethality in severe or total ischemia. However, it seems likely that Ca^{2+} ions are the only lethal factors.

ELECTROLYTE CHANGE OCCURRING AS A CONSEQUENCE OF REPERFUSION OF ISCHEMIC MYOCARDIUM

Restoration of arterial flow after 15 to 18 min of severe ischemia in the dog, i.e., at a time when the ATP levels are about 35% of control and when the adenine nucleotide pool has been depleted to about 50% of control (22), produces little change in tissue structure, water, or electrolytes (29). Rather, the cells survive and function returns. This sequence of events comprises the definition of reversible myocyte injury (12).

The dramatic changes which occur after irreversibly injured cells are reperfused are demonstrated best after 40 min of severe ischemia *in vivo*, because this period of ischemia produces a high proportion of cell death (about 72% of the cells) in the posterior papillary muscle (10) without enough vascular damage to interfere with reperfusion of the tissue (15). Prior to reperfusion of tissue injured by 40 min of ischemia, the contents of high-energy phosphates are very low and anaerobic glycolysis has virtually stopped (13). Although the tissue is indistinguishable from control myocardium by routine techniques of light microscopy, it shows striking ultrastructural alterations (9,10) in the mitochondria, nuclei, myofibrils, and in portions of the plasmalemma of the affected cells.

Reperfusion of arterial blood for only 2 min following 40 min of ischemia, induces a dramatic change in the structure of the affected cells (3,15,16,28), an appearance which now usually is termed *contraction-band necrosis* (Fig. 1). Large contraction bands comprised of 4 to 10 sarcomeres are prominent with myofibrillar disruption in between. The cells are swollen. Subsarcolemmal blebs, which often exhibit large breaks in the plasmalemma, are common. The mitochondria of cells with contraction bands contain granular densities of Ca phosphate. Even at this early time, the contraction bands are readily detectable by light microscopy and permit the diagnosis of contraction-band necrosis.

The changes in tissue water are shown in Fig. 2. Note that the episode of

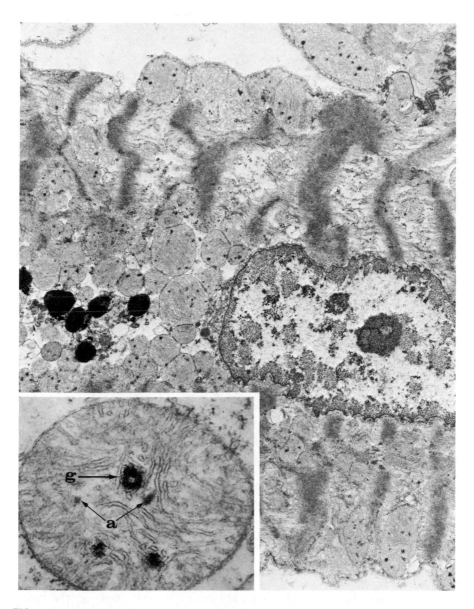

FIG. 1. A myocardial cell is shown here after 40 min of *in vivo* ischemia followed by 20 min of reperfusion with arterial blood. Numerous dense contraction bands are present. Peripheral condensation of nuclear chromatin also is apparent, and the mitochondria appear swollen. They contain both amorphous and granular matrix densities. The insert on the *lower left* shows a higher power view of characteristic granular densities of Ca²⁺ phosphate in mitochondria of these cells. Both amorphous (a) and granular densities (g) are present. (Osmium tetroxide fixation; magnification: × 12,600, inset × 40,500.) Reprinted from ref. 9, with permission.

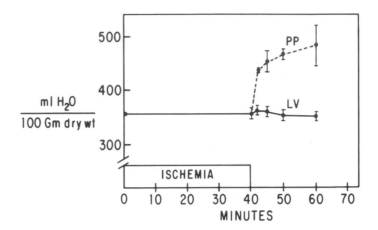

FIG. 2. Plot of total tissue water (TTW) of severely ischemic posterior papillary muscle (PP) after varying intervals of ischemia in contrast to the TTW of nonischemic anterior superior left ventricle (LV) of the same dog hearts. The TTW plotted is the mean of groups of 4 dogs after 40 min of ischemia and 2, 5, 10, and 20 min of reflow. Note the enormous increase in water in the PP after only 2 min of reperfusion. The 0, 2, 5, and 10 min *points* are from ref. 29; the 20 min *point* is from ref. 26.

permanent ischemia induced no detectable increase in water, presumably because there was too little collateral arterial flow available to provide any new tissue water, i.e., edema. However, failure of cell volume control became obvious immediately when irreversibly injured cells were provided with access to the essentially infinite plasma pool of the arterial blood reperfusing the damaged tissue. Moreover, most of the edema developed during the first 2 min of reperfusion (29). As one would expect, increases in tissue Na^+, Cl^-, and decreases in tissue K^+ and Mg^{2+} are associated with the increased H_2O shown in Fig. 2. The edema results in subsarcolemmal blebs and vacuoles in the cells, one of which is illustrated in Fig. 11 in ref. 9. The structural evidence that the edema is primarily intracellular is quite striking.

CALCIUM DURING REPERFUSION

The concentration of tissue Ca^{2+} increases 8 to 10 times over control during the early phase of reperfusion (29). The actual Ca^{2+} accumulated is far more than can be accounted for by edema alone and is due chiefly to the active accumulation of Ca^{2+} in mitochondria (25,26) in the form of characteristic granular densities (Fig. 1) of Ca phosphate probably complexed as hydroxyapatite. This granular appearance is not invariably present. Sometimes they appear as needle-like crystals of Ca^{2+} phosphate (see Fig. 30 B of ref. 9).

It seems likely that the Ca^{2+} phosphate deposition in these mitochondria is equivalent to cation loading in isolated mitochondria *in vitro*. Accordingly, it is instructive to review the requirements for massive Ca^{2+} loading in isolated myocardial mitochondria; these include aerobic conditions, substrate, inorganic phosphate, Ca^{2+}, and ATP (18). We assume that the mitochondrial requirements are similar when myocytes are reperfused with arterial blood *in vivo*. This means that a portion of the electron transport system of the mitochondria of ischemic cells must be intact and that the ATP available in the myocytes or synthesized by the damaged myocyte at the time of reperfusion must be adequate to support massive cation loading. Finally, since cation loading occurs in preference to oxidative phosphorylation (18), massive loading of Ca phosphate in the mitochondria of the affected cells results in depressed mitochondrial ATP synthesis even though O_2 and substrate are present. We suspect, therefore, that mitochondria provided with O_2 by arterial reflow make very little high-energy phosphate when abundant intracellular Ca^{2+} and inorganic phosphate are present.

Studies with radioactive Ca^{2+} have shown that the source of the new Ca^{2+} in myocytes early in the phase of irreversible ischemia is the plasma reperfusing the heart, and that most of the accumulation occurs in the first 10 min of reperfusion (26). The mean increase in the radioactive Ca^{2+} content of the damaged muscle over control nonischemic muscle is approximately 18 to 20 times. Attempts to prevent Ca^{2+} accumulation by perfusing the tissue with blood containing zero Ca^{2+} have been unsuccessful because the reperfused myocytes separate from one another at the intercalated disk (24). In permanent ischemia, on the other hand, because of low collateral flow, very little radioactive Ca^{2+} appears in the zone of low-flow ischemia (26) if the plasma is labeled with $^{45}Ca^{2+}$ immediately after occlusion of the artery.

In Fig. 3, the major changes found in reversible and in the early and late phases of irreversible injury are summarized along with the effect of reperfusion. Note that successful reperfusion late in the irreversible phase (90–180 min) results in contraction bands, but no Ca^{2+} accumulation (9,15). The best available explanation for the lack of Ca^{2+} accumulation is mitochondrial failure secondary to changes in the terminal electron transport system or to lack of adequate supplies of ATP and ADP to support massive loading (18). Capillaries and small blood vessels also become focally necrotic at about the same time; reperfusion of areas with vascular damage is not possible. This leads to the so-called "no-reflow" phenomenon (15). In such areas, neither contraction bands nor Ca^{2+} accumulation appear (15).

The role Ca^{2+} may play in severe ischemia followed by reperfusion is shown in Fig. 4. After severe ischemia of sufficient duration to induce the irreversible state, reperfusion with arterial blood provides an abundant source of Ca^{2+} which enters the sarcoplasm through routes not yet surely identified. The increased $[Ca^{2+}]_i$ results in massive cation loading of the mitochondria; the loading results in depressed production of high-energy phosphates by oxidative phosphorylation and acceleration of the appearance of necrosis. The sarcoplasmic Ca^{2+} concentration increases because of the excessive rate of influx and because the sarcoplasmic ATP is too low to support Ca^{2+} transport functions of the SR and the mitochondria as well as the Na^+,K^+-ATPase (sodium pump) of the cell membrane. It is not now known if the low high-energy phosphate content of the ischemic cell causes the plasmalemmal alterations; the only evidence available is temporal,

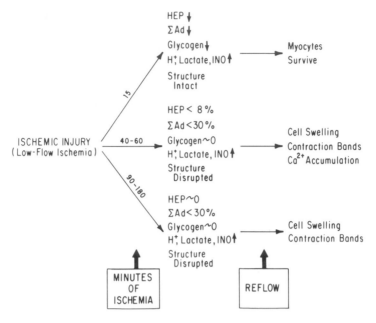

FIG. 3. Diagram depicting the sequence of events occurring in myocytes injured by varying periods of ischemia followed by reperfusion of arterial blood. An episode of low-flow ischemia of 15 min duration results in a decrease in tissue high-energy phosphate (HEP), total adenine nucleotides (ΣAd), and glycogen, while H^+, lactate, and inosine (INO) all increase. These myocytes are reversibly injured and survive if reperfused with arterial blood. The chemical changes are similar, but more marked after 40 to 60 min of ischemia, at which time the injury is irreversible. Moreover, significant structural changes now are detectable. The sarcolemma is focally disrupted and amorphous matrix densities are present in virtually all the mitochondria of the affected cells. In addition, the irreversibly injured tissue is in rigor mortis (contracture-rigor). Reperfusion of tissue early in the irreversible phase of injury is associated with accumulation of massive quantities of mitochondrial Ca^{2+} phosphate, marked edema, and with formation of contraction bands in the myofibrils, while successful reperfusion of tissue after 90 to 180 min of ischemia results only in contraction bands and edema. After late reperfusion, massive cation loading of mitochondria does not occur. (From ref. 11.)

i.e., there is a close association between low cellular high-energy phosphates for a period of 20 to 30 min and the appearance of sarcolemmal defects and cell death.

The above analysis (Fig. 4) is based on the assumption that the severely ischemic myocytes are irreversibly injured prior to reperfusion and accumulate Ca^{2+} as a consequence of membrane damage, damage being manifest as increased permeability or as breaks in the plasmalemma (6,12).

CALCIUM OVERLOADING OF CELLS

On the other hand, it is clear that Ca^{2+} loading may be the primary event leading to cell death in certain other forms of myocyte injury. Thus, toxic

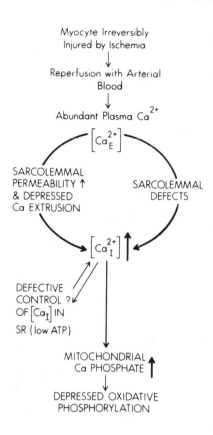

FIG. 4. Diagram summarizing the probable relationships of [Ca²⁺]ᵢ shifts in contraction-band necrosis of the type found in acute ischemic injury. (From ref. 7.)

doses of isoproterenol result in the development of foci of contraction-band necrosis which are indistinguishable from those seen in reperfused irreversibly injured myocardium. The fact that necrosis can be prevented by the Ca²⁺ channel blocker verapamil suggests that increased [Ca²⁺]ᵢ is the lethal mediator in this form of injury (2). In addition, it has been shown that Ca²⁺ accumulation is an early sign of irreversible injury in hepatocytes in *d*-galactosamine (1) and CCl₄ poisoning (23). Both these toxins result in membrane damage; however, in *d*-galactosamine poisoning, Farber et al. (1) hypothesize that the membrane damage is not necessarily lethal, and that the hepatocytes would survive the deleterious effects of *d*-galactosamine on the cell membrane if Ca²⁺ entry could be prevented.

Once excess Ca²⁺ has entered the cytoplasm of oxygenated cells, it can produce lethal effects by numerous routes. A few of the potential mechanisms are shown in Fig. 5. For example, cell death might result from interference with aerobic energy production because of massive loading of the mitochondria with Ca²⁺ phosphate. Alternatively, stimulation of endogenous membrane phospholipases by Ca²⁺ could result in membrane damage leading to further Ca²⁺ entry. The situation is extraordinarily complex and probably will not be resolved quickly.

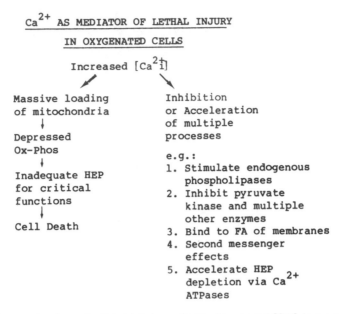

FIG. 5. Diagram showing potential deleterious effects of increased $[C^{2+}]_i$ in oxygenated cells. Inhibition of aerobic metabolism would have disastrous effects on production of high-energy phosphate and could lead to cell death by the mechanism shown on the *left side* of the diagram. However, other potentially serious deleterious effects of Ca^{2+} also are possible. Such effects are listed on the *right-hand side* of the figure. FA: fatty acids; HEP: high energy phosphates.

SUMMARY

It is uncertain how or whether alterations in intracellular Ca^{2+} are related to the development of irreversibility in permanent severe ischemia. Increases in $[Ca^{2+}]_i$ to the micromolar range are theoretically possible and could contribute to the deleterious effects of ischemia by, e.g., accelerating depletion of high-energy phosphates or by activating endogenous phospholipases.

Reperfusion of myocardium reversibly injured by ischemia is not associated with detectable changes in tissue Ca^{2+}, while reperfusion of myocardium which just has entered the phase of irreversible injury is associated with explosive cell swelling, contraction-band formation, and massive loading of the mitochondria with Ca^{2+} phosphate (contraction-band necrosis). The massive loading is the result of entry of plasma Ca^{2+} into the sarcoplasm of the myocyte. The damaged plasmalemma of the irreversibly injured cells is considered to be the chief route of entry, but other mechanisms of entry have not been ruled out. These observations have led to the hypothesis that changes in the sarcoplasmic Ca^{2+} ion concentration do not cause myocyte death in ischemia, but rather, that Ca^{2+}, O_2, and other substances in the arterial blood reperfusing the affected tissue accelerate the appearance of signs of lethal injury (necrosis) in myocytes which were dead prior to reperfusion.

ACKNOWLEDGMENTS

This work was supported in part by research grants from the National Heart, Lung and Blood Institute #HL23138 and #HL27416.

REFERENCES

1. Farber, J. L., El-Mofty, S. K., Schanne, F. A. X., Alco, J. J., Jr., and Serroni, A. (1977): *Arch. Biochem. Biophys.*, 178:617–624.
2. Fleckenstein, A. (1971): *Calcium and the Heart*, edited by P. Harris and L. Opie, pp. 135–188. Academic Press, New York.
3. Herdson, P. B., Sommers, H. M., and Jennings, R. B. (1965): *Am. J. Pathol.*, 46:367–386.
4. Hill, J. L., and Gettes L. S. (1980): *Circulation*, 61:68–78.
5. Hirche, H., Franz, C., and Bös, L. (1979): *Brain and Heart Infarct II*, edited by K. J. Zülch, W. Kaufmann, K.-A. Hossman, and V. Hossman, pp. 104–111. Springer-Verlag, Berlin.
6. Jennings, R. B. (1975): *Acta Med. Scand. (Suppl.)*, 587:83–92.
7. Jennings, R. B. (1982): *Proceedings of a Symposium for Pharmacologists, Physiologists and Medical Practitioners*, edited by W. Nayler. Abbott Laboratories, Queensboro, England (*in press*).
8. Jennings, R. B., Crout, J. R., and Smetters, G. W. (1957): *AMA Arch. Pathol.* (*Chicago*), 63:586–592.
9. Jennings, R. B., and Hawkins, H. K. (1980): *Degradative Processes in Heart and Skeletal Muscle*, edited by K. Wildenthal, pp. 295–346. Elsevier, New York.
10. Jennings, R. B., Hawkins, H. K., Lowe, J. E., Hill, M. L., Klotman, S., and Reimer, K. A. (1978): *Am. J. Pathol.* 92:187–214.
11. Jennings, R. B., Hawkins, H. K., Lowe, J. E., Hill, M. L., and Reimer, K. A.: (1980): *Proceedings of the Fourth US-USSR Symposium on Myocardial Metabolism*, Tashkent, U.S.S.R., pp. 351–371. DHEW Publication No. 80–2017 (*in press*).
12. Jennings, R. B., and Reimer, K. A. (1981): *Am. J. Pathol.*, 102:241–255.
13. Jennings, R. B., Reimer, K. A., Hill, M. L., and Mayer, S. E. (1981): *Circ. Res.*, 49:892–900.
14. Jennings, R. B., Sommers, H. M., Kaltenbach, J. P., and West, J. J. (1964): *Circ. Res.*, 14:260–269.
15. Kloner, R. A., Ganote, C. E., and Jennings, R. B. (1974): *J. Clin. Invest.*, 54:1496–1508.
16. Kloner, R. A., Ganote, C. E., Whalen, D., and Jennings, R. B. (1974): *Am. J. Pathol.*, 74:399–414.
17. Leaf, A. (1973): *Circulation*, 48:455–458.
18. Lehninger, A. L. (1970): *Biochem. J.*, 119:129–138.
19. Nayler, W. G., Poole-Wilson, P. A., Williams, A. (1979): *J. Mol. Cell. Cardiol.*, 11:683–706.
20. Neely, J. R., and Morgan, H. E. (1974): *Annu. Rev. Physiol.*, 36:413–459.
21. Reimer, K. A., and Jennings, R. B. (1979): *Lab. Invest.*, 40:633–644.
22. Reimer, K. A., Hill, M. L., and Jennings, R. B. (1981): *J. Mol. Cell. Cardiol.*, 13:229–239.
23. Reynolds, E. S., and Ree, H. J. (1971): *Lab. Invest.*, 25:269–278.
24. Rocco, M. B., Reimer, K. A., and Jennings, R. B. (1979): *Circulation*, 59 and 60:II–216.
25. Shen, A. C., and Jennings, R. B. (1972): *Am. J. Pathol.*, 67:417–440.
26. Shen, A. C., and Jennings, R. B. (1972): *Am. J. Pathol.*, 67:441–452.
27. Shine, K. I., Douglas, A. M., and Ricchiuti, N. V. (1978): *Circ. Res.*, 43:712–720.
28. Sommers, H. M., and Jennings, R. B. (1964): *Lab. Invest.*, 13:1491–1503.
29. Whalen, D. A., Jr., Hamilton, D. G., Ganote, C. E., and Jennings, R. B. (1974): *Am. J. Pathol.*, 74:381–398.

Calcium Antagonists and Cardiovascular Disease, edited by L. H. Opie.
Raven Press, New York © 1984.

Chapter 9

Enzyme Loss and Calcium Exchange in Ischemic or Hypoxic Myocardium

P. A. Poole-Wilson

Cardiothoracic Institute, London W1N 2DX, England

The definitive diagnosis of myocardial infarction in patients is made from changes of the electrocardiogram and the detection of increased myocardial enzymes in the blood (55). Enzymes are released from necrosing myocardial tissue, and the reduction of the tissue content of enzymes can be used in the dog to delineate an area of infarction and to study the effect of drug interventions on infarct size (42). Infarct size can also be estimated by obtaining serial measurements of enzyme activity in blood (49). The method has many problems (15,46); nevertheless, in man, measurements of infarct size at necropsy correlate with the size estimated from blood enzyme profiles (7). The extent of necrosis is related to mortality (4,49) and other sequelae of myocardial infarction (29,44). Such an association could be anticipated since, in the extreme examples of small and large infarcts, the pattern of enzyme release will be different and the clinical consequences are well known (29). Where there is controversy is in the detection of minor myocardial infarcts and the significance of small rises in plasma enzymes. The problem has great clinical implications since, on the basis of enzyme measurements, patients with chest pain are classified as having had a myocardial infarct, prolonged ischemic pain, or coronary artery disease, with all the attached social and medical consequences.

Creatine kinase (CK) is detectable in the blood of normal man at rest. The isoenzyme (CKMB) is presumed to arise almost exclusively from heart muscle. CKMB is raised in the blood of marathon runners (3,51) and competitive swimmers after exercise (52). The appearance of CKMB may be due to increased physiological release of enzymes from the myocardium or other tissues (14), or to damage to the heart (51). Studies in dogs show that, even under control conditions, enzymes specific to the heart are substantially more concentrated in cardiac lymph than in the coronary sinus (50). Enzymes appear to be released from the normal heart. Numerous *in vivo* and *in vitro* studies of enzyme release and tissue content in the heart have been undertaken during and after periods of hypoxia or ischemia. Current knowledge is presented in a recent book (35). The clinical question as to the significance of small rises in plasma enzymes will only be resolved when it is known how enzymes move from the intracellular to extracellular fluid under control conditions, and how enzymes are released from cells undergoing pathological changes.

TRANSPORT OF ENZYMES ACROSS THE MYOCARDIAL CELL MEMBRANE

In theory, cytosolic proteins which are not bound to any intracellular structure could pass through a cell membrane by several mechanisms (Table 1). Most cell membranes have turnover rates of approximately 24 to 48 hr (17,47). The repair and replacement of damaged or aged membranes will almost inevitably result in small quantities of intracellular fluid being released to the extracellular space. In the myocardium, such a process may be the reason for the release of enzymes under normal conditions and for the increased release of enzymes under stressful conditions (50). Destruction of myocardial cells is unlikely since myocardial cells do not divide, and the amount of enzyme released over years would be so large that a macroscopic loss of cardiac tissue would be apparent; this is not observed.

RELEASE OF ENZYMES UNDER PATHOLOGICAL CONDITIONS

Under pathological conditions, myocardial enzymes have been widely used as an indicator of cell necrosis or "irreversible damage." Enzymes have been measured during and after periods of hypoxia or ischemia (35), but the release of enzymes is related to ultrastructural changes in the sarcolemma and to the recovery of mechanical function only in broad terms. During global ischemia the release of enzymes cannot be studied, but during hypoxia detailed investigations have been undertaken. In a series of experiments, Hearse and colleagues (31,33,34) and Feuvray and de Leiris (16) showed that during hypoxia some enzyme was released in the initial 60 min, but that no ultrastructural damage to the sarcolemma occurred. Between 120 and 360 min a second larger efflux of enzymes was apparent, and at this time structural damage was evident. On reoxygenation, further sudden release of enzyme occurred.

TABLE 1. *Possible mechanisms for transsarcolemmal movement of proteins*

Exocytosis (efflux due to coalescence of an intracellular vesicle and the cell membrane)
Endocytosis (influx due to coalescence of an extracellular vesicle and the cell membrane)
Outward budding
Transient "slits or tears"
Localized pores or "holes"
Specific transport mechanism
Gross disruption of the cell membrane

TABLE 2. *Possible causes of damage to heart muscle on reperfusion or reoxygenation*

Cause of damage (refs.)	Effect (refs.)

Lack of energy
  ATP deficiency (10,28,38)
  NAD deficiency (40)
	Integrity of cell membrane
	Repair of cell membrane
	Maintenance of cellular functions

Mechanical effects	Contracture causing disruption (19) Cell swelling against matrix No reflow phenomenon (26)
Membrane damage	Mitochondria (30,43) Sarcolemma Phospholipases (12) Proteases Leukotrienes Acyl esters (39) Lysophosphoglycerides (48) Oxygen radicals (22,27) Acidosis (5) Ca²⁺ on membrane stability (20) Na⁺-Ca²⁺ exchange (21)

Similarities have been drawn between enzyme release in reoxygenation and after the Ca^{2+} paradox (32). On reperfusion of ischemia, a similar release of enzymes has been reported (30) and has been related to discontinuities observed in the sarcolemma (36,37). Many theories have been put forward to account for the sudden loss of enzymes and influx of Ca^{2+} which occurs at the moment of reperfusion or reoxygenation. It should be noted that the occurrence of these events, sometimes confusingly referred to as an "exacerbation of damage," is a hurdle which must be cleared in order for the tissue to recover; failure to reperfuse or reoxygenate will inevitably lead to tissue necrosis, and damage to the tissue after reperfusion or reoxygenation increases with the duration of ischemia or hypoxia. Possible causes of cell damage are listed in Table 2. Ultimately, a cell will break down and release all cytosolic enzymes into the extracellular fluid. The central question is how are these enzymes released during the early period of hypoxia (34), and in particular on reoxygenation or reperfusion.

EVIDENCE THAT THE SARCOLEMMA IS NOT DISRUPTED

The simplest hypothesis for events at the time of reperfusion or reoxygenation would be that the sarcolemma developed discontinuities or "holes" (36,37), or that the sarcolemma was grossly disrupted, for example, by tearing itself apart due to contracture (19). Discontinuities of the sarcolemma can be demonstrated by electron microscopy. A problem arises as to whether these represent true defects in the membrane or are a consequence of the fixation process, preparation of the specimen, or the plane in which the specimen has been cut. Our own work does not support the concept that enzyme loss early during hypoxia or reoxygenation is due to disruption of the membrane (8,9,24). The distribution volume of the extracellular marker ^{51}Cr-EDTA (ethyldisminetetraacetate) (MW = 343) can be followed continuously with great accuracy in myocardial tissue (20). At the time of reoxygenation (24) or reperfusion (8,9), although enzymes are released and Ca^{2+} enters the cell, the distribution volume of ^{51}Cr-EDTA is unchanged. Furthermore, the sudden influx of Ca^{2+} can be inhibited by the presence of a small divalent ion such as Ni^{2+} (25) suggesting that the Ca^{2+} influx also is not due to cell disruption. The study of Burton et al. (11) came to similar conclusions. The integrity of the cell membrane was assessed by the detection of intracellular deposition of La^{3+}. La^{3+} was not found intracellularly during more than 1 hr of hypoxia and intracellular La^{3+} deposition appeared to precede irreversible damage as assessed by ultrastructural changes.

The amount of enzyme released on reoxygenation is small even when severe contracture has developed during the period of hypoxia. In our experiments (23), it amounts to approximately 2% of the total tissue enzyme content after 30 min hypoxia and 30 min reoxygenation. A substantial contracture had developed and mechanical recovery of the muscle was almost absent. By comparison, when the cell membrane was disrupted by a detergent, or after the Ca^{2+} paradox, 66% of the tissue enzyme appeared in the effluent (24). Similar findings have been reported by others (32). Conrad et al. (13) attempted to determine the significance of a small efflux of enzymes be relating the loss to net loss of K^+. In general, there was a relationship suggesting that enzyme release did indicate a minor amount of cell necrosis. However, in their experiments where muscles were made hypoxic for short periods, enzyme was lost without a net loss of K^+. A relationship between enzyme loss and K^+ loss does not exclude the possibility that a proportion of the enzyme loss was by a mechanism other than cell disruption. It is possible to argue that in our experiments (8,24) and those of Conrad et al. (13) Ca^{2+} influx and a rise of resting tension are present in most cells, whereas the release of enzymes was from only a few cells which had been totally disrupted. That proposition cannot be entirely discounted, but other explanations are also possible.

A typical experiment is shown in Fig. 1. The release of enzyme is shown as an accumulated total. During the short period of hypoxia (Fig. 1), the rate of enzyme loss is constant. On reoxygenation, Ca^{2+} immediately enters the cell and is followed a few minutes later by the efflux of enzyme. The time lag might be due to delay in the diffusion of a large protein molecule out of the tissue, but that explanation is unlikely since there is no time delay when Ca^{2+} is reintroduced after a period of Ca^{2+}-free perfusion (the Ca^{2+} paradox).

A HYPOTHESIS

A possible hypothesis is that it is the inward movement of Ca^{2+} itself which brings about the small enzyme loss. Ca^{2+} is known to alter the fragility of the cell membrane (20) and to increase outward budding of the membrane of red

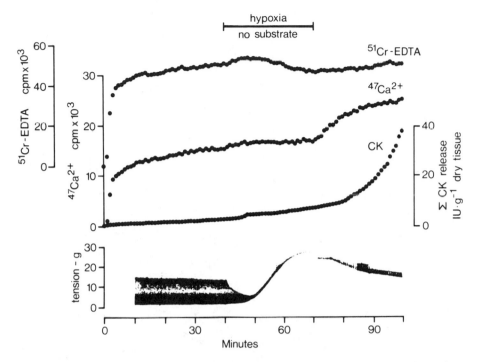

FIG. 1. Interventricular septum of rabbit heart. The technique used is described in ref. 8. ⁵¹Cr-EDTA did not enter the cell during hypoxia or on reoxygenation. The increase and then fall in counts of ⁵¹Cr-EDTA during hypoxia was a consequence of the mechanical changes in the heart. Note the sudden uptake of ⁴⁷Ca²⁺ on reoxygenation. The release of creatine kinase (CK) followed several minutes later; the amount released was small. The release of CK was expressed as a cumulative amount.

blood cells (18). Ca²⁺ also activates phospholipases (54) and proteases (2). Phospholipases may liberate lysophosphoglycerides from the cell membrane, and these reduce membrane stability. The mechanism initiating the sudden influx of Ca²⁺ on reoxygenation remains uncertain (Table 2).

If Ca²⁺ did increase turnover of the cell membrane and outward budding, the process only need transfer approximately 2% of the intracellular fluid to the extracellular spore in a period of 30 min reoxygenation in order to account for the observed enzyme loss. The anatomical presence of a bud on the cell surface would be a reasonably rare event. Outward budding in red cells has been reported in the presence of bile salts (6), with time on standing (53), and in the absence of substrate (41). It is possible to observe abnormalities in the cell membrane of hypoxic myocardium compatible with such a concept. A freeze-fracture picture of a vesicle apparently budding from the cell membrane is shown in Fig. 2. An elaborate quantitative study would be necessary to establish the significance of such a phenomenon. Enzymes could also be lost through other physiological changes in membrane structure (18).

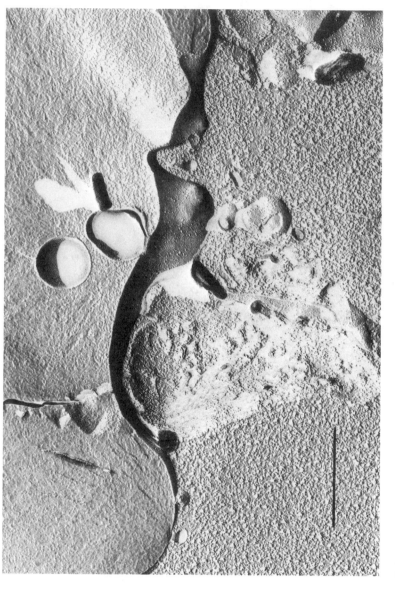

FIG. 2. A freeze-fracture electron micrograph of the rabbit interventricular septum after 30 min hypoxia and 30 min reoxygenation. The fracture plane crosses from the extracellular space (*top*) across the cell membrane (*middle*) to the interior of the cell (*bottom*). A vesicular structure appears to protrude from the cell membrane into the extracellular space. A cut across another vesicle is seen in the extracellular space. (Magnification: × 52,000. Scale bar, 0.5 μm.)

CONCLUSION

The detection of large quantities of intracellular myocardial enzymes in the effluent from the heart or in the blood of man undoubtedly does indicate myocardial cell necrosis. However, the significance of small changes in plasma enzymes is less certain. Enzyme loss can be brought about by increased turnover of cell membranes and outward budding; such phenomena may account for the rise of cardiac enzymes observed in marathon runners and competitive swimmers. The possibility exists that minor elevations of cardiac enzymes in man with coronary artery disease do not indicate a small amount of inevitable cell necrosis associated with irreversible destruction of the cell membrane, but rather a pathophysiological process associated with ischemia from which the myocardial cell would still potentially recover. If the exact mechanism of membrane damage were known, an effective therapeutic intervention might be possible.

REFERENCES

1. Allan, D., and Michell, R. H. (1977): *Biochem. J.,* 166:495–499.
2. Anderson, D. R., Davis, J. L., and Carraway, K. L. (1977): *J. Biol. Chem.,* 252:6617–6623.
3. Apple, F. S. (1981): *N. Engl. J. Med.,* 305:764–765.
4. Baughman, K. L., Maroko, P. R., and Vatner, S. F. (1981): *Circulation,* 63:317–323.
5. Billah, M. M., Finean, J. B., Coleman, R., and Michell, R. H. (1977): *Biochim. Biophys. Acta,* 465:515–526.
6. Billington, D., and Coleman, R. (1978): *Biochim. Biophys. Acta,* 509:33–47.
7. Bleifeld, W., Mathey, D., Hanrath, P., Buss, H., and Effert, S. (1977): *Circulation,* 55:303–311.
8. Bourdillon, P. D. V., and Poole-Wilson, P. A. (1981): *Cardiovasc. Res.,* 15:121–130.
9. Bourdillon, P. D., and Poole-Wilson, P. A. (1982): *Circ. Res.,* 50:360–368.
10. Brichnell, O. L., Daries, P. S., and Opie, L. H. (1981): *J. Mol. Cell. Cardiol.,* 13:941–945.
11. Burton, K. P., Hagler, H. K., Templeton, G. H., Willerson, J. T., and Buja, L. M. (1977): *J. Clin. Invest.,* 60:1289–1302.
12. Chien, K. R., Pfau, R. G., and Farber, J. L. (1979): *Am. J. Pathol.,* 97:505–529.
13. Conrad, G. L., Rau, E. E., and Shine, K. I. (1979): *J. Clin. Invest.,* 64:155–161.
14. Editorial (1978): *Lancet,* 2:718–719.
15. Editorial (1978): *Lancet,* 2:1082–1083.
16. Feuvray, D., and de Leiris, J. (1975): *J. Mol. Cell. Cardiol.,* 7:307–314.
17. Finean, J. B., Coleman, R., and Michell, R. H. (1978): *Membranes and Their Cellular Functions,* 2nd ed. Blackwell, Oxford.
18. Frank, J. S., Langer, G. A., Nudd, L. M., and Seraydarian, K. (1977): *Circ. Res.,* 41:702–714.
19. Ganote, C. E., and Kaltenbach, J. P. (1979): *J. Mol. Cell. Cardiol.,* 11:389–406.
20. Gordon, L. M., Saverheber, R. D., and Esgate, J. A. (1978): *J. Supramol. Struct.,* 9:299–326.
21. Grinwald, P. M. (1982): *J. Mol. Cell. Cardiol.,* 14:359–365.
22. Guarnierei, C., Flamigni, F., and Calderera, C. M. (1980): *J. Mol. Cell. Cardiol.,* 12:797–808.
23. Harding, D. P. (1982): *Calcium Fluxes and Myocardial Hypoxia.* Ph. D. thesis, London University.
24. Harding, D. P., and Poole-Wilson, P. A. (1980): *Cardiovasc. Res.,* 14:435–445.
25. Harding, D. P., and Poole-Wilson, P. A. (1981): *J. Mol. Cell. Cardiol.,* 13(Suppl. 1):37.
26. Harris, P. (1975): *Eur. J Cardiol.,* 3:157–163.
27. Hess, H. L., Okabe, E., and Kontos, H. A. (1981): *J. Mol. Cell. Cardiol.,* 13:767–772.
28. Higgins, T. J. C., Bailey, P. J., and Allsopp, D. (1981): *J. Mol. Cell. Cardiol.,* 13:1027–1030.

29. Hillis, L. D., and Braunwald, E. (1977): *N. Engl. J. Med.,* 296:971–978; 1034–1041; 1093–1096.
30. Hearse, D. J. (1977): *J. Mol. Cell. Cardiol.,* 9:605–616.
31. Hearse, D. J., and Humphrey, S. M. (1975): *J. Mol. Cell. Cardiol.,* 7:463–482.
32. Hearse, D. J., Humphrey, S. M., and Bullock, G. R. (1978): *J. Mol. Cell. Cardiol.,* 10:641–668.
33. Hearse, D. J., Humphrey, S. M., and Chain, E. B. (1973): *J. Mol. Cell. Cardiol.,* 5:395–407.
34. Hearse, D. J., Humphrey, S. M., Feuvray, D., and de Leiris, J. (1976): *J. Mol. Cell. Cardiol.,* 8:759–778.
35. Hearse, D. J., and de Lieris, J. (editors) (1979): *Enzymes in Cardiology. Diagnosis and Research.* Wiley, New York.
36. Jennings, R. B., Ganote, C. E., and Reimer, K. A. (1975): *Am. J. Pathol.,* 81:179–198.
37. Jennings, R. B., Hawkins, K. H., Lowe, J. E., Hill, M. L. Klotman, S., and Reimer, K. (1978): *Am. J. Pathol.,* 92:187–214.
38. Jennings, R. B., and Reimer, K. A. (1981): *Am. J. Pathol.,* 102:241–255.
39. Katz, A. M., and Messineo, F. C. (1981): *Circ. Res.,* 48:1–16.
40. Klein, H. H., Schaper, J., Puschmann, S., Nienaber, C., Kreuzer, H., Schaper, W. (1981): *Basic Res. Cardiol.,* 76:612–621.
41. Lutz, H. U., Barber, R., and McGuire, R. F. (1976): *J. Biol. Chem.,* 251:3500–3510.
42. Maroko, P. R., Kjekshus, J. K., Sobel, B. E., Watanabe, T., Covell, J. M., Ross, J., and Braunwald, E. (1971): *Circulation,* 43:67–82.
43. Nakanishi, T., Nishioka, K., and Jarmankani, J. M. (1982): *Am. J. Physiol.,* 242:H437–H449.
44. Opie, L. H. (1980): *Am. Heart J.,* 100:355–372.
45. Poole-Wilson, P. A., Bourdillon, P. D., and Harding, D. P. (1979): *Basic Res. Cardiol.,* 74:604–610.
46. Roe, C. R., and Starmer, C. F. (1975): *Circulation,* 52:1–5.
47. Siekevitz, P. (1972): *Annu. Rev. Physiol.,* 34:117–140.
48. Snyder, D. W., Crafford, W. A., Jr., Glashow, J. L., Rankin, D., Sobel, B. E., and Corr, P. B. (1981): *Am. J. Physiol.,* 241:H700–H707.
49. Sobel, B. E., Bresnahan, G. F., Shell, W. E., and Yoder, R. D. (1972): *Circulation,* 46:640–648.
50. Spieckermann, P. G., Nordbeck, H., and Preuse, C. J. (1979): *Enzymes in Cardiology,* edited by D. J. Hearse and J. de Leiris, pp. 81–91. Wiley, New York.
51. Stansbie, D. S., Aston, J. P., Powell, N. H., and Willis, N. (1982): *Lancet,* 1:1413–1414.
52. Strauss, R. H., Lott, J. A., Bartels, R., Fox, E., and Whitcomb, M. E. (1982): *N. Engl. J. Med.,* 306:1180.
53. Weed, R. I., and Reed, C. F. (1966): *Am. J. Med.,* 41:681–98.
54. Weglicki, W. B., Waite, B. M., and Stam, A. C. (1972): *J. Mol. Cell. Cardiol.,* 4:195–201.
55. WHO International Collaborative Study, Regional Office for Europe (1976): Myocardial infarction community registers. *Copenhagen: WHO (Public Health in Europe No. 5).*

Calcium Antagonists and Cardiovascular Disease, edited by L. H. Opie.
Raven Press, New York © 1984.

Chapter 10

Calcium Antagonists and Eperimental Myocardial Ischemia and Infarction

Joël de Leiris, Vincent Richard, and Sophie Pestre

Laboratoire de Physiologie Animale, Université Scientifique et Médicale de Grenoble, Grenoble, France

Since the pioneering work of Fleckenstein and co-workers (11), Ca^{2+} antagonists have attracted considerable interest for their beneficial effects in the treatment of several forms of cardiovascular disease (37). Although Ca^{2+} antagonists have been used clinically mainly as antianginal and antiarrhythmic agents, these drugs may also be of value in the treatment of acute myocardial infarction and for cardiac preservation during cardiac surgery (16).

In this chapter, we will consider the effect of Ca^{2+} antagonists in experimental myocardial ischemia and infarction. Firstly, some characteristics of the main experimental models used to study myocardial ischemia and infarction will be briefly described. Secondly, some of the recent results obtained with Ca^{2+} antagonists using some of these models will be reviewed. Finally, we will discuss the possible mode of action of these drugs in these particular conditions.

PRODUCTION OF MYOCARDIAL ISCHEMIA AND INFARCTION

Complete occlusion of a coronary artery, generally the left anterior descending artery (LAD), is the most commonly used method for the production of myocardial infarction in the open-chest anesthetized dog, pig, or baboon under artificial respiration. Occlusion can also be accomplished in the closed-chest state, e.g., by introducing a bolus of mercury or graded microspheres into the coronary circulation, or by electrically inducing a thrombus formation. Another possibility is to place surgically a hydraulic occluder on a coronary artery and to allow the animal to recover from the surgery. With this technique, the vessel is occluded in the unanesthetized state. Progressive constriction of a coronary artery may also be obtained by means of ameroid material. Johns and Olson (17) have described a technique for ligation of coronary arteries in small animals. After a light anesthesia with ether, a left intercostal thoracotomy is performed without artificial respiration, and the left coronary artery is rapidly ligated at 1 to 2 mm from its origin. The heart is then placed back in the chest with the whole procedure being accomplished in less than 5 min. Operative and postoperative mortality is about 25%. Histochemical analysis indicates that the margins of the infarct are sharply demarcated and are remarkably constant from one animal to another, especially in mice and rats.

In both *in situ* or *in vitro* models of myocardial ischemia (5,33), one of the major difficulties in determining the efficacy of pharmacological interventions designed to limit the final extent of myocardial necrosis has been the available indices for quantifying infarct size. In a wide variety of species, the degree of myocardial enzyme depletion (most often, creatine kinase) is generally considered to be well correlated with infarct size (measured morphometrically). In isolated hearts, the release of intracellular enzymes into the coronary effluent has been used to assess the severity and extent of myocardial damage (26). Other experimental techniques for measuring infarct size include histochemical staining, electronmicroscopy, hemodynamic and mechanical measurements, and electrophysiology (for instance epicardial ECG). Direct visualization of infarcted myocardium is also possible with the use of radioindicators. Finally, metabolic studies have been generally based on rapid sequential or simultaneous multiple biopsies followed by the analysis of metabolic markers, such as ATP, creatine phosphate, lactate, and glycogen. However, biopsy studies are often limited by various factors (13).

Despite the limitations of the techniques and models used to investigate myocardial infarction, a number of these have been used to assess the efficacy of various drugs and treatments in ischemic conditions.

IN SITU STUDIES OF MYOCARDIAL ISCHEMIA AND INFARCTION

In 1975, Smith et al. (31) reported that when open-chest anesthetized dogs received intravenous verapamil 15 min *after* ligation of the LAD (distal to the origin of its first diagonal branch), this drug produced a highly significant reduction of epicardial ST-segment elevation and prevented the hemodynamic deterioration seen in the control animals. This effect could be due to verapamil-induced bradycardia, since it was abolished by pacing (2). However, Reimer et al. (27) indicated that verapamil was effective in reducing infarct size in dogs *only* when administered *prior* to coronary occlusion. Such conflicting conclusions illustrate the difficulty of studies designed to assess myocardial protection with Ca²⁺ antagonists. Indeed, as in most experimental studies, differences exist in (a) experimental conditions (species under investigation, model of ischemia, permanent or temporary occlusion, and site of ligation), (b) criteria used to quantify the degree of ischemia and protection, and (c) nature of the drug used, route of administration, dosage, and whether the treatment is given prior to or after induction of ischemia. It is, therefore, difficult to have a clear, precise, and logical view of the possible protective effect of Ca^{2+} antagonists in myocardial ischemia, let alone the precise mode of action of these drugs in ischemic myocardium.

Some published results describing the use of various Ca^{2+} antagonists in experimental conditions of myocardial ischemia or infarction are listed in Table 1. In most cases, myocardial injury, assessed by various parameters, is reduced when drugs are given *before* induction of myocardial ischemia. However, it must be noted that Geary et al. (12) reported a lack of effect of nifedipine when given 1 hr *before* LAD occlusion in the baboon. They proposed that the failure of nifedipine to reduce infarct size in baboons, in contrast to the dog in which pretreatment with this drug significantly reduced myocardial injury, could result from the difference in coronary collateral flow between the dog and the baboon, the latter species having minimal coronary collaterals.

When given *after* coronary occlusion, Ca^{2+} antagonists do not always protect myocardial tissue (1,19,28). However, verapamil given 15 min after LAD occlusion produced a highly significant reduction in ST-segment elevation and prevented the hemodynamic deterioration seen in the control animals (31). Similarly, Ribeiro et al. (28) reported a marked decrease in reperfusion ventricular tachycardia or fibrillation under the effect of verapamil administered 20 min after LAD occlusion, whereas nifedipine had no significant effect. Moreover, when given 1 hr after permanent occlusion of LAD, verapamil was found to limit infarct size, assessed by autoradiographic measurements using ^{99m}Tc labeled microspheres (8). This technique allows delineation of the mass of necrotic or jeopardized tissue from normal myocardium. These results suggest that, in some instances, Ca^{2+} antagonists may reduce myocardial necrosis even when administered late in the ischemic episode, a condition which more closely resembles the therapeutic delay occurring in the clinical management of myocardial infarction. However, it must be noted that if given *after* coronary occlusion, the major site of action of Ca^{2+} antagonists will most likely not be the severely ischemic tissue, but more probably the nonischemic myocardium (with reduction of myocardial contractility, and hence of myocardial O_2 consumption) and/or the vascular system (with systemic vasodilatation and afterload reduction, and vasodilatation of coronary collateral vessels supplying the mildly ischemic zone). It should be noted that in most cases where a protective effect of a Ca^{2+} antagonist given *after* coronary artery occlusion has been demonstrated, this has been with verapamil. This could be due to the particular electrophysiological effect of this drug (16).

It must be stressed that the relationship between dose and effects has to be considered in interventions designed to protect the ischemic myocardium. Indeed, using nifedipine at two different doses (bolus injection over 15 min at 13 or 1 $\mu g \cdot kg^{-1}$ in the dog with permanent LAD occlusion), Selwyn et al. (29) reported a beneficial effect of the lower dose used, whereas the higher dose tended to increase infarct size as assessed by ECG alterations, ^{81m}Kr scintigraphy, and creatine kinase release. Similar results have been reported when

TABLE 1. Effect of various calcium antagonists in the protection of the myocardium from ischemic injury in different experimental conditions

Drug	Mode of administration and dosage	Species	Conditions	Criteria used to assess myocardial injury	References: favorable effect claimed	References: no or unfavorable effect
Bepridil	1 mg · kg⁻¹ i.v. before occlusion	Dog	Temporary LADᵃ occlusion	Regional myocardial blood flow	Berdeaux et al. (3)	
Bepridil	5 mg · kg⁻¹ i.v. before occlusion	Dog	LAD permanent occlusion	Ventricular ectopic beats; incidence of ventricular fibrillation	Marshall and Muir (23)	
Diltiazem	0.2 mg · kg⁻¹ i.v. 10 min after occlusion	Dog	Ligation of 3–5 small branches of LAD	ATP content; mitochondrial function	Weishaar and Bing (35)	
Diltiazem	20 mg · kg⁻¹ i.p. 30 min before ligation	Rat	Permanent occlusion of left coronary artery	Tissue creatine kinase activity	Flaim and Zelis (10)	
Diltiazem	100 µg · kg⁻¹ · min⁻¹ i.v. infusion 20 min before ligation and continued until 60 min after ligation	Rat	Permanent occlusion of left coronary artery	Tissue succino-dehydrogenase activity; high-energy phosphates	Zamanis et al. (36)	
Diltiazem	0.02 mg · kg⁻¹ · min⁻¹ 5, 25, or 45 min before ligation	Dog	Simultaneous occlusion of LAD and circumflex	Ventricular fibrillation latency	Clusin et al. (7)	
Diltiazem	Loading dose: 0.75 mg · kg⁻¹ 15 min before occlusion followed by i.v. infusion (600 µg · kg⁻¹ · hr) for 4 hr	Dog	Occlusion of circumflex	Histochemical measurements	Bush et al. (6)	
Nifedipine	Loading dose: 3 µg · kg⁻¹ i.v. followed by i.v. infusion (0.5 µg · kg⁻¹ · min⁻¹) for 10 min	Dog	Permanent LAD occlusion	Collateral flow; regional muscle shortening	Henry et al. (15)	
Nifedipine	13 µg · kg⁻¹ i.v. 30 min after occlusion	Dog	Permanent LAD occlusion	ECG; creative kinase release		Selwyn et al. (29)
Nifedipine	1 µg · kg⁻¹ i.v. 30 min after occlusion	Dog	Permanent LAD occlusion	ECG; creative kinase release	Selwyn et al. (29)	
Nifedipine	5–50 µg · kg⁻¹ i.v. 15 min before ligation	Rat	Permanent occlusion of left coronary artery	Early postinfarction ventricular fibrillation	Fagbemi and Parratt (9)	

Drug	Animal	Procedure	Dose	Measurement	Reference
Nifedipine	Dog	Temporary occlusion of LAD	Loading dose: 100 μg · kg^{-1} i.v. 20 min after ligation, followed by i.v. infusion (3 μg · kg^{-1} · min^{-1}) for 25 min	Occurrence of ventricular tachycardia or fibrillation, regional myocardial blood flow	Ribeiro et al. (28)
Nifedipine	Baboon	Temporary occlusion of LAD	Loading dose: 5 μg · kg^{-1} i.v. 1 hr before occlusion followed by i.v. infusion (30 μg · kg^{-1} · hr)	Postreperfusion histology	Geary et al. (12)
Verapamil	Dog	Permanent LAD occlusion	Loading dose: 0.2 mg · kg^{-1} i.v. 15 min after occlusion followed by i.v. infusion (0.005 mg · kg^{-1} · min^{-1}) for 2 hr	Epicardial ST-segment elevation; hemodynamic parameters	Smith et al. (31)
Verapamil	Dog	Temporary occlusion of circumflex	Loading dose i.v. followed by i.v. infusion. Total dose: 0.8–3.5 mg · kg^{-1}	Histology	Reimer et al. (27)
Verapamil	Dog	Permanent LAD occlusion	0.2–0.7 mg · kg^{-1} i.v. beginning 5 hr after CK elevation	Regional myocardial blood; tissue creatine kinase activity	Karlsberg et al. (19)
Verapamil	Rhesus monkey	Permanent LAD occlusion	0.5 mg · kg^{-1} i.v. 30 min after ligation	Histochemistry (NBT staining)	Anand et al. (1)
			12 mg · kg^{-1} daily per os (for 10 days before ligation)		Anand et al. (1)
Verapamil	Dog	Permanent LAD occlusion	Loading dose: 0.2 mg · kg^{-1} i.v. 1 hr after ligation followed by i.v. infusion (0.01 mg · kg^{-1} · min^{-1}) for 7 hr	Autoradiography (^{99m}Tc labeled microspheres)	De Boer et al. (8)
Verapamil	Dog	Temporary LAD occlusion	Loading dose: 0.2 mg · kg^{-1} i.v. 20 min after ligation followed by i.v. infusion (0.01 mg · kg^{-1} · min^{-1}) for 25 min	Occurrence of ventricular tachycardia of fibrillation	Ribeiro et al. (28)
Verapamil	Dog	Temporary LAD occlusion	I.v. infusion (10 μg · kg^{-1} · min^{-1}) 30 min prior and during ischemia	Mechanical performance	Sherman et al. (30)

[a] LAD, left anterior descending coronary artery.

TABLE 2. *Effect of intravenous diltiazem infusion (administered pre- or postligation) on infarct size[a]*

Group (no.)	Infarct size[b]	Significance[c]
Control ($n = 12$)	38.0% ± 1.2	—
Pretreatment ($n = 11$)	21.6% ± 2.7	$p < 0.01$
Postligation treatment ($n = 10$)	40.3% ± 2.1	ns

[a] Forty-eight hours after left coronary artery occlusion.
[b] Infarct size is expressed as a percentage of total ventricular mass.
[c] Results are expressed as mean ± SEM. ns: not significant.

dogs with permanent LAD occlusion were treated with bepridil (1 or 3 mg · kg⁻¹) (3). Such results suggest that large doses of Ca^{2+} antagonists which markedly dilate normal coronary vessels, may induce a fall in resistance to blood flow in these vessels which, in turn, compete with the ability of collateral vessels to do the same.

Although the regulation of collateral perfusion in the ischemic myocardium is still incompletely understood, it is generally thought that the increase in collateral flow occurs via a drop in vascular resistance at the level of collaterals supplying the ischemic bed. However, another possible mechanism could be related to a decreased external compression of the vascular bed (extracoronary component of coronary resistance) (15).

In addition, Henry et al. (14) showed that nifedipine failed to increase flow in the most severely ischemic part of the myocardium. This may explain why, in some studies, improvement in perfusion of the ischemic area was not found (4).

Using a model of permanent coronary occlusion in the rat, we have estimated myocardial infarct size by histochemistry 48 hr after left coronary artery ligation (36). In rats receiving an intravenous infusion of diltiazem (100 μg · kg⁻¹ · min⁻¹) given for 20 min before and during 60 min after ligation, myocardial necrosis was significantly reduced (Table 2) and metabolic status improved. However, when diltiazem infusion was started 10 min *after* coronary occlusion (V. Richard and J. de Leiris, *unpublished results*), no significant effect of the drug was found as assessed by both histochemistry and metabolite measurements. In this highly reproducible experimental model, diltiazem is effective in reducing infarct size only when administered *before* ligation. Using a similar experimental model (10), a single injection of diltiazem (20 mg · kg⁻¹ i.p., 30 min prior to surgery) significantly preserved total myocardial creatine kinase activity and reduced infarct size in left ventricle. However, the validity of these results should be questioned because of the very high incidence of mortality in both treated and untreated groups (about 75%).

IN VITRO STUDIES OF MYOCARDIAL ISCHEMIA

In the isolated heart preparation, the peripheral vascular system of the intact animal is eliminated. Therefore, in these conditions, any beneficial effect of

Ca^{2+} antagonists against ischemic damage can be attributed to the action of the drug on the heart itself. In addition to the reduction or prevention of the intracellular accumulation of Ca^{2+} occurring under ischemic conditions, Ca^{2+} antagonists may (a) reduce the amount of cardiac work and, therefore, reduce O_2 demand by their negative inotropic action, which is particularly evident *in vitro;* (b) improve the perfusion of ischemic areas of the myocardium during regional ischemia, both effects which may lead to a better preservation of myocardial energy; and (c) reduce the incidence of early ventricular arrhythmias possibly resulting from Ca^{2+}-dependent slow-response action potentials (see Chapters 26, 27, 28; *this volume*). A few of these studies relate to regional ischemia, whereas the great majority relate to models of global ischemia.

In a very elegant model of coronary vasospasm, with or without additional coronary occlusion (21), it was reported that in isolated, Langendorff-perfused rabbit heart, nifedipine at a concentration of 0.3 to $0.45 \cdot 10^{-7}$ M delayed the development of energy imbalance and reduced the final degree of reduced nicotinamide adenine dinucleotide (NADH) fluorescence in response to occlusion, an effect attributed either to an increase in collateral flow after occlusion, or to an energy-conserving action of the drug due to reduction of contractility, heart rate, or basal metabolism. On the other hand, during acute regional myocardial ischemia in isolated Langendorff-perfused rat heart, verapamil ($1.5 \cdot 10^{-7}$ M), nifedipine (10^{-6} M), and diltiazem (5.10^{-6} M) afforded substantial protection against ventricular fibrillation (32). The mechanism whereby Ca^{2+} antagonists mediate protection against ventricular fibrillation appears particularly complex due to the heterogeneous action of these drugs (reduction of heart rate, preservation of high-energy phosphate, coronary vasodilation, reduction in tissue cyclic AMP, reduction in transmembrane Ca^{2+} influx, and, in some cases, nonspecific effects on other membrane systems such as the fast Na^+ channel) (32).

In isolated working rat heart, submitted to 25 min of global no-flow normothermic ischemia, verapamil (10^{-7} M) added to the perfusion fluid 5 min *before* the onset of ischemic conditions resulted in an improved postischemic recovery of cardiac function, a better preservation of total adenine nucleotides and ATP, and creatine phosphate contents, and a reduced cellular Ca^{2+} compared with untreated hearts (34). The addition of verapamil at the onset of reperfusion did not improve cardiac function or metabolic content. The beneficial effect of verapamil, when present throughout the ischemic period, was due to a decrease in energy demand during ischemia and to the resulting preservation of the total adenine nucleotide pool, rather than to other Ca^{2+}-dependent processes.

Nayler et al. (24) reported that pretreatment of rabbits with verapamil or nifedipine (2 mg $\cdot$ kg^{-1} s.c. for 5 days) markedly improved the resistance of isolated heart to a 90-min period of total whole-heart ischemia as shown by a significant increase in recovery of developed tension during reperfusion (about 75% as compared with 24% in control hearts). In these experiments, treated hearts also exhibited higher ATP and creatine phosphate content, and a smaller accumulation of Ca^{2+} after 30 min of reperfusion. Similar results were obtained by Jolly et al. (18) studying the effect of a 45-min period of global low-flow ischemia ($0.1 \text{ ml} \cdot \text{min}^{-1} \cdot \text{g}^{-1}$ wet wt) in isolated guinea pig hearts in the presence of diltiazem ($8 \cdot 10^{-7}$ to $2.5 \cdot 10^{-5}$ M) in the perfusion fluid. Moreover, these authors observed that in the diltiazem group, the active form of pyruvate dehydrogenase was decreased less by ischemia than in the untreated group. An increase in pyruvate dehydrogenase (PDH) activity has been suggested as being responsible for the beneficial effect of dichloroacetate during ischemia (26). When administered at a lower concentration, diltiazem ($4 \cdot 10^{-7}$ M) was also found (35) to protect isolated rat heart against longer periods (120 min) of global low-flow ischemia induced by means of a one-way valve in the aortic outflow tract (final ischemic coronary flow: less than 10% of the preischemic value). In blood-perfused isolated cat heart, diltiazem given prior to a period of 60 to 90 min of global ischemia prevented the loss of compliance and the intramitochondrial Ca²⁺ accumulation occurring in untreated hearts at the time of reperfusion; and the recovery of ATP during reperfusion was significantly improved (6).

In isolated working rat hearts submitted to 30 min of global normothermic low-flow ischemia ($0.2 \text{ ml} \cdot \text{min}^{-1}$), the new Ca²⁺ antagonist, bepridil ($5 \text{ mg} \cdot \text{kg}^{-1}$ i.v.), given 10 min before excision of the heart significantly improved the post-ischemic recovery of cardiac work, aortic output and ATP, total adenine nucleotide, and creatine phosphate content (Table 3) (S. Pestre and J. de Leiris, *unpublished data*).

All these experimental results indicate that *Ca²⁺ antagonists are able to improve the resistance of isolated hearts to ischemia.* One of the most frequently proposed mechanisms for such a beneficial effect relates to the potent negative inotropic and chronotropic effects of Ca²⁺ antagonists *in vitro*. In contrast, therapeutic doses of these drugs do not appear to appreciably depress the heart in the

TABLE 3. *Effect of pretreatment with bepridil on postischemic recovery of various functional or metabolic parameters[a]*

Measurement	Control[b]	Bepridil[b]
Cardiac work (% of preischemic value)	33 ± 10	66 ± 7[c]
Aortic output (% of preischemic value)	27 ± 9	67 ± 8[c]
Coronary flow (% of preischemic value)	79 ± 7	84 ± 8[c]
ATP (μmoles g dry wt^{-1})	12.4 ± 0.7	16.6 ± 0.5[c]
Total adenine nucleotides (μmoles g dry wt^{-1})	17.2 ± 0.6	25.6 ± 0.5[c]
Creatine phosphate (μmoles g dry wt^{-1})	23.8 ± 1.0	29.5 ± 1.5[c]

[a] Bepridil ($5 \text{ mg} \cdot \text{kg}^{-1}$) is administered i.v. 10 min before excision of the heart. After 30 min of control atrial perfusion, isolated hearts are submitted to 30 min of global low-flow (0.2 ml min^{-1}) normothermic ischemia, followed by 30 min of reperfusion. Values given are measured after 30 min of reperfusion (means $\pm$ SEM).

[b] Control: $n = 6$; bepridil: $n = 6$.

[c] Significantly different from controls $p < 0.05$ (S. Pestre and J. de Leiris, *unpublished results*).

intact organism (16). This discrepancy has been generally attributed to *in vivo* reflex sympathetic discharges masking the direct negative action of the drug. It must be pointed out, however, that concentrations which induce negative inotropic effects *in vitro* largely exceed the peak therapeutic plasma levels of the free drug. Thus, it is likely that the protective effect of Ca^{2+} antagonists in ischemia *in vivo* does not primarily depend on the negative inotropic effect of these drugs, whereas, *in vitro,* such an effect could become predominant. It cannot be excluded that Ca^{2+} antagonist-induced *in vivo* vasodilation may trigger a sympathetic discharge which, in turn, neutralizes the negative inotropic and chronotropic effects of the drug.

CONCLUDING COMMENTS

In the previous sections, we have reviewed some of the experimental studies concerning the effect of Ca^{2+} antagonists during ischemic conditions both *in vivo* or *in vitro*. The first conclusion of such a short review is that no clear-cut interpretation of results is emerging. This is due to many factors including: nature of the drug, species under investigation, dose, mode of administration, drug given prior to or after induction of the ischemic process, *in vivo* or *in vitro* experimental model, criteria used to assess myocardial damage, duration of ischemic conditions, and other variables.

There is generally no simple explanation for the protection afforded by Ca^{2+} antagonists in ischemic heart muscle. One exception is where the ischemic process is caused by localized coronary spasm. In the presence of spasm, Ca^{2+} antagonists particularly effective in smooth muscle, such as nifedipine, should exert a marked effect because they will bring about coronary vasodilation (25).

Myocardial injury during ischemia or infarction is thought to be associated with a cytosolic accumulation of Ca^{2+} (20). Most of the Ca^{2+} antagonists have been shown to prevent the massive overloading with Ca^{2+} which is thought to cause myocardial cell necrosis. However, the ischemia-induced cytosolic Ca^{2+} overload appears to be a very complex process which is not necessarily dependent only on entry of Ca^{2+} through slow channels (25). Although the precise mechanism of the protective effect of Ca^{2+} antagonists in ischemic conditions is unknown, there are several alternative, and perhaps related, mechanisms which could be involved:

1. Electrophysiological studies on the ischemic myocardium indicate that the early postinfarction *ventricular arrhythmias* are reentry in origin, mediated by slow-response action potentials in which the current may be carried by Ca^{2+} ions (22). If this is the case then Ca^{2+} antagonists may exert their beneficial effect by blocking such action potentials, so preventing the development of severe ventricular arrhythmias or fibrillation resulting from experimental coronary artery ligation.

2. Ca^{2+} antagonists may *increase blood flow* in the ischemic myocardium by improvement of coronary collateral flow. Such an effect may be beneficial

with respect to both high-energy phosphate stores which are critical for the survival of the cardiac cell and electrophysiologic performance of the ischemic myocardium, the latter effect reducing the incidence of severe ventricular arrhythmias or fibrillation (16).

3. *Myocardial O_2 demand* may be reduced by Ca^{2+} antagonists because they reduce afterload and cardiac work (at least *in vitro*). Thus, the energy deficit would be less marked and cellular function better preserved.

Although several Ca^{2+} antagonists appear to be effective in protecting myocardial cells against ischemia, a question is still unresolved: Is the protection afforded by these drugs of a permanent or temporary nature? In other words, do these agents protect myocardial cells or do they only delay the onset of irreversible tissue damage?

ACKNOWLEDGMENTS

Much of the original work reported in this chapter was supported by a grant from INSERM (contract no. 805010) and by the laboratories DAUSSE. The help of Dr. Deborah Harding in rereading the manuscript is gratefully acknowledged.

REFERENCES

1. Anand, I. S., Sharma, P. L., Chakravati, R. N., and Wahi, P. L. (1980): *Adv. Myocardiol.,* 2:425–433.
2. Berdeaux, A., Coutte, R., Giudicelli, J. F., and Boissier, J. R. (1976): *Eur. J. Pharmacol.,* 39:287–294.
3. Berdeaux, A., Kantelip, J. P., Eschaliera, A., Giudicelli, J. F., and Duchene-Marullaz, P. (1980): *J. Pharmacol.,* 11:391–409.
4. Bruckner, N. B., Keller, H. E., Mittmann, U., and Wirth, R. H. (1980): *Arzneim. Forsch./ Drug Res.,* 30:780–784.
5. Bush, L. R., Yuk-Ping, L., Shlafer, M., Jolly, S. R., and Lucchesi, B. R. (1981): *J. Pharmacol. Exp. Ther.,* 218:653–661.
6. Bush, L. R., Romson, J. L., Ash, J. L., and Lucchesi, B. R. (1982): *J. Cardiovasc. Pharmacol.,* 4:285–296.
7. Clusin, W. T., Bristow, M. R., Baim, D. S., Schroeder, J. S., Jaillon, P., Brett, P., and Harrison, D. C. (1982): *Circ. Res.,* 50:518–526.
8. DeBoer, L. W., Strauss, H. W., Kloner, R. A., Rude, R. E., Davis, R. F., Maroko, P. R., and Braunwald, E. (1980): *Proc. Natl. Acad. Sci. USA,* 77:6119–6123.
9. Fagbemi, O., and Parratt, J. R. (1981): *Eur. J. Pharmacol.,* 75:179–185.
10. Flaim, S. F., and Zelis, R. (1981): *Pharmacology,* 23:281–286.
11. Fleckenstein, A., Tritthart, H., Fleckenstein, B., Herbst, A., and Grun, G. (1969): *Pfluegers Arch. ges. Physiol.,* 307:R25.
12. Geary, G. G., Smith, G. T., Suehiro, G. T., and McNamara, J. J. (1982): *Am. J. Cardiol.,* 49:331–337.
13. Hearse, D. J., and Yellon, D. M. (1981): *Am. J. Cardiol.,* 47:1321–1334.
14. Henry, P. D., Shuchleib, R., Borsa, L. J., Roberts, R., Williamson, J. R., and Sobel, B. E. (1978): *Circ. Res.,* 43:372–380.
15. Henry, P. D., Shuchleib, R., Clark, R. E., and Perez, J. E. (1979): *Am. J. Cardiol.,* 44:817–824.
16. Henry, P. D. (1980): *Am. J. Cardiol.,* 46:1047–1058.
17. Johns, T. N. P., and Olson, B. J. (1954): *Ann. Surg.,* 140:675–682.

18. Jolly, S. R., Menahan, L. A., and Gross, C. J. (1981): *J. Mol. Cell. Cardiol.*, 13:359–372.
19. Karlsberg, R. P., Henry, P. D., Ahmed, S. A., Sobel, B. E., and Roberts, R. (1977): *Eur. J. Pharmacol.*, 42:339–346.
20. Katz, A. M., and Reuter, H. (1979): *Am. J. Cardiol.*, 44:188–190.
21. Kissin, I., and Kilpatrick, J. V. (1982): *J. Cardiovasc. Pharmacol.*, 4:111–115.
22. Lazzara, R., El-Sherif, N., Hope, R. R., and Sherlag, B. J. (1978): *Circ. Res.*, 42:740–749.
23. Marshall, R. J., and Muir, A. W. (1981): *Br. J. Pharmacol.*, 73:471–479.
24. Deleted in proof.
25. Nayler, W. G., Ferrari, R., and Williams, A. (1980): *Am. J. Cardiol.*, 46:242–248.
26. Nayler, W. G., and Poole-Wilson, P. A. (1981): *Basic Res. Cardiol.*, 76:1–15.
27. Opie, L. H., and de Leiris, J. (1979): In: *Enzymes in Cardiology: Diagnosis and Research*, edited by D. J. Hearse and J. de Leiris, pp. 481–502. Wiley, Chichester.
28. Reimer, K. A., Lowe, J. E., and Jennings, R. B. (1977): *Circulation*, 55:581–587.
29. Ribeiro, L. G., Brandon, T. A., Debauche, T. L., Maroko, P. R., and Miller, R. (1981): *Am. J. Cardiol.*, 48:69–74.
30. Selwyn, A. P., Welman, E., Fox, K., Horlock, P., Pratt, T., and Klein, M. (1979): *Circ. Res.*, 44:16–23.
31. Sherman, L. G., Liang, C. S., Boden, W. E., and Hood, W. B. (1981): *Circ. Res.*, 48:224–232.
32. Smith, H. J., Singh, B. N., Nisbet, H. D., and Norris, R. M. (1975): *Cardiovasc. Res.*, 9:569–578.
33. Thandroyen, F. T. (1982): *J. Mol. Cell. Cardiol.*, 14:21–33.
34. Waldenstrom, A., and Hjalmarson, A. (1979): In: *Enzymes in Cardiology: Diagnosis and Research*, edited by D. J. Hearse and J. de Leiris, pp. 379–398. Wiley, Chichester.
35. Watts, J. A., Koch, C. D., and Lanoue, K. F. (1980): *Am. J. Physiol.*, 238:H909–H916.
36. Weishaar, R. E., and Bing, R. J. (1980): *J. Mol. Cell. Cardiol.*, 12:993–1009.
37. Deleted in proof.
38. Zamanis, A., Verdetti, J., and de Leiris, J. (1982): *J. Mol. Cell. Cardiol.*, 14:53–62.
39. Zsoter, T. S. (1980): *Am. Heart J.*, 99:805–810.

Calcium Antagonists and Cardiovascular Disease, edited by L. H. Opie.
Raven Press, New York © 1984.

Chapter 11

Coronary Artery Spasm and Calcium Ions

Hirofumi Yasue

Division of Cardiology, Shizuoka City Hospital, Shizuoka City 420, Japan

Ischemic heart disease is myocardial impairment due to an imbalance between coronary blood flow and myocardial requirements caused by changes in the coronary circulation. This includes the syndromes of angina pectoris and myocardial infarction, as well as some arrhythmias and sudden death. Until recently, the pathogenesis of ischemic heart disease was considered to be solely related to the fixed coronary artery obstruction due to coronary atherosclerosis (8).

In recent years, a large body of information has come forth indicating that coronary artery spasm also may play an important role in the pathogenesis of many clinical conditions of ischemic heart disease (4,15,27). Coronary artery spasm has now been firmly established as the pathogenetic mechanism underlying variant angina. It has also been associated with other types of resting angina, some of exertional angina, some of acute myocardial infarction, and various arrhythmias including ventricular fibrillation. It may also be responsible for some instances of sudden death.

However, the mechanism(s) by which coronary artery spasm occurs has not been elucidated. There are still some controversies concerning the definition of coronary artery spasm. *Coronary artery spasm is here defined as a transient constriction of a large (epicardial) coronary artery resulting in myocardial ischemia.* Because it is established that variant angina is caused by coronary artery spasm, it is important to know the clinical features of variant angina to understand the pathophysiology of coronary artery spasm.

CIRCADIAN VARIATION OF EXERCISE CAPACITY IN PATIENTS WITH VARIANT ANGINA

Variant angina is angina occurring at rest and associated with ST-segment elevation in the electrocardiogram (18). The attacks appear most often from midnight to early morning when patients are at rest, and are usually not provoked by exercise in the daytime.

We performed treadmill exercise tests both in the early morning and in the afternoon of the same day in patients with variant angina (26). All patients had been tested on a treadmill at least once before the study. They were kept in bed in the fasting state until 5:00 A.M. to 8:00 A.M., when they were taken by wheelchair to the ECG room, where they exercised on a motor-driven treadmill under constant monitoring of ECG. In all patients this procedure repeatedly induced attacks of chest pain associated with ST-segment elevation. The treadmill exercise test was repeated between 3:00 P.M. and 4:00 P.M. of the same day. The patients had strolled around the wards between the morning and the afternoon.

In the early morning, mild exercise could induce attacks, but, in the afternoon, vigorous exercise did not provoke attacks except in patients with severe organic stenosis of a large coronary artery, or in patients who had spontaneous attacks in the afternoon as well as in the morning. Thus, there is circadian variation of exercise capacity in most patients with variant angina.

EFFECTS OF VARIOUS DRUGS ON EXERCISE-INDUCED ATTACKS IN PATIENTS WITH VARIANT ANGINA

In 34 patients with variant angina we examined the effects of propranolol (β-adrenergic blocking agent), diltiazem (Ca^{2+} antagonist), nifedipine (Ca^{2+} antagonist), and phentolamine (α-adrenergic blocking agent) on the attacks induced by treadmill exercise (29). Propranolol 80 mg, diltiazem 90 mg, and nifedipine 20 mg were given orally 2 hr before, and phentolamine 0.2 mg/kg body wt was injected intramuscularly 5 min before the treadmill exercise. The treadmill exercise tests were repeated at the same hour of the day within one week, and the order of the administration of these drugs was randomized. The effects of these drugs on the attacks were judged as "completely suppressed" when exercise-induced ST-segment elevation was completely suppressed, as "partially

TABLE 1. *Effects of various drugs on the attacks induced by treadmill exercise in patients with variant angina[a]*

ST-Segment elevation[b]	Propranolol		Diltiazem		Nifedipine		Phentolamine	
	No.	(%)	No.	(%)	No.	(%)	No.	(%)
++	0	(0.0)	26	(76.5)	20	(87.0)	11	(42.3)
+	6	(17.6)	8	(23.5)	3	(13.0)	10	(38.5)
0	14	(41.2)	0	(0.0)	0	(0.0)	3	(11.5)
−	14	(41.2)	0	(0.0)	0	(0.0)	2	(7.7)
Total	34	(100.0)	34	(100.0)	23	(100.0)	26	(100.0)

[a] $n = 34$.
[b] ++: ST-segment elevation completely suppressed; +: ST-segment elevation improved by more than 0.1 mV; 0: ST-segment elevation changed by less than 0.1 mV; −: ST-segment elevation aggravated by more than 0.1 mV.

suppressed" when ST-segment elevation was suppressed by more than 0.1 mV, as "not affected" when ST-segment elevation changed by less than 0.1 mV, and as "aggravated" when ST-segment elevation was aggravated by more than 0.1 mV on the lead showing maximum ST-segment elevation one minute after exercise.

Table 1 shows our results. Propranolol, which reduces myocardial O_2 demand and which has been widely used for the treatment of exertional angina, did not suppress the attacks completely in any of the 34 patients. It aggravated the attacks in 14 of the 34 patients (41.2%). In contrast, diltiazem suppressed the attacks completely in 26 of the 34 patients (76.5%), and nifedipine in 20 of the 23 patients (87.0%), and both drugs partially suppressed the attacks in the remaining patients. Phentolamine suppressed the attacks completely in 11 of the 26 patients (42.3%), and partially in 10 of them (38.5%). These results

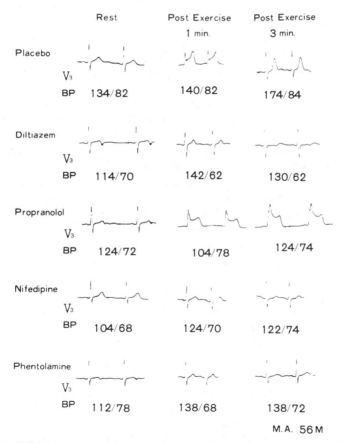

FIG. 1. Effects of diltiazem, propranolol, nifedipine, and phentolamine on the treadmill exercise-induced attack. Propranolol aggravated the attack, whereas diltiazem, nifedipine, and phentolamine suppressed it (see text for details). BP, blood pressure. (From ref. 29.)

strongly suggest that coronary artery spasm was induced by exercise and that α-adrenergic receptors play a role in producing coronary spasm.

Figure 1 shows a representative case. Diltiazem, nifedipine, and phentolamine completely suppressed the attack with ST-segment elevation in the anterior leads. Propranolol, however, aggravated the attack, although the drug suppressed the exercise-induced increase in heart rate.

We performed coronary arteriography before and after arm exercise, and after giving nitroglycerin in 15 patients with variant angina in the early morning. In 11 of them, we could induce the attack by arm exercise in the catheterization laboratory. Coronary arteriography indicated that in all patients spasm of a large coronary artery supplying the area of myocardium showing ST-segment elevation on the ECG appeared during the attacks and disappeared along with the attacks after nitroglycerin administration.

Thus, coronary artery spasm may be induced by exercise and is probably a cause of exercise-induced attacks in patients with variant angina.

CIRCADIAN VARIATION OF TONE OF THE LARGE CORONARY ARTERIES IN PATIENTS WITH VARIANT ANGINA

We compared coronary arteriograms taken in the early morning with those taken in the afternoon in patients with variant angina (26). In the early morning, the tone of the large coronary artery was increased and its diameter was small. Under such conditions, even mild exercise could induce coronary spasm resulting in the attack, and the administration of nitroglycerin dilated the artery markedly. In the afternoon, however, the large coronary artery was usually already dilated and its tone was low on the control coronary arteriograms. Exercise could induce few spasms, and no attacks occurred except in patients with severe organic stenosis in whom only slight degree of constriction of the artery occluded the artery and resulted in the attack.

To record quantitatively the difference in the tone of the large coronary artery observed in the early morning and afternoon, we measured the diameter of the large coronary arteries on both the control coronary arteriograms and the coronary arteriograms taken after nitroglycerin administration (26,27). The percentage increase in diameter of the large coronary artery after nitroglycerin administration was significantly higher in the early morning than in the afternoon ($p < 0.001$), which indicates that the tone of the large coronary artery is increased in the early morning compared with the afternoon.

Thus, there is circadian variation in the tone of the large coronary arteries which seems to have an intimate relation with circadian variation of exercise capacity in most patients with variant angina.

There are also daily, weekly, and monthly variations in exercise capacity in most patients with variant angina. It may be concluded that the presence of variability of exercise threshold for the development of angina strongly suggests that coronary artery spasm plays a role in the pathogenesis of the angina.

AUTONOMIC NERVOUS SYSTEM AND CORONARY ARTERY SPASM

Coronary arteries are innervated by both the sympathetic and parasympathetic nervous system (11), and it is known that the activity of the parasympathetic nervous system is increased in the night when the patient is sleeping and is decreased during physical activity in the daytime. The increased activity of the parasympathetic nervous system causes reduction in heart rate, blood pressure, and myocardial contractility, all of which lead to decreased myocardial O_2 (metabolic) demands. Decreased metabolic demands cause constriction of large coronary arteries (13). Moreover, acetylcholine, the parasympathetic neurotransmitter, directly constricts large coronary arteries in human beings (9). Increased parasympathetic nervous activity may then increase the tone of the large coronary artery in the night. Indeed, injection of methacholine, a parasympathomimetic agent, induces coronary spasm and anginal attacks in some patients with variant angina, and this response is suppressed by atropine, a parasympathetic blocking agent (22). Atropine also suppresses the attacks of variant angina in some patients (22,24).

Stimulation of α-adrenergic receptors results in coronary vasoconstriction (6,14), and large coronary arteries are richly supplied with α-adrenergic receptors (21). Stimulation of α-adrenergic receptors by injection of epinephrine after β-adrenergic receptor blockade by propranolol induces coronary artery spasm and anginal attacks in patients with variant angina (23). Phentolamine, an α-adrenergic blocking agent, suppresses the exercise-induced attacks in patients with variant angina (Table 1), and phenoxybenzamine, another α-adrenergic blocking agent, also suppresses the attacks in patients with variant angina (24). Cold pressor test (19) and/or the Valsalva maneuver (straining), which cause sympathetic discharge, induce the attacks in patients with variant angina.

The tone of the large coronary arteries is increased in the early morning, probably because parasympathetic nervous activity is still high. Under such conditions, even a slight degree of sympathetic discharge, as caused by mild exercise, may lead to coronary artery spasm and anginal attacks by way of α-adrenergic stimulation. It is reported that the attacks of variant angina are often associated with rapid eye movement periods of sleep (17), and it is known that during rapid eye movement periods the enhanced parasympathetic nervous activity is often and suddenly replaced by the enhanced sympathetic nervous activity (this is called "autonomic storm"); atropine suppresses rapid eye movement periods (12). It is quite probable that sudden sympathetic discharge during periods of rapid eye movement may induce coronary artery spasm and anginal attacks in patients with variant angina.

On the other hand, the tone of the large coronary arteries is decreased in the afternoon probably because parasympathetic nervous activity is low. Under such conditions, even strenuous exercise may not induce coronary spasm and anginal attack.

It is thus quite probable that both the sympathetic and the parasympathetic nervous systems play important roles in the production of coronary artery spasm.

However, sympathetic (α-adrenergic) or parasympathetic stimulation is not the sole factor responsible for coronary artery spasm. The nearer the time of α-adrenergic stimulation is to the time zone of spontaneous attacks, which is usually from midnight to early morning, the easier it is for the sympathetic stimulation to induce coronary artery spasm (27). It should also be noted that coronary artery spasm may occur in denervated coronary arteries (3).

Thus, even slight degrees of sympathetic discharge caused by such activities as walking, straining at stool or urination, cleaning teeth or shaving, exposure to cold, or smoking, may induce coronary artery spasm in the early morning. However, in the afternoon, even a higher degree of sympathetic discharge, such as caused by strenuous exercise, may not induce spasm. Pharmacological agents such as epinephrine or methacholine can easily induce coronary artery spasm in low doses in the early morning, but may not induce spasm even in larger doses in the afternoon.

Thus, there is circadian variation in the reactivity of the large coronary arteries to the adrenergic stimulation, which is probably related to circadian variation of the tone of the large coronary arteries (27). There are also daily, weekly, or monthly variations in the reactivity of the large coronary artery to adrenergic stimulation.

VASOACTIVE SUBSTANCES AND CORONARY ARTERY SPASM

Various vasoactive substances or agonists influence and regulate coronary artery tone and may play an important role in the production of coronary artery spasm. The role of catecholamines, as norepinephrine or epinephrine, and that of acetylcholine have already been mentioned.

Prostaglandins

Platelets release arachidonic acid from membrane phospholipids and convert it to an unstable derivative, thromboxane $(TX)A_2$, which then causes vasoconstriction and platelet aggregation (5). Endothelial cells of the arteries also convert arachidonic acid or an unstable endoperoxide precursor released by platelets into prostaglandin $(PG)I_2$ (prostacyclin) which is a potent vasodilator and inhibitor of platelet aggregation (5). The balanced production of these two compounds is thought to regulate vascular tone and blood fluidity. The suggestion that TXA_2 may provoke coronary artery spasm in human beings has attracted great interest. Elevated levels of its inactive hydration product, TXB_2, have been found in coronary sinus blood during attack in patients with variant angina (20). However, it is not yet determined whether platelet production of TXA_2 is a cause or a result of anginal attack of variant angina. Production of PGI_2 is decreased during the attacks of variant angina (20). Large doses of aspirin, which inhibit the production of both TXA_2 and PGI_2, aggravate variant angina (16). Thus, interaction of TXA_2 and PGI_2 may be important for the production of coronary artery spasm.

Histamine

Histamine is a naturally occurring biogenic amine that is found in abundance in the heart. Ginsburg and co-workers have shown that in the proximal portion of the isolated human coronary artery, histamine generates a greater contractile response than either norepinephrine or acetylcholine (9). Furthermore, they provoked coronary artery spasm by the injection of histamine in patients with variant angina (10). Thus, histamine may play a role in the production of coronary artery spasm.

Other vasoactive substances such as angiotensin, serotonin, or vasopressin, may also play a role in regulating coronary artery tone and producing spasm.

CORONARY ATHEROSCLEROSIS AND CORONARY ARTERY SPASM

Variant angina may develop in patients with almost normal coronary arteries and with atherosclerotic changes involving one, two, or three vessels.

We examined coronary arteriograms of 126 patients with variant angina. We defined coronary artery disease as fixed arteriographic narrowing greater than 50% of luminal diameter. Of the 126 patients with variant angina, 37 (29.3%) had almost normal coronary arteries, 66 (52.4%) had one-, 16 (12.7%) two-, and 7 (5.6%) had three-vessels disease. Spasm usually appeared at the proximal portion and at the site of atherosclerotic stenosis of a large coronary artery, but there were some exceptions. Out of the 48 almost normal coronary arteries involved in spasm, 33 (68.7%) were the right coronary artery, 12 (25.0%) the left anterior descending coronary artery, and 3 (6.3%) the left circumflex artery. Thus, spasm occurs more often in the right coronary artery than in the left coronary artery when the artery is almost normal. These observations indicate that there are no specific organic lesions for variant angina.

However, most patients with variant angina are over the age of 40 (as were 127 out of the 131 patients in our series) and have significant atherosclerotic stenosis of large coronary arteries (89 out of the 126 patients had organic stenosis of more than 50% of the luminal diameter in their coronary arteries in our series). Furthermore, spasm usually appears at the site of atherosclerotic stenosis. This seems to indicate that spasm does not occur in the young and normal coronary artery and is somehow related to atherosclerosis (27).

It is known that proliferation of smooth muscle cell is essential in the pathogenesis of atherosclerosis. It seems probable that all coronary arteries which develop spasm may be in various stages of atherosclerosis, although some of them may appear normal angiographically. Coronary arteries can themselves synthesize PGI_2 which causes vasodilatation, and it is reported that the local synthesis of PGI_2 is disturbed in the presence of atherosclerosis. Reduced production of PGI_2 may then contribute to abnormal contraction of coronary artery or spasm. A recent report (30) indicates that atherosclerotic coronary arteries are more sensitive to α-adrenergic stimulation and ergonovine than are normal coronary arteries.

CALCIUM IONS AND CORONARY ARTERY SPASM

Coronary artery spasm may be regarded as an abnormal contraction of smooth muscle cells of coronary artery. Thus, factors which influence intracellular Ca^{2+} will play an important role in the production of coronary artery spasm.

The role of the autonomic nervous system in the pathogenesis of coronary artery spasm has already been mentioned. The sympathetic and parasympathetic nerves stimulate α-adrenergic and muscarinic receptors respectively, and thus increase intracellular Ca^{2+} by both increasing the membrane permeability to Ca^{2+} through receptor-operated channels and releasing Ca^{2+} from intracellular stores (2).

Other vasoactive substances such as histamine, PGs, serotonin, and angiotensin also seem to cause contraction of vascular smooth muscle by the same mechanism (2) and may play a role in the production of coronary artery spasm.

The smooth muscle cells of the coronary artery involved in spasm may have increased membrane permeability to Ca^{2+} because spasm can be suppressed by Ca^{2+} antagonists such as nifedipine, diltiazem, or verapamil which block the Ca^{2+} channels and thus suppress the entry of Ca^{2+} into the cell (27). The membrane permeability may be influenced by various factors. Fleckenstein and his co-workers showed that alkaline solutions cause contraction of an isolated dog coronary artery, and that this response is abolished in the absence of Ca^{2+} in the extracellular fluids (7). They postulated that hydrogen ions compete with Ca^{2+} for the same active sites at the transmembrane Ca^{2+}-transport system. We examined the effects of changes in pH (hydrogen ion concentration), Ca^{2+} concentration, and diltiazem (a Ca^{2+} antagonist) on the vascular tone of the isolated rabbit coronary artery (28). As shown in Fig. 2A, stepwise increase in pH from 7.0 to 8.0 of the bath fluid caused a pH-dependent increase in vascular tone. Figure 2B shows the relationship between pH in the extracellular bath fluid and maximum tension developed in seven experiments. Increased vascular tone in response to high pH was minimal without Ca^{2+} in the bath fluid, and addition of Ca^{2+} to the bath fluid produced dose-dependent increase in vascular tone (Fig. 3). Diltiazem suppressed increased coronary vascular tone induced by high pH. These results strongly suggest that extracellular Ca^{2+} is essential for increased vascular tone caused by high pH. Thus, it can be inferred that increased extracellular pH principally causes increased membrane permeability to Ca^{2+}, thereby increasing intracellular Ca^{2+} which is essential for the contraction of vascular smooth muscle. It may be concluded that *vasoconstriction occurs if the extracellular Ca^{2+} concentration increases or hydrogen ion concentration decreases* (i.e., the pH rises), whereas vasodilatation is produced by opposite changes. Diltiazem seems to decrease coronary vascular tone by interfering with transmembrane influx of Ca^{2+} or decreasing membrane permeability to Ca^{2+}.

We examined whether coronary artery spasm and anginal attack could be induced by hyperventilation and Tris-buffer infusion, which decrease hydrogen

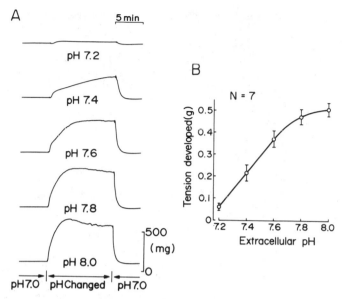

FIG. 2. Effects of varying the extracellular pH on the tone of isolated rabbit coronary artery. **A:** Experimental records. Stepwise increase in pH from 7.0 to 8.0 of the bath fluid caused pH-dependent increase in vascular tone and earlier development of maximum tension. **B:** Relationship between pH in the extracellular bath fluid and maximum tension developed during a 10-min period in seven experiments conducted as shown in **A.** Each *point* on the curve represents the mean of seven experiments (mean ± SEM). (From ref. 28.)

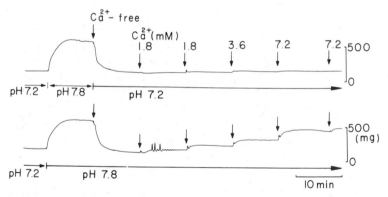

FIG. 3. Experimental records of effects of varying Ca^{2+} concentration on the tone of coronary artery preparations exposed to Ca^{2+}-free solutions at pH 7.2 and pH 7.8. (From ref. 28.)

ion concentration (25). In 8 out of the 9 patients with variant angina, attacks occurred during this procedure or within 5 min after it ended. Coronary artery spasm appeared after the procedure and disappeared after the administration of nitroglycerin in all of the 4 patients in whom coronary arteriography was performed. The oral administration of 90 mg of diltiazem 2 hr before, completely

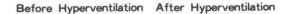

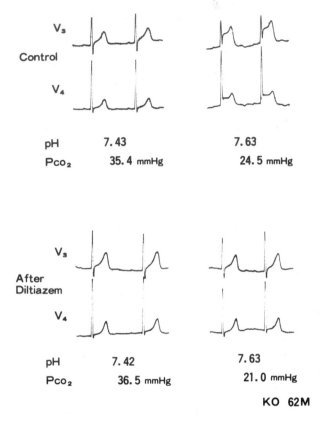

FIG 4. Electrocardiogram, arterial pH, and Pco_2 before (*left*) and after (*right*) the hyperventilation plus Tris-buffer infusion in a patient with variant angina. Arterial blood pH rose from 7.43 to 7.63, and anginal attack associated with ST-segment elevation in the chest leads appeared after the hyperventilation plus Tris-buffer infusion (*upper panel*). However, after the administration of diltiazem, the same procedure did not induce the attack although the degree of the change in the arterial blood pH was almost the same (*lower panel*).

suppressed the attack induced by this procedure in all of the 5 patients who received this drug. Figure 4 shows a representative case. Anginal attack associated with ST-segment elevation in the chest leads in the ECG appeared immediately after hyperventilation was stopped. Arterial blood pH rose from 7.43 to 7.63 as a result of this procedure (*upper panel*). However, after the administration of diltiazem, the same procedure did not induce the attack, although the degree of change in the arterial blood pH was almost the same (*lower panel*). Thus, the hydrogen ion concentration plays a role in the production of coronary artery spasm.

Hydrogen ion production decreases at rest particularly in the night when metabolism decreases, and increases after exercise during the day when metabolism increases. This may partly explain the reason why the attacks of variant angina occur most often at rest in the night and are rarely provoked by exercise in the daytime.

Diseases such as atherosclerosis may also affect the membrane permeability to Ca^{2+}. Spasm appears mostly in patients with coronary atherosclerosis (27), usually at the site of atherosclerotic stenosis, and is rarely seen in the young and normal coronary artery (27). Experimental studies in the dog show that atherosclerotic coronary arteries are more sensitive to the effects of Ca^{2+} than normal arteries.

CONCLUSIONS

Coronary artery spasm occurs most often at rest, particularly from midnight to early morning and is usually not provoked by exercise in the daytime. There is circadian variation in the tone of the large coronary artery, the tone being increased in the early morning and decreased in the afternoon. The activity of the autonomic nervous system and metabolism seem to play an important role in the regulation of coronary artery tone and, thus, in the production of coronary artery spasm.

It is assumed that coronary artery spasm is an abnormal contraction of smooth muscle of coronary artery caused by an increase of intracellular Ca^{2+}. Autonomic nervous system, vasoactive substances such as norepinephrine, epinephrine, acetylcholine, histamine, serotonin, or PGs, and ions (hydrogen or magnesium) may play a role in the production of coronary artery spasm by affecting intracellular Ca^{2+}. Local factors in the coronary artery such as atherosclerosis or receptor density may also play a role in producing spasm. However, the exact mechanism by which these factors affect intracellular Ca^{2+} still remains to be elucidated. Ca^{2+} antagonists such as nifedipine, diltiazem, and verapamil probably suppress coronary artery spasm by blocking the entry of Ca^{2+} into the cell. We should also consider the possibility that besides intracellular Ca^{2+} concentration, other mechanisms might play a role in the production of coronary artery spasm independent of changes of intracellular Ca^{2+} (1).

REFERENCES

1. Adelstein, R. S., Conti, M. A., Hathaway, D. R., and Kole, C. B. (1978): *J. Biol. Chem.,* 253:8347–8350.
2. Bolton, T. B. (1979): *Physiol. Rev.,* 59:606–718.
3. Buda, A. J., Fowlles, R. E., Schroeder, J. S., Hunt, S. A., Cipriano, P. R., Stinson, E. B., and Harrison, D. C. (1981): *Am. J. Med.,* 70:1144–1149.
4. Conti, C. R., Feldman, R. L., and Pepine, C. J. (1982): *Am. Heart J.,* 103:584–588.
5. Dusting, G. J., Moncada, S., and Vane, J. R. (1979): *Prog. Cardiovasc. Dis.,* 11:405–430.
6. Feigl, E. O. (1967): *Circ. Res.,* 20:262–271.
7. Fleckenstein, A., Nakayama, K., Fleckenstein-Grun, G., and Byon, Y. K. (1976): In: *Ionic Actions on Vascular Smooth Muscle,* edited by E. Betz, pp. 117–123. Springer-Verlag, Berlin.

8. Friedberg, C. K. (1972): *Circulation,* 46:1037–1047.
9. Ginsburg, R., Bristow, M. R., Harrison, D. C., and Stinson, E. B. (1980): *Chest,* 78 (Suppl.):180–186.
10. Ginsburg, R., Bristow, M. R., Kantrowitz, N., Baim, D. S., Harrison, D. C. (1981): *Am. Heart J.,* 102:819–821.
11. Hirsch, E. F., and Borghard-Erdle, A. M. (1962): *Arch. Pathol.,* 73:101–117.
12. Jouvet, M. (1969): *Science,* 163:32–35.
13. Macho, P., Hintze, T. H., and Vatner S. F. (1981): *Circ. Res.,* 49:594–599.
14. MacRaven, D. R., Mark, A. L., Abboud, F. M., and Mayer, H. E. (1971): *J. Clin. Invest.,* 50:773–778.
15. Maseri, A., and Chierchia, S. (1980): *Chest,* 78 (Suppl.): 210–215.
16. Miwa, K., Kanbara, H., and Kawai, C. (1981): *Am. J. Cardiol.,* 47:1210–1214.
17. Murao, S., Harumi, K., Katayama, S., Mashima, S., Shimomura, K., Murayama, M. (1972): *Jpn. Heart J.,* 13:295–303.
18. Prinzmetal, M., Kennamer, R., Merliss, R., Wada, T., and Bor, N. (1959): *Am. J. Med.,* 27:375–388.
19. Raizner, A. E., Chahine, R. A., and Ishimori, T. (1980): *Circulation,* 62:925–932.
20. Tada, M., Kuzuya, T., Inoue, M., Kodama, K., Mishima, M., Yamada, M., Inui, M., and Abe, H. (1981): *Circulation,* 64:1107–1115.
21. Toda, N. (1981): *Circ. Res.,* 49:1228–1236.
22. Yasue, H., Touyama, M., Shimamoto, K., Kato, H., Tanaka, S., and Akiyama, F. (1974): *Circulation,* 50:534–539.
23. Yasue, H., Touyama, M., Kato, H., Tanaka, S., and Akiyama, F. (1976): *Am. Heart J.,* 91:148–155.
24. Yasue, H., Omote, S., Takizawa, A., Nagao, M., Miwa, K., and Tanaka, S. (1978): *Jpn. Circ. J.,* 42:1–10.
25. Yasue, H., Nagao, M., Omote, S., Takizawa, A., Miwa, K., and Tanaka, S. (1978): *Circulation,* 58:56–62.
26. Yasue, H., Omote, S., Takizawa, A., Nagao, M., Miwa, K., and Tanaka, S. (1979): *Circulation,* 59:938–948.
27. Yasue, H. (1980): *Chest,* 78 (Suppl.):216–223.
28. Yasue, H., Omote, S., Takizawa, A., Nagao, M., Nozaka, K., and Nakajima, H. (1981): *Am. Heart J.,* 102:206–210.
29. Yasue, H, Omote, S., Takizawa, A., and Nagao, M. (1982): In: *What Is Angina?,* edited by D. G. Julian, K. I. Lie, L. Wilhelmsen, A. B. Molndal, Hassle, pp. 102–111.
30. Yokoyama, M., Goldman, M., and Henry, P. D. (1978): *Circulation,* 58 (Suppl. 11):57(abstract).

Calcium Antagonists and Cardiovascular Disease, edited by L. H. Opie.
Raven Press, New York © 1984.

Chapter 12

Critical Distinctions in the Modification of Myocardial Cell Injury

David J. Hearse

The Heart Research Unit, Rayne Institute, St. Thomas' Hospital, London SE1, England

The measurement and manipulation of myocardial injury has attracted the attention of cardiologists for many decades (21). Despite this, myocardial protection remains controversial (18,29) and characterized by a number of misconceptions which this article attempts to identify and discuss.

The literature contains many attractive terms: "tissue salvage," "tissue protection," "jeopardized cells," "reversible and irreversible injury," "infarct size reduction," "reoxygenation-induced injury," and "stunned myocardium." Unfortunately, many of these are insufficiently specific or are inappropriately used. The problem is compounded by the inadequacy, or inappropriate interpretation, of many indices of injury and protection (19).

An example of the above problem would be a dog heart study in which the administration of a drug, following coronary ligation, is shown to reduce the area of necrosis as indicated by tetrazolium staining after 6 hr of ischemia. Although such a study may be heralded as an example of tissue protection and infarct size reduction, rarely is it demonstrated that the "salvaged" tissue returns to normal contractile function or that protection is sustained, i.e., that drug treatment has truly reduced the *extent,* as opposed to merely *delayed* the development, of injury. Similarly, many studies have claimed that certain interventions or reperfusion can exacerbate injury without questioning whether there is a true increase in the extent of injury or whether there is merely an acceleration in the rate of development of a predetermined level of injury. It could be argued that the great success of myocardial protection during cardiac surgery, and its relative failure during evolving infarction, is due in part to better appreciation and exploitation of the above distinctions in the surgical field. Since it will be argued that much of the current confusion relates to inappropriate use of terminology, the following section presents definitions critical to the arguments developed in this article.

DEFINITIONS

Oxygen Deprivation

Two forms of O_2 deprivation exist: ischemia and hypoxia, and although often used interchangeably, they are different in their origins and consequences (17, 28,34).

Ischemia

Ischemia represents an imbalance between the myocardial demand for, and the vascular supply of, coronary flow (23). Not only does this create a deficit of O_2, substrates and energy, but it also results in an insufficient capacity for the removal of toxic metabolites such as lactate, CO_2, and protons. Total cessation of coronary flow is not a prerequisite of ischemia; such cessation rarely occurs clinically, and even under experimental conditions, with multiple coronary artery occlusions, the collateral circulation (27,36) may provide substantial perfusion to the ischemic zone. Similarly in global ischemia, such as during cardiac surgery, noncoronary collateral flow (4) may provide significant blood flow to the myocardium.

Reperfusion

Reperfusion represents the complete or partial restoration of flow after regional or global ischemia; it is not only an experimental phenomenon but occurs under a number of pathological and clinical circumstances. On a short-time scale, reperfusion occurs after the relief of coronary spasm, a process which may generate transient periods of ischemia lasting seconds or minutes. On a slightly longer time scale, reperfusion occurs during cardiac surgery after global ischemia lasting minutes or hours. Extending the time scale further, the advent of thrombolytic or mechanical procedures for the localized disruption of coronary occlusions results in reperfusion of tissue which may have been ischemic for hours or days. Another example of reperfusion after extended ischemia is coronary artery bypass surgery. Finally, reperfusion may occur after seconds or days of ischemia through the action of collateral vessels, either by the recruitment of preexisting vessels or by the growth of new vessels (27,36).

Hypoxia

Whereas O_2 delivery in ischemia is limited by flow, in anoxia or hypoxia it is limited by the removal of all or some of the O_2 dissolved in the coronary supply. Thus, while the Po_2 is reduced, coronary flow, substrate delivery, and metabolite removal may be normal or even elevated.

Reoxygenation

Reoxygenation is achieved by partial or total restoration of Po_2 and may be without effect upon coronary flow or delivery and removal of substrates and metabolites. While of less interest than ischemia and reperfusion, hypoxia and reoxygenation do occur clinically. Sudden changes in Po_2 may be observed during altitude changes, respiratory arrest, hyperbaric and O_2 therapy, pulmonary embolism, and in the correction of various defects in hemoglobin O_2-binding characteristics.

Manipulation of Myocardial Injury

Numerous interventions are able to alter injury as assessed by markers such as enzyme leakage, the electrocardiogram, or morphology. These alterations are often loosely referred to as "reducing" or "increasing" injury. However, these terms are imprecise and have led to extensive misinterpretation particularly in relation to "infarct size reduction." It is essential to distinguish between altering the *extent* as opposed to the *rate* of injury development.

Modifying the Rate of Development of Injury

Changes in the *rate* of injury, i.e., a slowing or acceleration of the time course of what *may be* a predetermined level of injury, are readily achievable, and this is exemplified by the use of cardioplegia and hypothermia during cardiac surgery (17). Hypothermia, for example, can slow ATP depletion such that rat hearts exposed to 30 min of zero flow ischemia at 37°C will fail to recover contractile function upon reperfusion, but hearts maintained at 10°C during ischemia will recover to greater than 90%. It must be stressed, however, that hypothermia only reduces the *rate* of development of injury since, in the absence of reflow, cell death is inevitable in a zero flow preparation; the cells are therefore "condemned" as opposed to "jeopardized" (see later).

Modifying the Extent of Development of Injury

Modifying the extent of development of injury requires that an intervention achieves a *sustained* reduction (or increase) in the degree of injury arising from a fixed ischemic insult. Whereas changes in the *rate* of development of injury are relatively easily achieved, a sustained reduction, which is essentially a prerequisite for infarct size limitation, is much more difficult to accomplish. *It could be argued that in the absence of reperfusion a severe reduction in flow (for example to 25% or less) must inevitably lead to cell death, and that no intervention has yet been described which can sustain normal contractile function in tissue deprived of flow to this extent.* Most studies can be criticized in that they are either of too short a duration, or that reperfusion was introduced too early to allow definitive proof of absolute tissue salvage.

Clinical Relevance of Delaying and Reducing Injury

Whereas an ability to reduce injury is more attractive than an ability to delay injury, the latter is not without application even in the field of regional ischemia. For example, thrombolytic procedures must be applied during the early stages of evolving infarction; any agent which acts to buy time may be of great importance if it is able to delay the onset of irreversible injury so as to allow the use of the technique or to give time for the growth of collateral vessels.

As already mentioned, delaying injury has found successful application during cardiac surgery. It is of interest to identify the reasons for this surgical success in contrast to the relative clinical failure of infarct size reduction. Important features of surgically induced ischemia are that it can be anticipated; it is of a fixed, relatively short duration; reperfusion can be instituted at will, and protective agents can be administered at the moment of, or before, the induction of ischemia. By contrast, in evolving infarction the duration of ischemia is not finite and cannot necessarily be reversed; the time of onset may be unknown, and rarely is it possible to administer drugs before or during early ischemia. An additional and important factor is that with surgical ischemia contractile activity is not required (its active suppression is an important component of the protection process), whereas in the case of infarction, the maintenance of pump function is essential. Finally, under surgical conditions the heart is far more accessible; the highly protective procedure of hypothermia can be applied and the ischemia is relatively uniform throughout the myocardium, a factor which may be of considerable importance in preventing various secondary problems arising from the heterogeneity of regional ischemia.

State of Tissue

The feasibility of modifying injury is critically determined by the state of the tissue at the time of treatment. In essence, it is important to ascertain if protection is possible and also if it is practicable.

Reversibility of Injury

O_2 deprivation initiates a sequence of progressively more severe cellular changes (24); initially, these are reversible such that reperfusion or reoxygenation results in a rapid and complete return of contractile function and normalization of any metabolic impairment. As the duration or severity of O_2 deprivation increases, cellular injury becomes more severe, and reperfusion or reoxygenation may not result in an immediate return of function. However, if injury is still reversible, then a full recovery should eventually occur although this may take some time; for example, after even brief periods of ischemia, the contents of adenine nucleotides may not return to normal for several hours or days (31). The term "stunned myocardium" has been applied to tissue in this state (3). Injury eventually becomes irreversible and here, by definition, reperfusion or reoxygenation cannot lead to recovery, thus cell death becomes an inescapable consequence. Clearly, protective agents must be used while the tissue is still in its phase of reversible injury and recovery is theoretically possible. However, it is important that recovery is also practicable; this requires the distinction between "jeopardized" and "condemned" tissue (18,39).

Jeopardized Tissue

With jeopardized tissue, cellular injury is reversible primarily because the *degree* of ischemia is not very severe, cells are receiving suboptimal flow, and, although their mechanical function may be severely impaired, they can remain in a viable condition for some time. Tissue salvage without reperfusion is, therefore, a practical consideration and contrasts with one in which the ischemia is severe but the injury is reversible only because the duration of elapsed ischemia is short. In this latter condition, the term condemned tissue is more appropriate.

Condemned Tissue

In condemned tissue, the cells are also reversibly damaged, but flow is greatly impaired and ischemia is very severe. In practical terms, without reperfusion, tissue salvage is not possible, and deterioration to irreversible injury and cell death is inevitable. It can be argued that in many dog studies with coronary ligation, flow in the ischemic zone is so low (less than 20%) that the affected cells are condemned and injury can only be delayed. Under these conditions, reperfusion after 4 or 6 hr may facilitate recovery, but after 12 or 24 hr it is likely to have little effect. Many studies of "antiinfarct" agents [as defined by Opie (29)] have incorporated reperfusion and functional assessment after 6 or less hr, which effectively prevents the critical distinction being made between reducing and delaying injury.

Meaning of Tissue Protection

Incorrect interpretation and inadequacy of many indices of injury have often led to inappropriate use of the term "protection." For example, many early influential studies of infarct size reduction used electrocardiographic or enzymatic assessments. Although these were the best procedures available at the time, it is now clear that indices such as ST-segment elevation or cumulative creatine kinase leakage are often imprecise and prone to serious artifacts. However, even when used carefully and correctly there is a further problem which could be called "the limitation of association."

Limitation of Association

Although a drug may reduce some index of injury such as ST-segment elevation or enzyme leakage, this cannot necessarily be equated with an increase in tissue viability. It may well indicate that a high level of injury is being reduced to a lower level, but if the tissue still remains irreversibly injured with no return of contractile function then the term "protection" would hardly seem appropriate.

Protection: A Physiological Versus a Biological Definition

It is proposed that true tissue protection must involve not only preventing the critical transition from reversible to irreversible injury, but also promoting the return of the physiological role of the organ, i.e., pump function. Often, in the past, changes in staining or metabolism have been equated with a return of physiological as well as biological function. Such associations may be quite unjustified as, indeed, are other often-made associations such as that between "intermediate" staining or "intermediate" metabolite depletion, and "intermediate" or reversible injury. It is difficult to find studies where drug treatment has achieved an unquestioned and *sustained* reduction of infarct size, while at the same time promoting a return of condemned or jeopardized cells to normal or near-normal contractile function.

Chronic Cell Injury

The interesting and yet unresolved possibility arises that tissue injury may be such that a cell is biologically alive in the sense that many of its metabolic characteristics, e.g., mitochondrial function, are normal but it is physiologically "dead" in that it remains acontractile. It is not inconceivable that protective interventions might prevent the process of necrosis while not evoking a return of contraction. Under such conditions, cells might exhibit misleadingly normal profiles for some indices of injury, e.g., tissue ATP content. *If* such a condition exists, it underscores the importance of contractile assessments of injury and protection, or at least the use of multiple, independent indices of injury and protection.

SEVERITY AND MODIFICATION OF MYOCARDIAL INJURY

In the preceding section, specific distinction has been made between reperfusion and any other intervention capable of influencing the progression of tissue injury. This distinction has been made because the consequences of reperfusion can be complex and controversial and also because, under some conditions such as severe ischemia, reperfusion might be argued to be the only procedure capable of effective and sustained protection. It can also be argued that, under some conditions, reperfusion may be specifically hazardous. These possibilities will now be discussed in the light of some of the definitions and distinctions made in the preceding sections.

Prediction of the feasibility of tissue protection and the outcome of reperfusion requires that the severity of ischemic injury be known, i.e., some assessment must be made of the complex interplay between the duration of ischemia and the extent of flow deprivation.

Severity of Injury: Problems of the FD × L Concept

It has been suggested (25,35) that the severity of ischemic injury, as reflected by the fall in tissue ATP content, can be best and simply predicted by the product of flow deprivation and duration of ischemia. A good correlation was reported for the relationship between ATP content and flow deprivation (FD) multiplied by the duration of the ischemia (L). Flow deprivation was calculated by the formula:

$$FD = 1 - \frac{\text{Blood flow in ischemic tissue}}{\text{Blood flow in normal tissue}}$$

This simple relationship necessitates, for example, that 60 min with coronary flow reduced by 50% will generate the same ATP depletion, and presumably ischemic injury, as 40 min with flow reduced by 75%. If this is to hold true then a prerequisite is that ATP depletion must be linear with time. Also inherent in the proposed FD × L relationship is the requirement that, even with very small flow reductions, ATP depletion must occur. A third characteristic of the FD × L and ATP relationship for the dog heart as presented by Kloner and Braunwald (25) is that because the maximum allowable value for FD is unity (zero flow), and the published correlation curve intercepts the FD × L axis at a value of 80, ATP depletion must be complete by 80 min under conditions of zero flow.

The present author (20) has proposed that a number of experimental and theoretical factors argue against the FD × L concept. Firstly, it has been the author's experience (15) that ATP depletion in a number of species, including the dog, is not linear with time. A consideration of the intracellular compartmentation of ATP and its complex equilibrium with several pools of creatine phosphate (which initially buffer ATP depletion until they themselves are depleted) would also argue against a linear decline. Secondly, the complex and conservative effects of contractile failure would also contribute to a complex profile for ATP depletion (16). In support of these arguments, the author has studied (20) the relationship between flow deprivation and ATP depletion in more than 700 biopsies from dog hearts after various durations of ischemia and concluded that three states of ischemic injury may exist (Fig. 1).

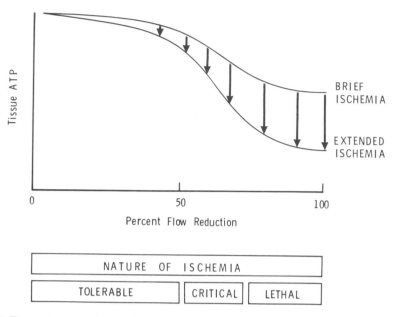

FIG. 1. Three phases in the relationship between tissue injury and the duration of ischemia and the degree of flow deprivation. A speculative theoretical curve indicating that tissue injury (as assessed by ATP depletion) is small and relatively time-independent under conditions of "tolerable" ischemia (residual flow greater than 50%). Under conditions of critical flow deprivation (probably in the range 60–80% flow reduction), ATP depletion and tissue injury are time-dependent and flow-dependent. In this relatively narrow flow band, tissue salvage by reperfusion or by metabolic manipulation is probably feasible but time-dependent. With lethal flow deprivation (flow less than 20%), the development of injury is time-dependent for only a short time, injury is very severe, and without early reperfusion the tissue must be considered as "condemned." For full details see text.

Three States of Flow Reduction and Ischemic Injury: "Tolerable," "Critical," and "Lethal"

The preceding studies (20) revealed that coronary flow could be reduced by up to 50 to 60% without any major fall in tissue ATP even if the reduction was maintained for 2 hr. In this state of *"tolerable" ischemia,* ATP is probably maintained by a combination of increased O_2 consumption per unit flow, reduced contractile performance, and more efficient substrate utilization (e.g., switching from fatty acid to glucose utilization). Thus, while contractility may be reduced, the tissue should remain free of major metabolic or morphological injury for long or indefinite periods. Consequently, reperfusion or other protective measures, such as substrate manipulation or the use of drugs such as coronary vasodilators, might reasonably be expected to afford real protection with a sustained improvement or even normalization of contractile performance.

In the second state of ischemic injury, with flow reductions of 60 to 80%, ATP levels declined and the greater the flow reduction and/or the greater the duration of ischemia, then the greater was the fall in ATP content. In this phase of *"critical" ischemia,* small changes in flow or duration could result in large changes in ATP content. It would seem reasonable to designate this tissue as jeopardized in that a small improvement in flow might halt the time-dependent decline in energy reserves and possibly convert the tissue to the time-independent state of tolerable ischemia. It may well be that in this relatively narrow band of flow deprivation, metabolic and pharmacological salvage (or considerable delays in the onset of irreversible injury) may be feasible. However, the time-dependency of the phase would necessitate that interventions be made as soon after the onset of ischemia as possible—perhaps within 1 to 2 hr with 80% reductions of flow and 6 to 12 hr with 60% reduction of flow. Similar arguments might apply to reperfusion where early introduction might result in substantial salvage.

The third state of injury can be designated as *"lethal" ischemia,* and here flow reductions of greater than 80% occur. In this phase, injury occurs very rapidly and has a complex time-dependency such that tissue ATP falls rapidly with time up to about 45 min. With increasing durations ATP declines more slowly, the tissue probably being in a state of irreversible injury. Thus, with flow deprivations of 80% or more (the condition usually observed in a dog or pig heart with coronary artery ligation), reperfusion probably represents the only means of achieving true and sustained protection for the bulk of the tissue, but for this to be effective it must be instituted very early after the onset of ischemia.

While the times of ischemia and extents of flow deprivation cited in the preceding paragraphs can only be approximate and are likely to vary between hearts, species, and models, the author proposes that, at present, the timely restoration of flow represents the only means of achieving a sustained recovery of contractile function in tissue which has been rendered severely ischemic. In less severely ischemic tissue, metabolic and pharmacological manipulations, in addition to slowing injury, are probably also able to reverse it.

Reperfusion: A Hazardous Process?

The obvious advantages of reperfusion have been somewhat overshadowed by the growing belief that, under some conditions, reperfusion may exacerbate ischemic injury. Although reperfusion can undoubtedly precipitate some undesirable side effects (9,14,22), it is the author's belief that the term "reperfusion-induced injury" is often inappropriately applied and, as with myocardial protection, often represents a failure to distinguish between modifying the *rate* and the *extent* of injury.

The myocardial response to reperfusion or reoxygenation is highly dependent upon the duration and severity of the preceding period of O_2 deprivation (Fig. 2). In the early stages of injury, reperfusion evokes a rapid return of normal function. With the possible exception of the induction of arrhythmias, reperfusion is clearly beneficial. As the duration of ischemia increases, more severe injury

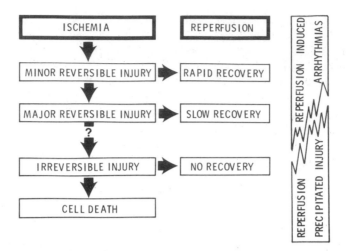

FIG. 2. Phases and consequences of O_2 depletion and repletion: Factors which must be considered when assessing whether reperfusion is beneficial or apparently detrimental to the ischemic myocardium.

occurs and reperfusion may not evoke an immediate return of function; however, if injury is still in its reversible phase, then a full recovery should eventually occur. With the possible exception of the induction of arrhythmias, reperfusion cannot be designated as injurious as without it functional recovery may not be possible. Tissue injury eventually becomes irreversible; here reperfusion cannot prevent cell death and tissue necrosis since, by definition, they are inescapable consequences of irreversible injury. Under these conditions, reperfusion might be expected to be of no consequence; however, such an analysis is prevented by numerous reports that reperfusion may cause a paradoxical and sometimes massive exacerbation of tissue injury. Consideration of such reports, however, allows alternative interpretation.

Enzymatic and Morphological Changes

The author (12) and others have reported that reoxygenation (and reperfusion) of tissue after an extended period of anoxia can result in a massive surge of enzyme leakage. Electron microscopy (13) of tissue taken one minute before and one minute after reoxygenation reveals the occurrence of dramatic additional injury, including cell swelling and disruption and contracture of myofibrils. Although reoxygenation has undoubtedly caused a large increase in the injury apparent at that time (probably by triggering uncontrolled uptake of Ca^{2+}), it is necessary to ask whether the effect has been to accelerate the rate of development of a "predestined" level of injury, or whether more injury has arisen than would have occurred if the ischemia had been maintained. Analysis of enzyme leakage and morphology after 6 hr of uninterrupted anoxia, and after 2 hr of anoxia and 4 hr of reoxygenation, reveals a remarkably similar picture suggesting perhaps that reoxygenation merely accelerates injury in a population of cells which were already irreversibly injured and destined to die. This interpretation gains support from studies of reoxygenation after brief periods of hypoxia. Under these conditions, there is no major exacerbation of injury and the tissue may return to normal contractile function. It is conceivable that the ability of reoxygenation to accelerate injury may mark the onset of irreversible injury.

Contractile Changes

Reperfusion can precipitate sudden increases in resting tension and the development of severe contracture. There is considerable evidence that Ca^{2+} overload (2), secondary to ATP deficiency, is a critical component of this effect. Again it is possible that reperfusion is able to *accelerate* an injurious process, but perhaps only when the point of irreversibility has been passed and recovery is no longer possible.

Reperfusion or reoxygenation after brief periods of ischemia or hypoxia, when injury is still in its reversible phase, can cause changes which might be designated as unfavorable. However, these changes are transient. An example is the assymetrical recovery of various contractile indices (1) during the early minutes of reperfusion where a marked prolongation of contraction occurs before any significant recovery of developed tension. This prolongation is characterized by an increase in half-relaxation time and time to peak tension; the relaxation process, however, gradually returns to control to coincide with a complete recovery of developed tension. The myocardium is therefore able to correct these reperfusion abnormalities which are of little importance when compared with the advantages of reperfusion.

Vascular Changes

Often associated with reperfusion injury is the "no-reflow" phenomenon (10). Although the no-reflow effect was thought to be an important factor in tissue injury, possibly determining the time limit beyond which the ischemic myocardium can no longer be salvaged, it now appears that the phenomenon is a relatively late event occurring after the onset of irreversible injury and that reperfusion of even necrotic tissue can occur. Again, we have a situation where the unfavorable effects of reperfusion may become operative after the onset of irreversibility.

Electrical Changes

Although the preceding sections have argued that reperfusion accelerates rather than increases injury, there is some evidence for specific injury caused by reperfusion. Serious arrhythmias are often associated with reperfusion (7); these are quite distinct from ischemia-induced arrhythmias and can prove lethal in otherwise viable tissue. The nature, severity, and mechanisms of reperfusion arrhythmias probably vary with the duration of preceding ischemia (8), serious rhythm disturbances being particularly likely after brief periods of ischemia, when cellular injury is still reversible and normal functional recovery is possible. Paradoxically, therefore, the recovery process can induce arrhythmias which, in themselves, can prove lethal to the tissue. Reperfusion arrhythmias after extended ischemia, when irreversible injury has occurred, are likely to be less severe, so again a somewhat paradoxical situation exists where reperfusion is no longer able to facilitate recovery, and at this time it becomes electrophysiologically benign.

WHAT PROSPECT FOR CALCIUM ANTAGONISTS IN THE MODIFICATION OF INJURY?

Since this book is devoted to Ca^{2+} antagonists, it is appropriate to consider to what extent these drugs may influence injury as defined in this chapter.

Calcium Antagonists and Ischemia

There is abundant evidence that Ca^{2+} antagonists can be beneficial in global ischemia. Verapamil has been shown to conserve myocardial ATP and enhance postischemic functional recovery in the rat (33), and in other similar studies (41) the drug reduced ischemia-induced Ca^{2+} overload. Nifedipine and diltiazem, in addition to verapamil, have been shown (43) to enhance the protective properties of cardioplegic solutions, although it was questioned if the drugs were as effective under the clinically relevant conditions of hypothermic (20°C) ischemic arrest. These studies, along with several others, can only be interpreted as having slowed the rate of development of injury such that the transition to irreversible injury was delayed beyond the time of reperfusion. There is no doubt that without reperfusion, these globally ischemic preparations would have eventually died, despite the presence of the Ca^{2+} antagonists. As stressed earlier, such a delaying action is not without value, and this is supported by the increasing use of nifedipine and other Ca^{2+} antagonists as an adjunct to cardioplegia in patients undergoing cardiac surgery (6).

In regional ischemia, as predicted in this chapter, the protective effects of Ca^{2+} antagonists are controversial. Geary et al. (11) claimed that nifedipine was unable to reduce infarct size in the baboon heart with 2 hr coronary artery occlusion. In view of the severe flow reduction in this model, the affected tissue could be designated as condemned and, therefore, although the drug may have delayed the onset of irreversibility, cell death eventually occurred, and at a time before the induction of reperfusion. In contrast, Reimer et al. (30) reported that verapamil substantially reduced necrosis in the dog with coronary artery ligation. In that study, hearts were subjected to 40 min of ischemia followed by 2 to 4 days of reperfusion. The most likely interpretation of these results is that the drug slowed injury such that, with the short ischemic duration used, the onset of irreversibility was delayed so allowing an improved recovery upon reperfusion. An alternative, but less likely, possibility is that in the dog heart with its extensive collateral supply, there were areas of "tolerable" or "critical" ischemia where a true reduction of tissue injury, independent of reperfusion, could have been achieved. Smith et al. (38) reported protective effects of verapamil upon hemodynamic and electrocardiographic indices in dog hearts with 2 hr regional ischemia. However, despite the absence of reperfusion in these studies, the short duration of ischemia makes it impossible to distinguish between a delay and an absolute reduction of injury. There are few studies of the effects of Ca^{2+} antagonists where regional ischemia is maintained for long periods. However, Zamanis et al. (45) studied the effect of diltiazem in the rat after coronary ligation for 48 hr, and Yellon et al. (44) studied verapamil in the dog heart with 24 hr of uninterrupted coronary occlusion. In both studies, a significant reduction of infarct size was reported. Although encouraging, these results do not provide definitive proof for an absolute reduction of injury since protection was assessed histochemically, and due to the problems of limitation of association discussed earlier, it is not possible to automatically equate histological salvage with a return of physiological function [it is noteworthy, however, that improved overall mechanical function was observed in the drug-treated group by Zamanis et al. (45)]. Furthermore, the absence of regional flow studies prevented the demonstration of possible areas of tolerable ischemia or drug-induced reflow in the areas which appeared to be salvaged.

As indicated in Fig. 3, current evidence suggests that Ca^{2+} antagonists can undoubtedly substantially delay the onset of irreversible injury in both global and regional ischemia. There is, however, much less evidence for the ability of these drugs to achieve a sustained reduction of injury in severely ischemic tissue unless early reperfusion is initiated. However, under conditions of mild ischemia there is some indication that permanent salvage may be feasible.

Calcium Slow-Channel Blockers and Reperfusion

The ability of Ca^{2+} antagonists to enhance recovery or reduce injury during reperfusion is far from clear. Some have claimed that these drugs, when applied *during reperfusion,* are unable to afford protection and are incapable of preventing Ca^{2+} overload. Thus, although Watts et al. (41) demonstrated beneficial effects during ischemia, they could not improve functional recovery, conserve ATP, or limit Ca^{2+} overload when verapamil was employed during the reperfusion of globally ischemic rat hearts. Similarly, Bourdillon and Poole-Wilson (2), using the isolated rabbit septum, were unable to improve recovery when verapamil was used during ischemia. In contrast, Weishaar and Bing (42) reported diltiazem to reduce reperfusion-induced injury (creatine kinase leakage) in the globally ischemic rat heart. Attempting to reconcile this report with

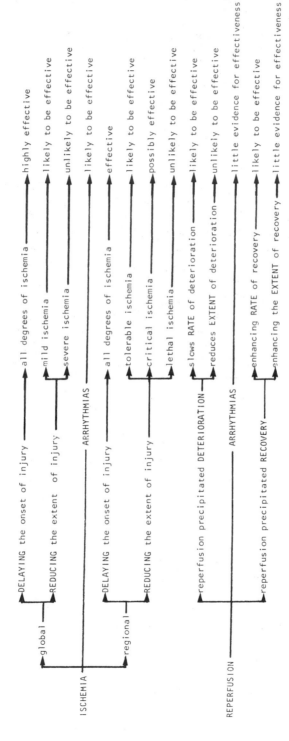

FIG. 3. Prospects for Ca²⁺ slow-channel blocking drugs in the modification of myocardial cell injury: An assessment of the potential for modifying various aspects of tissue injury during myocardial ischemia and reperfusion. For explanation and supporting literature, see text.

the preceding studies, two points should be considered. Firstly, measuring a drug-induced *reduction* of damage after relatively moderate ischemia [Watts et al. (41), 25 min of ischemia] is not necessarily comparable to measuring a drug-induced reduction in the *exacerbation* of injury seen after prolonged ischemia [Weishaar and Bing (42), 120 min of ischemia]. Secondly, in the study of Weishaar and Bing, reperfusion was only maintained for 15 min, making it impossible to ascertain, for example, if enzyme leakage, which was still high in both control and diltiazem-treated groups, would eventually achieve the same level. In other words, diltiazem may have merely delayed the expression, or overridden the acceleration, of injury induced by the readmission of O_2.

The full interpretation of a number of other studies of Ca^{2+} slow-channel blockers and reperfusion is limited by drug inclusion *during* the ischemic phase of the study; at the present time, however, the consensus concerning the evidence is that while these drugs may influence the rate of recovery when used during reperfusion they are unlikely to be able to alter the ultimate extent of injury.

Calcium Antagonists and Arrhythmias

The ability of Ca^{2+} antagonists to influence ischemia- and reperfusion-induced arrhythmias has been separated from preceding sections since, as argued earlier in this chapter, arrhythmias might occupy a unique position in the spectrum and interpretation of tissue injury. The role of these drugs is controversial. In some studies (5) verapamil has been shown to reduce vulnerability to ventricular fibrillation in the dog heart both during ischemia (10 min) and reperfusion. However, since the drug was administered 15 min before coronary artery occlusion and terminated after 2 min of reperfusion, it is not possible to ascertain whether the protective effects during reperfusion were primary effects or secondary to the action of the drug during the preceding ischemia. In other studies (37), however, diltiazem or nifedipine administered prior to coronary artery occlusion in dogs did not reduce the incidence of reperfusion-induced ventricular fibrillation. It was speculated that this failure might result from differences in the electrophysiological actions of different Ca^{2+} antagonists. Such a conclusion might be drawn from another study (32) where clear protective effects were shown for verapamil against reperfusion-induced arrhythmias in the dog, whereas nifedipine exerted very little effect. One important aspect of the last study that aids in the separation of the effect of these drugs upon ischemia and reperfusion is that drug treatment was initiated just before the onset of reperfusion. Drug treatment was also initiated just prior to reperfusion in a pig heart study (40) and a dog heart study (26). However, whereas the former was able to demonstrate protective effects with nifedipine, the latter was unable to show any significant effects with verapamil. Whether this lack of agreement reflects differences in methods of study, Ca^{2+} slow-channel blockers, or species remains to be elucidated.

Although there is considerable evidence that Ca^{2+} slow-channel blocking drugs can exert a beneficial effect upon ischemia-induced rhythm disturbances, probably by their delaying action on ischemic injury and their ability to prevent specific conduction abnormalities, their effect upon reperfusion-induced arrhythmias is debatable (see Chapters 26–28, *this volume*). The present conflict of results undoubtedly underlines the electrophysiological differences between ischemia- and reperfusion-induced arrhythmias and also highlights differences in the specificity and electrophysiological site of action of this diverse group of drugs.

CONCLUDING COMMENTS

This chapter has sought to make critical distinctions which the author believes to be vital if we are to successfully understand, and appropriately treat, myocardial injury. Emphasis has been placed on the differences between ischemia and hypoxia, and between reperfusion and reoxygenation. The vital difference between modifying the rate of development as opposed to the ultimate extent of injury has been repeatedly highlighted, as has been the importance of defining the state of tissue injury in relation to the practical feasibility of its modification. The appropriate application of the term "protection" has been urged, since the incorrect use of this term, together with inappropriate models and markers of tissue injury, has contributed to much of the current confusion relating to myocardial protection. Reperfusion has been deliberately separated from other protective interventions such as pharmacological and biochemical manipulation of the ischemic cell, since it is argued that in some instances, e.g., severe ischemia, it remains the only proven means of achieving a sustained return to normal cellular function. Since reperfusion occupies a central role in tissue protection, it was considered appropriate to reassess possible detrimental effects of reperfusion, as well as the obvious beneficial effects; again the author endeavored to identify critical distinctions and widespread misconceptions. In the light of these points, and in relation to the subject of this book, a number of studies dealing with the protective properties of Ca^{2+} antagonists have been reviewed in an attempt to assess the extent to which we are currently able to modify myocardial tissue injury.

REFERENCES

1. Bing, O. H. L., Brooks, W. W., and Messer, J. V. (1976): *J. Mol. Cell. Cardiol.*, 8:205–215.
2. Bourdillon, P. D., and Poole-Wilson, P. A. (1982): *Circ. Res.*, 50:360–368.
3. Braunwald, E., and Kloner, R. A. (1982): *Circulation*, 66:1146–1149.
4. Brazier, J., Hottenrott, C., and Buckberg, G. D. (1975): *Ann. Thor. Surg.*, 19:426–442.
5. Brooks, W. W., Verrier, R. L., and Lown, B. (1980): *Cardiovasc. Res.*, 14:295–302.
6. Clark, R. E., Christlieb, I. Y., Ferguson, T. B., Weldon, C. S., Marbarger, J. P., Biello, D. R., Roberts, R., Ludbrook, P. A., and Sobel, B. E. (1981): *J. Thor. Cardiovasc. Surg.*, 82:848–859.
7. Corr, P. B., Penkoske, P. A., and Sobel, B. E. (1978): *Br. Heart J.*, 40:62–70.
8. Cox, D. A., Verrier, R., Baugham, K., Lown, B., and Vatner, S. F. (1981): *Am. J. Cardiol.*, 47:461.

9. Danforth, W. H., Nagle, S., and Bing, R. J. (1960): *Circ. Res.*, 8:965–971.
10. Fabiani, J. N. (1976): *Heart Bull.*, 7:134–142.
11. Geary, G. G., Smith, G. T., Suehiro, G. T., and McNamara, J. J. (1982): *Am. J. Cardiol.*, 49:331–338.
12. Hearse, D. J., Humphrey, S. M., and Chain, E. B. (1973): *J. Mol. Cell. Cardiol.*, 5:395–407.
13. Hearse, D. J., Humphrey, S. M., Nayler, W. G., Slade, A., and Border, D. (1975): *J. Mol. Cell. Cardiol.*, 7:315–324.
14. Hearse, D. J. (1977): *J. Mol. Cell. Cardiol.*, 9:605–616.
15. Hearse, D. J., Garlick, P. B., and Humphrey, S. M. (1977): *Am. J. Cardiol.*, 39:986–993.
16. Hearse, D. J. (1979): *Am. J. Cardiol.*, 44:1115–1121.
17. Hearse, D. J., Braimbridge, M. V., and Jynge, P. (1981): *Protection of the Ischemic Myocardium: Cardioplegia.* Raven Press, New York.
18. Hearse, D. J., and Yellon, D. (1981): *Am. J. Cardiol.*, 47:1321–1334.
19. Hearse, D. J. (1983): *Eur. Heart J.* (*Suppl. C*)4:43–48.
20. Hearse, D. J., Crome, R., Yellon, D., and Wyse, R. (1983): *Cardiovasc. Res.,* 17:452–458.
21. Hillis, L. D., and Braunwald, E. (1977): *N. Engl. J. Med.,* 296:971–978; 1034–1041; and 1093–1096.
22. Jennings, R. B., Sommers, H. M., Smyth, G. A., Flack, H. A., and Linn, H. (1960): *Arch. Pathol.,* 70:68–78.
23. Jennings, R. B. (1970): *J. Mol. Cell. Cardiol.,* 1:345–349.
24. Jennings, R. B., and Ganote, C. E. (1976): *Circ. Res.,* (Suppl. 1)38:80–91.
25. Kloner, R. A., and Braunwald, E. (1980): *Cardiovasc. Res.,* 14:371–395.
26. Naito, M., Michelson, E. L., Kmetzo, J. J., Kaplinksy, E., and Dreifus, L. S. (1981): *Circulation,* 63:70–79.
27. Newman, P. E. (1981): *Am. Heart J.,* 102:431–445.
28. Opie, L. H. (1976): *Circ. Res.,* (Suppl. 1)38:52–74.
29. Opie, L. H. (1980): *Am. Heart J.,* 100:355–372; 531–552.
30. Reimer, K. A., Lowe, J. E., and Jennings, R. B. (1977): *Circulation,* 55:581–587.
31. Reimer, K. A., Hill, M. L., and Jennings, R. B. (1981): *J. Mol. Cell. Cardiol.,* 13:229–239.
32. Ribeiro, L. G. T., Brandon, T. A., Debauche, T. L., Maroko, P. R., and Miller, R. R. (1981): *Am. J. Cardiol.,* 48:69–74.
33. Robb-Nicholson, C., Currie, W. D., and Wechsler, A. S. (1978): *Circulation,* (Suppl. 1) 58:119–124.
34. Rovetto, M. J., Whitmer, J. T., and Neely, J. R. (1973): *Circ. Res.,* 32:699–711.
35. Rude, R. E., De Boer, L. W. V., Ingwall, J. S., Kloner, R. A., Hale, S. L., Davis, M., Maroko, P. R., and Braunwald, E. (1980): *Am. J. Cardiol.,* 45:415.
36. Schaper, W. (1971): *The Collateral Circulation of the Heart.* North-Holland, Amsterdam.
37. Sheehan, F. H., and Epstein, S. E. (1982): *Am. Heart J.,* 103:973–977.
38. Smith, H. J., Singh, B. N., Nisbet, H. D., and Norris, R. M. (1975): *Cardiovasc. Res.,* 9:569–578.
39. Sobel, B. E., and Shell, W. E. (1973): *Circulation,* 47:215–216.
40. Verdouw, P. D., Hartog, J. M., ten Cate, F. J., Schamhardt, H. C., Bastiaans, O. L., van Bremen, R. H., Serruys, P. W., and Hugenholtz, P. G. (1981): *Progr. Pharmacol.,* 4:91–100.
41. Watts, J. A., Koch, C. D., and LaNoue, K. (1980): *Am. J. Physiol.,* 238:H909–H916.
42. Weishaar, R. E., and Bing, R. J. (1980): *J. Mol. Cell. Cardiol.,* 12:993–1009.
43. Yamamoto, F., Manning, A. S., Braimbridge, M. V., and Hearse, D. J. (1982): *Circulation,* (Suppl. 2)66:150.
44. Yellon, D. M., Hearse, D. J., Maxwell, M. P., Chambers, D. E., and Downey, J. M. (1983): *Am. J. Cardiol.,* 51:1409–1413.
45. Zamanis, A., Verdetti, J., and de Leiris, J. (1982): *J. Mol. Cell. Cardiol.,* 14:53–62.

Calcium Antagonists and Cardiovascular Disease, edited by L. H. Opie.
Raven Press, New York   1984.

Chapter 13

Calcium as a Risk Factor for Coronary Atherosclerosis

William C. Roberts

Pathology Branch, National Heart, Lung and Blood Institute, National Institutes of Health, Bethesda, Maryland 20205

Several years ago I examined the heart at necropsy of a patient in whom massive calcific deposits were present in the mitral valve anulus and coronary arteries and small deposits in the tricuspid valve anulus and in both pulmonic and aortic valve cusps. Primarily on the basis of these calcific deposits, I predicted that the patient had been about 90 years of age. When clinical information was provided, however, it was learned that the patient had been only 44 years old and had died from consequences of primary hyperparathyroidism. Because I had never missed a patient's age by nearly half a century on the basis of the cardiac examination at necropsy, a search was made of reports describing the heart at necropsy in patients with chronic hypercalcemia. Essentially none were found. Accordingly, the necropsy files of the National Institutes of Health were searched for patients with chronic hypercalcemia and 18 in whom the serum Ca^{2+} level was known to be unequivocally elevated for ≥ 1 year were found. The findings in these 18 patients were reported in detail elsewhere (3) and will be commented on here.

VALVULAR CALCIFICATION

Analysis of the 18 necropsy patients described with chronic hypercalcemia clearly demonstrates an increased frequency of cardiac calcific deposits including an accelerated amount (compared to controls) of coronary arterial atherosclerosis. Of the 18 patients, calcific deposits were present in the mitral valve anuli in 10, 2 of whom also had calcific deposits in the tricuspid valve anuli and in both pulmonic and aortic valve cusps. All 10 patients with mitral anular calcific deposits also had calcific deposits in the coronary arteries: in atherosclerotic plaques (intima) in all 10 and in the media ("medial calcinosis") as well in 4 patients.

Although calcific deposits are well known to occur in the mitral anular region in elderly persons living in the Western world, they are definitely infrequent in all areas of the world in patients less than 65 years of age (except in patients with the Marfan or Hurler syndromes). Of the 18 patients described with chronic hypercalcemia, 10 had mitral anular Ca^{2+} and all were relatively young (range 35–58 years, mean 46 years), and none had either the Marfan or Hurler syndromes.

The occurrence of calcific deposits in the tricuspid valve anulus is rare, but 2 of the 18 patients described had such deposits. Of the few previously reported patients with tricuspid valve anular deposits, all had severely increased right ventricular systolic pressures and right ventricular hypertrophy. The latter were absent in all the 18 patients reported herein.

Calcific deposits on the aortic aspects of the aortic valve cusps also are commonly seen in elderly patients in the Western world, frequently in association with mitral anular Ca^{2+} (2). Three of the 18 patients, all of whom had much larger mitral anular calcific deposits, had calcific deposits in the aortic valve cusps but each was relatively young (aged 43, 45, and 47, respectively).

An extremely rare site of calcific deposits is the pulmonic valve, and all previously reported such patients had pulmonic valve stenosis. Two of the 18 patients had calcific deposits on the arterial aspects of each pulmonic valve cusp.

ARTERIAL CALCINOSIS

Although calcific deposits in coronary atherosclerotic plaques are common in persons with coronary atherosclerosis, particularly elderly persons and those with diabetes mellitus, calcific deposits in the media of a coronary artery have been reported only once previously (1). Of the 18 patients with chronic hypercalcemia, 5 had medial calcinosis, 4 of whom also had calcific deposits in intimal atherosclerotic plaques.

Calcific deposits within individual myocardial fibers (dystrophic calcification) is observed fairly frequently in patients with chronic renal failure, hypervitaminosis D, and in those with prolonged low cardiac output syndromes after cardiac operations. It was found in 7 of the 18 patients with chronic hypercalcemia, all of whom had associated cardiac valvular or anular calcific deposits.

In addition to the cardiac calcific deposits in 12 of the 18 patients, in at least 11 patients calcific deposits were observed in one or more blood vessels outside the heart and in one or more other body organs, including kidney, lung, and stomach. Thus, the cardiac calcific deposits in these patients are simply part of a systemic calcific process.

MECHANISMS

Although the exact mechanism of the calcific deposition in the 18 patients is unclear, chronic hypercalcemia is clearly the common link in all 18, and therefore it is reasonable to believe that it played the major role in causing the unusual and often extensive cardiovascular calcific deposits. It is also reasonable to believe that the cause of the vascular and nonvascular calcific deposits in the 18 patients was the same.

Although surely playing a major role in producing the vascular calcific deposits, chronic hypercalcemia is not the only factor because one-third of the 18 patients had no vascular or nonvascular calcific deposits. Comparison of a number of factors between the 10 patients with cardiac valvular and extensive coronary calcific deposits (group I), and the 8 patients without cardiac valvular deposits (2 of whom had minimal coronary deposits) (group II), disclosed no significant differences in ages at death (46 versus 43 years), duration of chronic hypercalcemia (5.9 versus 3.6 years), frequency of systemic hypertension (8 of 10 versus 6 of 8), cause of the hypercalcemia, or the mean values of the peak serum Ca^{2+} levels, but significant differences in the mean total serum cholesterol levels (216 versus 163 mg/dl; $p < 0.01$) and the mean heart weights (426 versus 320 g; $p < 0.05$). The differences in the mean cholesterol levels support the thesis that elevation of these levels not only may lead to atherosclerosis, but also that its elevation may play a large role in causing calcific deposits in other portions of the heart, particularly mitral anulus and aortic valve cusps.

SUMMARY

Irrespective of the precise mechanism of the vascular calcific deposits, it is clear that chronic hypercalcemia is detrimental to the vascular system and that its effect, at least in adults, is worsened by the presence of hypercholesterolemia, and possibly also by the presence of systemic hypertension. Additional support for the role of hypercalcemia in causing vascular and nonvascular calcific deposits comes from studies of chronic hypervitaminosis D in infants and children, and from its association with the congenital syndrome of peculiar elfin faces, mental retardation, and supravalvular aortic stenosis. The present study also strongly suggests that chronic hypercalcemia is a "risk factor" to premature coronary atherosclerosis, especially in patients with an elevated serum cholesterol (3).[1]

REFERENCES

1. Lachman, A. S., Spray, T. I., Kerwin, D. M., Shugall, G. I., and Roberts, W. C. (1977): *Am. J. Med.*, 63:615–622.
2. Roberts, W. C. (1983): *Am. J. Cardiol.*, 51:1005–1028.
3. Roberts, W. C., and Waller, B. F. (1981): *Am. J. Med.*, 71:371–384.

---

[1] *Editor's note:* An increased serum Ca^{2+} may be an independent risk factor for the production of hypertension [Kesteloot and Geboers (1982): *Lancet*, 1:813–815].

Calcium Antagonists and Cardiovascular Disease, edited by L. H. Opie. Raven Press, New York © 1984.

Chapter 14

Where Do Calcium Antagonists Act?

C. J. Cohen, R. A. Janis, D. G. Taylor, and A. Scriabine

Miles Institute for Preclinical Pharmacology, New Haven, Connecticut 06509

Ca^{2+} antagonists may be defined as drugs that potentially inhibit Ca^{2+} dependent processes or regulatory mechanisms without exerting their primary effect at some other known sites, such as ion channels other than Ca^{2+} channels or receptors for neurotransmitters. Within this definition, Ca^{2+} antagonists can be subdivided as shown in Fig. 1. Most of the Ca^{2+} antagonists used at present in the clinic are believed to reduce the availability of intracellular Ca^{2+} by decreasing Ca^{2+} entry into vascular smooth muscle or myocardial cells. Facilitation of Ca^{2+} efflux or stimulation of uptake into storage sites by Ca^{2+} antagonists is conceivable and should be considered as additional possible mechanisms of action. A decrease of cellular actions of Ca^{2+} without a reduction in the availability of Ca^{2+} to the cytosol is now recognized as at least one of the mechanisms of action of trifluoperazine (58) and methylenedioxyindenes (73).

This chapter will deal with some new information and viewpoints on the sites and mechanisms of action of Ca^{2+} channel inhibitors as revealed by recent ligand-binding, hemodynamic, and electrophysiological studies. Attempts will be made to provide at least partial answers to the following questions: (a) How have ligand-binding studies helped to elucidate the site and mechanism of action

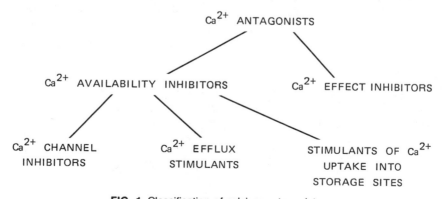

FIG. 1. Classification of calcium antagonists.

of Ca^{2+} antagonists? (b) What are the possible intracellular sites of action of Ca^{2+} antagonists and are they of any therapeutic relevance? (c) Do the clinically useful Ca^{2+} antagonists uncouple excitation-contraction coupling in vascular smooth muscle by blocking Ca^{2+} channels? (d) Is there more than one type of Ca^{2+} channel in vascular smooth muscle? (e) What is the basis for organ selectivity in the action of these drugs? (f) What are the important hemodynamic effects of these drugs in animals and humans?

It is hoped that a critical review of our present knowledge will stimulate further research in this important field.

LIGAND-BINDING STUDIES

A number of subclasses of organic Ca^{2+} channel inhibitors can be identified based on their structures, for example: (a) dihydropyridines, such as nifedipine, nitrendipine, and nimodipine; (b) verapamil and gallopamil (D600); (c) diltiazem and structurally related compounds; (d) flunarizine, lidoflazine, and cinnarizine. The qualitative differences in pharmacological effects of these various subclasses (39,62) suggest that different groups of agents exert their effects by acting at different sites, and/or by different mechanisms of action. Using radioactive ligands for neurotransmitter receptors, it has been established that both verapamil and gallopamil inhibit the binding of several neurotransmitters, including ligands for α_1- and α_2-adrenoceptors (2,26,69). The recent availability of [³H]dihydropyridines provides a new dimension to studies of the sites of action of Ca^{2+} channel inhibitors. Direct evidence as to whether the different subclasses act at different sites can now be obtained.

Early studies established that K^+-induced contraction of smooth muscle is usually very sensitive to nifedipine, whereas agonist-induced contraction of some smooth muscles (even when it is highly dependent on extracellular Ca^{2+}) and cardiac twitch tension, are often less sensitive to nifedipine and other dihydropyridines (23,48,75). These results suggested that ligand-binding studies might detect both low- and high-affinity [³H]nitrendipine-binding sites in smooth muscle membranes, whereas only a low-affinity site would be detected in cardiac muscle membranes. In contrast, only a single high-affinity dihydropyridine-binding site (dissociation constant of 0.1 to 1 nM) has been consistently found in both smooth (8,9,17,50,104) and cardiac muscle membranes (4,5,9,19,20,46,49,65,77,104), as well as in membranes from brain (20,30,64).

The affinities obtained for the binding of nitrendipine (8,9,50,104) and nimodipine (50) to smooth muscle membranes are in good agreement with their potency for inhibition of contraction. In contrast, the dissociation constant of these ligands for cardiac membranes is approximately the same as that for smooth muscle membranes, but the concentration required for half maximal inhibition of cardiac contraction is at least 100 times greater (24,90). The reason for the large discrepancy between the apparent affinity of these blocking agents for their binding site in isolated membranes and intact cardiac muscle may be due to covalent or conformational changes in the binding site that are associated with the isolation of cardiac, but not smooth, muscle membranes. Alternately, low-affinity binding sites of reasonable density may be present in cardiac membranes but have not been reported. Even for ileal smooth muscle, where there is an excellent correlation between binding and contractile data (8,9), the question of whether the binding site is on the Ca^{2+} channel itself, or on an associated regulatory protein, must be answered.

Since the site of action of these drugs is believed to be Ca^{2+} channels in the sarcolemma (see later), the localization of the binding site is important. Studies with canine ventricular membranes indicated that dihydropyridines bind to sarcolemmal membranes, but not to a purified subfraction of sarcoplasmic reticulum, nor to mitochondrial membranes (77). In contrast, another report suggests that the terminal cisternae may contain significant numbers of binding sites for nitrendipine (105).

The effect of structurally unrelated drugs on the high-affinity nitrendipine-binding site can also help to elucidate the identity of the dihydropyridine-binding site. Verapamil, gallopamil, lidoflazine, flunarizine, tiapamil, and prenylamine appear to act at an allosteric site to inhibit nitrendipine-binding (8,19,20,64). In this regard, it will be of interest to determine if dihydropyridines block cardiac Ca^{2+} channels by acting at the cytosolic side of the membrane, as has been reported for gallopamil (42). Diltiazem (at 0.1–10 μM) has been found to either not effect [³H]nitrendipine-binding (20) or to increase it (8,17,64). The results of these studies and others have led to the hypothesis (64) that all of the above-mentioned non-dihydropyridine Ca^{2+} channel inhibitors bind to a common site which is allosterically linked to the nitrendipine binding site.

OTHER BIOCHEMICAL STUDIES

Many biochemical effects of Ca^{2+} channel inhibitors on the sarcolemma have been detected. For example, nimodipine, and to a lesser extent, nitrendipine, stimulate the Na^+,K^+-ATPase of isolated smooth muscle membranes (71), raising the possibility that *Na⁺ pump stimulation* may contribute to the smooth muscle relaxant effect of these agents. Flaim (23) and Hermsmeyer (41) have also proposed that some of these drugs may stimulate electrogenic ion pumps. Nifedipine (60) and diltiazem (23) were found to reduce intracellular Na^+ in blood vessels, also supporting the view that these drugs may stimulate the Na^+ pump. In very high concentrations, some of these compounds also stimulate Ca^{2+}-ATPase and Ca^{2+} uptake of isolated skeletal and cardiac muscle sarcoplasmic reticulum (13). Still another potential intracellular effect of these Ca^{2+} antagonists is the inhibition of Na^+-induced Ca^{2+} release from heart mitochondria, which was observed with micromolar concentrations of diltiazem and higher concentrations of other Ca^{2+} antagonists (92). The relevance of the above findings to the therapeutic sites of action of these compounds remains to be defined.

Calmodulin

It has been proposed that *calmodulin* may represent the site of action of dihydropyridines (11) as well as other Ca^{2+} channel inhibitors. If calmodulin is the final common Ca^{2+} receptor for smooth muscle contraction, then its blockade would inhibit contraction independent of the mechanism by which Ca^{2+} was elevated, as do phenothiazines (74) and other calmodulin antagonists (52). However, in low concentrations, most Ca^{2+} channel inhibitors do not inhibit calmodulin (21) or associated regulatory and contractile proteins in smooth muscle, as indicated by their inability to block agonist-induced contraction in rabbit aorta (23), and the inability of some dihydropyridines to block Ca^{2+}-induced contraction in skinned muscle preparations (24,81). Furthermore, the interaction of phenothiazines with calmodulin is less structurally selective (76,101) than is the interaction of dihydropyridines with their receptor. Several other proposals have been made regarding the ability of these drugs to block intracellular Ca^{2+} mobilization (23) or to block the intracellular effects of Ca^{2+} (102). More research is needed to evaluate the importance of the above biochemical mechanisms for the effect of these drugs in intact cells.

UNCOUPLING OF EXCITATION AND CONTRACTION IN VASCULAR SMOOTH MUSCLE

Verapamil, nifedipine, and diltiazem block Ca^{2+} channels in cardiac muscle (40) and the electrical spiking activity that is apparently due to inward Ca^{2+} currents in smooth muscle (35,88). These drugs also block excitation-contraction coupling in both cardiac and smooth muscle. A popular hypothesis is that blockade of Ca^{2+} channels accounts for inhibition of tension development in both cardiac and smooth muscle. This idea has been directly tested in cardiac muscle by simultaneously measuring tension and Ca^{2+} currents under voltage clamp (12). In heart, Ca^{2+} current is closely correlated with phasic contraction, but not with tonic tension occurring during maintained depolarization (14). Tonic tension is insensitive to verapamil or gallopamil (18,103). Tonic tension produced by a high extracellular K^+ can be eliminated by removing external Ca^{2+}, but the effect seems to involve Na^+-Ca^{2+} exchange rather than elimination of Ca^{2+} current (12,14). Due to technical limitations, it has not been possible to measure Ca^{2+} currents under voltage clamp in vascular smooth muscle. Since the time- and voltage-dependence of Ca^{2+}-channel gating is unknown for these cells, we do not know whether channel blockade can fully account for drug effects.

Inhibition of vasoconstriction produced by a high extracellular K^+ has often been used as a measure of Ca^{2+} channel blockade (23). Ca^{2+} channels are assumed to be involved because the high K^+ depolarizes the cells, increases $^{45}Ca^{2+}$ uptake, and the contractions are eliminated by removing external Ca^{2+} (51). The studies in heart discussed previously indicate that inhibition of high K^+ contractions need not represent blockade of Ca^{2+} channels. If Ca^{2+} channels are responsible for generating maintained tension in vascular smooth muscle, a mechanism distinct from that which maintains tonic tension in cardiac muscle must be involved.

Studies of vasoconstriction produced by a high extracellular K^+ indicate a maintained influx of Ca^{2+} during depolarization. *K^+-induced vasoconstriction* can be initiated by adding Ca^{2+} to a preparation that has been depolarized for a long time (93). K^+ depolarization increases Ca^{2+} influx for many minutes, and pharmacological inhibition of this influx is correlated with inhibition of tension development (75,95; see ref. 53 for an alternate viewpoint). Many Ca^{2+} channel inhibitors, like nimodipine, not only prevent K^+-induced vasoconstriction, but also relax an artery in the continued presence of high K^+ (89). If relaxation is caused by blockade of voltage-dependent Ca^{2+} channels, then continued Ca^{2+} influx through these channels must be necessary for maintenance of tension. Studies in other tissues establish a precedent for maintained conduction through Ca^{2+} channels (33,57), and Coraboeuf (15) has noted its possible importance in vascular smooth muscle. The existence of a maintained Ca^{2+} current suggests that an outward current is present to repolarize the cells and deactivate the Ca^{2+} channels. A drug that enhances this outward current should produce vasodilatation by hyperpolarizing the cell and thereby closing Ca^{2+} channels. The vasodilator 2-nicotinamidoethyl nitrate increases membrane conductance and hyperpolarizes vascular smooth muscle, which is consistent with an enhanced outward current rather than a decreased inward current (27).

Contractions of vascular smooth muscle initiated by neurotransmitters and autacoids have varying sensitivities to the Ca^{2+} channel inhibitors. In some cases, particularly rabbit aorta, tension development persists in the absence of external Ca^{2+} (93). These contractions, apparently triggered by the release of intracellular Ca^{2+}, are relatively insensitive to the Ca^{2+} channel inhibitors. Transmitter-induced contractions that are highly dependent on external Ca^{2+} influx are more likely to be inhibited by low concentrations of the Ca^{2+} channel inhibitors. The relative importance of Ca^{2+} influx for the inititation of transmitter-induced contractions differs in various vascular beds and even within branches of an artery (93). Conflicting claims have been made that only α_1- or only α_2-adrenoceptors mediate contractions sensitive to the Ca^{2+} channel inhibitors (16,97). At present, it appears that vasoconstriction mediated by either type of receptor can be antagonized by these drugs.

The concept of "pharmacomechanical coupling" was introduced to account for those contractions produced by neurotransmitters that do not change the membrane potential (10,51). A second class of Ca^{2+} channels has been invoked that is not potential-dependent, but *"receptor-operated."* The ability of drugs to antagonize the contractions produced by neurotransmitters has been attributed to blockade of these channels (23,94). However, electrophysiological support for the notion of multiple Ca^{2+} channels is lacking because no membrane Ca^{2+} conductance has been correlated with the putative receptor-operated channels.

The block of Ca^{2+}-dependent action potentials in vascular smooth muscle by the Ca^{2+} channel inhibitors indicates that these drugs can reduce a phasic entry of Ca^{2+} into the cells. There have been two serious concerns about the physiological importance of this action. First, action potentials are often elicited in arteries only under special conditions that reduce the membrane K^+ conductance (35,51), and it was not clear that the action potentials occur under physiological conditions. Second, the theory of pharmacomechanical coupling suggests that some cells do not depolarize in response to nerve stimulation because the application of neurotransmitters does not always alter the membrane potential. Recent studies have addressed both of these concerns. It was found that pharmacomechanical coupling results from the activation of nonjunctional α-adrenoceptors in mesenteric arterioles, saphenous artery, and ear artery (44,45,47,83). However, *excitatory junction potentials* are produced in response to nerve stimulation or the application of norepinephrine to the neuromuscular junction. Some earlier measurements of membrane potential distant from the neuromuscular junction did not record the excitatory junction potentials because of electrotonic decay of the potential change. The excitatory junction potentials are accompanied by contractions and can summate to elicit an action potential (44,83). The action potentials are more sensitive to the Ca^{2+} channel inhibitors than are the excitatory junction potentials (7,84), suggesting that the two electrical events are produced by different membrane conductances. Hence, neuromuscular transmission in arteries seems to involve electrical activity and Ca^{2+} channel activation; the efficacy of the Ca^{2+} channel inhibitors may depend on their ability to inhibit this activity.

In order to account for the various effects of the Ca^{2+} channel inhibitors on vascular smooth muscle, a variety of types of Ca^{2+} channels has been invoked that differ in their affinity for the drugs. While there is a firm electrophysiological basis for *multiple types of Ca^{2+} channels* in some tissues (25), no comparable evidence is available for smooth muscle. Ligand-binding studies also do not support the theory of multiple Ca^{2+} channels. This may reflect technical limitations of these techniques, but the possibility that there is only one population of Ca^{2+} channels should not be ignored. Several possibilities should be considered that offer alternatives to multiple populations of Ca^{2+} channels. Neurotransmitters may modify the gating of Ca^{2+} channels so that the number of Ca^{2+} channels that are open at some membrane potentials is altered. This is a well-established phenomenon in cardiac muscle and nerve (33,91). Neurotransmitters could activate Ca^{2+} channels without changing the membrane potential by shifting the voltage-dependence of channel activation to more negative potentials. In addition, some neurotransmitter-induced contractions that depend on external Ca^{2+} may not represent activation of Ca^{2+} channels, as discussed previously. The Ca^{2+} channel inhibitors also may not have unique binding affinities for the channels. Rather, the binding could depend on the state of the channel, and this may be altered by external Ca^{2+}, K^+, or protons, or by neurotransmitters. The block of Na^+ channels by local anesthetics is known to be modified in this way (43), and some of the Ca^{2+} channel inhibitors also seem to interact with the mechanisms that control channel opening in cardiac muscle (72). The idea of variable binding affinities, known as the *modulated receptor hypothesis* in the literature of Na^+ channel blockers, has been very useful in accounting for the tissue specificity and therapeutic usefulness of some antiarrhythmic agents (3). By way of analogy, some tissues may show preferential sensitivity to the Ca^{2+} channel inhibitors because more of their Ca^{2+} channels are in a high-affinity state for the drug.

INTEGRATED HEMODYNAMIC RESPONSE

Most excitable mammalian cells possess Ca^{2+} channels, and therefore many neuroendocrine and muscular sites are available where Ca^{2+} channel inhibitors can alter state and function (10,33,91). In isolated organ studies, the Ca^{2+} channel inhibitors alter cardiac contraction and automaticity, and vascular tone. In the intact animal or humans, the net hemodynamic effects produced by these drugs probably represent a composite of direct actions on the vasculature and on the heart, as well as reflex actions on the vasomotor center which control vessel tone and cardiac function. Generally, the hemodynamic response pattern consists of a decrease in total peripheral resistance, and an increase in cardiac output with less myocardial O_2 consumption (22,39,40,82).

The *decrease in total peripheral resistance* results from dilatation of virtually all major vascular beds; namely, the coronary, cerebral, skeletal muscle, mesenteric, and renal (22). Of the Ca^{2+} channel inhibitors most widely used, nifedipine is most potent, followed by diltiazem and verapamil (22,66,82,98,99). Although the vasodilatation is ubiquitous, there are substantial differences in the magnitude of vasorelaxation between individual organ beds. The coronary, cerebral, and skeletal muscle vascular beds are highly sensitive to these drugs, with the mesenteric and renal beds being less sensitive (22,37,99). Within the coronary bed, electrophysiological studies have revealed that verapamil blocked action potentials elicited by smooth muscle cells from both large and small diameter coronary vessels (6). In contrast, adenosine and nitroglycerin blocked action potentials in either the large or small vessels, but not both, thereby demonstrating a difference between the classes of vasodilators at the electrophysiological level (6,34). Although the renal bed is dilated relatively little by most Ca^{2+} channel inhibitors, autoregulatory responses in anesthetized dogs are effectively antagonized by these drugs (70).

Recently, a new dihydropyridine derivative, nimodipine, has been shown to selectively inhibit serotonin-induced contractions in cerebral vascular muscle strips, but not serotonin-induced contractions in peripheral (saphenous) arterial strips. It was hypothesized that the vascular selectivity of nimodipine was due to heterogeneity of the receptor-operated channel in the two types of vessels (89). Studies in dog, cat, and primate have verified the *cerebral vasodilator actions of nimodipine* while exerting only minimal actions on other vascular beds (36,56,85).

The *venous actions* of the Ca^{2+} channel inhibitors are less well characterized than the arterial actions. Nifedipine and verapamil were shown to inhibit spontaneous contractions of isolated portal venous strips (29,96,97). Interestingly, vasoconstriction produced by norepinephrine in splanchnic veins is attenuated by Ca^{2+} channel inhibitors, whereas contractions in cutaneous veins are far less sensitive to these drugs (96,97). In humans, nifedipine usually produces a slight decrease or no change in left ventricular end-diastolic pressure (59,78,79,82,). Hagemann et al. (32) demonstrated that nifedipine increased the transfusion blood volume needed to elevate blood pressure back to pre-drug levels in the dog. They concluded that nifedipine, indeed, acted predominantly on the arterial vasculature, but that a certain degree of venous pooling occurred due to an effect of nifedipine on capacitance vessels. In contrast, other studies showed that venous capacity was decreased somewhat, and that venous return was increased by nifedipine (31,37,63). The disparity in the data and the heterogeneity of the responsiveness of veins isolated from different organs suggests that actions of the Ca^{2+} channel inhibitors on the venous system are quite complex and that further experimentation is needed.

With regard to *actions on the heart,* isolated tissue studies have shown that the Ca^{2+} channel inhibitors exert negative chronotropic and inotropic actions (39,40,62,). Also, *in vitro* and local administration of the agents predominantly have a slowing effect on sinus and atrioventricular node automacity and conduction, but have little direct effect on atrial and ventricular muscle, or on the His-Purkinje system (1,39,40,54,80). In studies examining the direct actions of nifedipine, verapamil, and diltiazem on atrioventricular conduction time in relation to changes in coronary blood flow, it was found that the threshold dose of nifedipine which produced coronary vasodilatation was about 10-fold less than the dose which prolonged atrioventricular conduction time (68). In contrast, there was no difference between the doses of verapamil and diltiazem which caused vasodilatation and prolongation of atrioventricular conduction. From this and other studies (37,39,40,82), the consensus is that the ratio of cardiac to vascular action is shifted to the vascular side for nifedipine, and toward the cardiac side for verapamil and diltiazem. Possible explanations for the differences between nifedipine and verapamil and diltiazem have focused primarily on different mechanisms of Ca^{2+} channel blockade and differences in the ability to block other ionic currents (39).

Unlike *in vitro* experiments, the Ca^{2+} channel inhibitors usually produce positive chronotropic and inotropic actions in whole-animal studies and man (31, 39,40,62). The disparity between the *in vitro* and *in vivo* data have led to the idea that the cardiac actions observed in the whole animal are baroreceptor reflex-mediated in response to the peripheral vasodilatation (40,55,62,82). However, despite the reflex increase in cardiac function, the reduction in afterload, coupled with a possible direct drug effect, results in a net reduction in myocardial

O_2 demand (40,59,78,79,82,100). It is also worth noting that differences in reflex sympathetic neural outflow possibly contribute to the organ selectivity of the Ca^{2+} channel inhibitors.

Although basic inferences have come from observing cardiac responses, more detailed information on the effects of many of the Ca^{2+} channel inhibitors on *baroreceptor reflexes* have only recently been published (28,38,61,62,67,86,87). In one study, nimodipine inhibited the baroreceptor reflex-induced vagal bradycardia elicited by pressor responses in dogs pretreated with propranolol. Verapamil and diltiazem also inhibited reflex vagal bradycardia, but at higher doses than nimodipine. Interestingly, nifedipine produced very little change in the reflex bradycardia in anesthetized dogs (87). Experiments in conscious dogs confirmed the inhibitory effects of verapamil and diltiazem, but in contrast to studies in the anesthetized dog, nifedipine also inhibited the reflex bradycardia responses (62). At least one site of action is thought to reside in sensory elements in the carotid sinus because: (a) The slope of the curve relating carotid sinus nerve discharge versus pressure change was reduced by verapamil and increased by nifedipine when applied topically onto the sinus area (38); (b) vagal bradycardia elicited by pressure elevations in the isolated carotid sinus were antagonized by nimodipine at the same doses that blocked the bradycardia produced by norepinephrine-induced pressor responses (87); and (c) vagal bradycardia evoked by electrical stimulation of afferent fibers in the carotid sinus nerve was not affected by nimodipine, thereby eliminating a central site of action and inhibition of efferent vagal transmission (87). The mechanism of action at the carotid sinus is not known, but it likely involves modification of Na^+ and/or Ca^{2+} currents. The effects of the Ca^{2+} channel inhibitors have not been investigated on other mechanoreceptor receptors, such as atrial, ventricular, and thoracic vessel receptors.

CONCLUSIONS

A classification of Ca^{2+} antagonists is presented. Ca^{2+} channel inhibitors can be viewed as a subclass of Ca^{2+} antagonists. The major mechanism of action of clinically useful Ca^{2+} antagonists is believed to be the blockade of Ca^{2+} entry into smooth and cardiac muscle rather than inhibition at intracellular sites. The blockade involves interaction of these drugs with specific binding sites, which are probably proteins associated with Ca^{2+} channels or Ca^{2+} channels themselves. Ca^{2+} channel inhibitors differ among themselves substantially in chemical structure and pharmacological profile. There is evidence that binding sites at the sarcolemmal membrane are different for dihydropyridines and non-dihydropyridine drugs of this class.

The basis for therapeutic success of Ca^{2+} channel inhibition is the organ and tissue selectivity of these drugs. Significant differences between drugs exist in the degree of uncoupling of excitation and contraction in cardiac muscle versus vascular or other smooth muscles and among various vascular beds.

Of particular importance, from the point of view of side-effects, is the relative ineffectiveness of some Ca^{2+} antagonists in blocking excitation-secretion coupling. The reasons for the organ and tissue selectivity of Ca^{2+} channel inhibitors are still controversial. Some investigators favor the concept that these drugs bind with different affinities to several populations of Ca^{2+} channels. Alternatively, drug binding to Ca^{2+} channels may be variable due to allosteric interactions between the drugs and the gating of a single type of channel.

In the whole animal, drug distribution and regulatory reflexes influence drug actions. These aspects should be considered in the assessment of the relative selectivity of Ca^{2+} channel inhibitors for various vascular beds.

REFERENCES

1. Antman, E. M., Stone, P. H., Muller, J. E., and Braunwald, E. (1980): *Ann. Int. Med.,* 93:875–885.
2. Atlas, D., and Adler, M. (1981): *Proc. Natl. Acad. Sci. USA,* 78:1237–1241.
3. Bean, B. P., Cohen, C. J., and Tsien, R. W. (1983): *J. Gen. Physiol.,* 81:613–642.
4. Bellemann, P., Ferry, D., Lübbecke, F., and Glossmann, H. (1981): *Arzneim. Forsch.,* 31:2064–2067.
5. Bellemann, P., Ferry, D., Lübbecke, F., and Glossmann, H. (1982): *Arzneim. Forsch.,* 32:361–363.
6. Berne, R. M., Belardinelli, L., Harder, D. R., Sperelakis, N., and Rubio, R. (1980): In: *Calcium-Antagonismus,* edited by A. Fleckenstein and H. Roskamm, pp. 208–220. Springer-Verlag, New York.
7. Blakely, A. G. H., Brown, D. A., Cunnane, T. C., French, A. M., McGrath, J. C., and Scott, N. C. (1981): *Nature,* 294:759–761.
8. Bolger, G. T., Gengo, P., Klockowski, R., Luchowski, E., Siegel, H., Janis, R. A., Triggle, A. M., and Triggle, D. J., (1983): *J. Pharmacol. Exp. Ther.,* 225:291–309.
9. Bolger, G. T., Gengo, P. J., Luchowski, E. M., Siegel, H., Triggle, D. J., and Janis, R. A. (1982): *Biochem. Biophys. Res. Commun.,* 104:1604–1609.
10. Bolton, T. B. (1979): *Physiol. Rev.,* 59:606–718.
11. Boström, S. L., Ljung, B., Mardh, S., Forsen, S., and Thulin, E. (1981): *Nature,* 292:777–778.
12. Chapman, R. A. (1979): *Prog. Biophys. Mol. Biol.,* 35:1–52.
13. Colvin, R. A., Pearson, N., Messineo, F. C., and Katz, A. M. (1982): *J. Cardiovasc. Pharmacol.,* 4:935–941.
14. Coraboeuf, E. (1974): *J. Mol. Cell. Cardiol.,* 6:215–225.
15. Coraboeuf, E. (1980): In: *4th International Adalat Symposium,* edited by P. Puech and R. Krebs, pp. 3–13. Excerpta Medica, Amsterdam.
16. De Mey, J., and Vanhoutte, P. M. (1981): *Circ. Res.,* 48:875–884.
17. DePover, A., Matlib, M. A., Lee, S. W., Dubé, G. P., Grupp, G., Grupp, I. L., and Schwartz, A. (1982): *Biochem. Biophys. Res. Commun.,* 108:110–117.
18. Einwachter, H. M., Haas, H. G., and Kern, R. (1972): *J. Physiol.,* 227:141–171.
19. Ehlert, F. J., Itoga, E., Roeske, W. R., and Yamamura, H. I. (1982): *Biochem. Biophys. Res. Commun.,* 104:937–943.
20. Ehlert, F. J., Roeske, W. R., Itoga, E., and Yamamura, H. I. (1982): *Life Sci.,* 30:2191–2202.
21. Epstein, P. M., Fiss, K., Hachisu, R., and Adrenyak, D. M. (1982): *Biochem. Biophys. Res. Commun.,* 105:1142–1149.
22. Flaim, S. F., and Kanda, K. (1982): In: *Calcium Blockers—Mechanisms of Action and Clinical Applications,* edited by S. F. Flaim and R. Zelis, pp. 179–192. Urban & Schwarzenberg, Baltimore.
23. Flaim, S. F. (1982): In: *Calcium Blockers—Mechanisms of Action and Clinical Applications,* edited by S. F. Flaim and R. Zelis, pp. 155–178. Urban & Schwarzenberg, Baltimore.

24. Fleckenstein, A. (1977): *Ann. Rev. Pharmacol. Toxicol.*, 17:149–166.
25. Fox, A. P., and Krasne, S. (1981): *Biophys. J.*, 33:145a (abstract).
26. Frelin, C., Vigne, P., and Lazdunski, M. (1982): *Biochem. Biophys. Res. Commun.*, 106:967–973.
27. Furukawa, K., Itoh, T., Kajiwara, M., Kitamura, K., Suzuki, H., Itol, Y., and Kuriyama, H. (1981): *J. Pharmacol. Exp. Ther.*, 218:249–259.
28. Goldman, W. F., and Saum, W. R. (1982): *Fed. Proc.*, 40:544.
29. Golenhofen, K., Hermstein, N., and Lammel, E. (1973): *Microvasc. Res.*, 5:73–80.
30. Gould, R. J., Murphy, K. M. M., and Snyder, S. H. (1982): *Proc. Natl. Acad. Sci. USA*, 79:3656–3660.
31. Gross, R., Kirchheim, H., and von Olshausen, K. (1979): *Arzneim. Forsch.*, 29:1361–1368.
32. Hagemann, K., Lochner, W., and Niehues, B. (1975): In: *2nd International Adalat Symposium*, edited by W. Lochner, W. Braasch, G. Kroneberg, pp. 49–54. Excerpta Medica, Amsterdam.
33. Hagiwara, S., and Byerly, L. (1981): *Annu. Rev. Neurosci.*, 4:69–125.
34. Harder, D. R., Belardinelli, L., Sperelakis, N., Rubio, R., and Berne, R. M. (1979): *Circ. Res.*, 44:176–182.
35. Harder, D. R. (1982): In: *Vascular Smooth Muscle: Metabolic, Ionic, and Contractile Mechanisms*, edited by M. F. Crass, III and C. D. Barnes, pp. 71–97. Academic Press, New York.
36. Harper, A. M., Craigen, L., and Kazda, S. (1981): *J. Cerebr. Blood Flow Metab.*, 1:349–356.
37. Hashimoto, K., Taira, N., Ono, H., Chiba, S., Hashimoto, K., Endoh, M., Kokubun, M., Kokubun, H., Iijima, T., Kimura, T., Kubota, K., and Ogura, K. (1975): In: *1st International Adalat Symposium*, edited by K. Hashimoto, E. Kimura, and T. Kobayashi, pp. 11–22. University of Tokyo Press, Tokyo.
38. Heesch, C. M., Thames, M. D., and Abboud, F. M. (1982): *Fed. Proc.*, 41:1116.
39. Henry, P. D. (1982): In: *Calcium Blockers—Mechanisms of Action and Clinical Applications*, edited by S. F. Flaim and R. Zelis, pp. 135–153. Urban & Schwarzenberg, Baltimore.
40. Henry, P. D. (1980): *Am. J. Cardiol.*, 46:1047–1058.
41. Hermsmeyer, K. (1983): In: *Calcium Entry Blockers, Adenosine, and Neurohumors: Recent Advances*, edited by G. F. Merrill and H. R. Weiss, pp. 51–62. Urban & Schwarzenberg, Baltimore.
42. Hescheler, J., Pelzer, D., Trube, G., and Trautwein, W. (1982): *Pfluegers Arch.*, 393:287–291.
43. Hille, B. (1978): In: *Biophysical Aspects of Cardiac Muscle*, edited by M. Morad, pp. 55–74. Academic Press, New York.
44. Hirst, G. D. S., and Neild, T. O. (1980): *Nature*, 283:767–768.
45. Hirst, G. D. S., and Neild, T. O. (1981): *J. Physiol. (Lond.)*, 313:343–350.
46. Holck, M., Thorens, S., and Haeusler, G. (1982): *Eur. J. Pharmacol.*, 85:303–315.
47. Holman, M. E. and, Surprenant, A. M. (1979): *J. Physiol. (Lond.)*, 287:337–351.
48. Janis, R. A. (1981): In: *The Mechanism of Gated Calcium Transport Across Biological Membranes*, edited by S. T. Ohnishi and M. Endo, pp. 101–110. Academic Press, New York.
49. Janis, R. A., Maurer, S. C., Sarmiento, J. G., Bolger, G. T., and Triggle, D. J. (1982): *Eur. J. Pharmacol.*, 82:191–194.
50. Janis, R. A., and Triggle, D. J. (1983): *J. Med. Chem.*, 26:775–785.
51. Johansson, B., and Somlyo, A. P. (1980): In: *Handbook of Physiology*, Vol. II, Section 2, edited by D. F. Bohr, A. P. Somlyo, and H. V. Sparks, Jr., pp. 301–323. American Physiological Society, Bethesda.
52. Kanamori, M., Naka, M., Asano, M., and Hidaka, H. (1981): *J. Pharmacol. Exp. Ther.*, 217:494–499.
53. Karaki, H., and Weiss, G. B. (1981): *Blood Vessels*, 18:28–35.
54. Kass, R. S., and Scheuer, T. (1982): In: *Calcium Blockers—Mechanism of Action and Clinical Applications*, edited by S. F. Flaim and R. Zelis, pp. 3–19. Urban & Schwarzenberg, Baltimore.
55. Kawai, C., Konishi, T., Matsuyama, E., and Okazaki, H. (1981): *Circulation*, 63:1035–1042.
56. Kazda, S., Garthoff, B., Krause, H. P., and Schlossmann, K. (1982): *Arzneim. Forsch.*, 32:331–338.
57. Lee, K. S., and Tsien, R. W. (1982): *Nature*, 297:498–501.
58. Levin, R. M., and Weiss, B. (1979): *J. Pharmacol. Exp. Ther.*, 208:454–459.
59. Lichtlen, P., Engel, H. J., Amende, I., Rafflenbeul, W., and Simon, R. (1976): In: *3rd Interna-*

tional Adalat Symposium, edited by A. D. Jatene and P. R. Lichtlen, pp. 14–29. Excerpta Medica, Amsterdam.

60. Mikkelsen, E., and Lederballe Pedersen, O. L. (1981): *Br. J. Pharmacol.*, 73:799–805.

61. Millard, R. W., Gabel, M., Fowler, N. O., and Schwartz, A. (1982): *Fed. Proc.*, 41:1632.

62. Millard, R. W., Lathrop, D. A., Grupp, G., Ashraf, M., Grupp, I. L., and Schwartz, A. (1982): *Am. J. Cardiol.*, 49:499–506.

63. Mostbeck, A., Partsch, H., and Peschi, L. (1975): In: *1st International Adalat Symposium*, edited by K. Hashimoto, E. Kimura, and T. Kobayashi, pp. 136–143. University of Tokyo Press, Tokyo.

64. Murphy, K. M. M., Gould, R. J., and Snyder, S. H. (1984): In: *Nitrendipine*, edited by A. Scriabine, S. Vanov, and K. Deck. Urban & Schwarzenberg, Baltimore.

65. Murphy, K. M. M., and Snyder, S. H. (1982): *Eur. J. Pharmacol.*, 77:201–202.

66. Nagao, T., Sato, M., Nakajima, H., and Kiyomoto, A. (1972): *Jpn. J. Pharmacol.*, 22:1–10.

67. Nakaya, H., Schwartz, A., and Millard, R. W. (1982): *Fed. Proc.*, 41:1688.

68. Narimatsu, A., and Taira, N. (1976): *Naunyn Schmiedebergs Arch. Pharmacol.*, 294:169–177.

69. Nayler, W. G., Thompson, J. E., and Jarrott, B. (1982): *J. Mol. Cell. Cardiol.*, 14:185–188.

70. Ono, H., Kokubun, H., and Hashimoto, K. (1974): *Naunyn Schmiedebergs Arch. Pharmacol.*, 285:201–207.

71. Pan, M., and Janis, R. A. (1982): *Biochem. Pharmacol.* (*in press*).

72. Pelzer, D., Trautwein, W., and McDonald, T. F. (1982): *Pfluegers Arch.*, 394:97–105.

73. Piascik, M. F., Rahwan, R. G., and Witiak, D. T. (1979): *J. Pharmacol. Exp. Ther.*, 210:141–146.

74. Prozialeck, W. C., and Weiss, B. (1982): *J. Pharmacol. Exp. Ther.*, 222:509–516.

75. Rosenberger, L. B., Ticku, M. K., and Triggle, D. J. (1979): *Can. J. Physiol. Pharmacol.*, 57:333–347.

76. Roufogalis, B. D. (1981): *Biochem. Biophys. Res. Commun.*, 96:607–613.

77. Sarmiento, J. G., Janis, R. A., Colvin, R. A., Triggle, D. J., and Katz, A. M. (1983): *J. Mol. Cell. Cardiol.*, 15:135–138.

78. Schulz, W., and Kaltenbach, M. (1981): *Cardiology*, 68 (Suppl. 2):200–208.

79. Serruys, P. W., Brower, R. W., Ten Katen, H. J., Bom, A. H., and Hugenholtz, P. G. (1981): *Circulation*, 63:584–591.

80. Singh, B. N., Nademanee, K., and Feld, G. (1982): In: *Calcium Blockers—Mechanisms of Action and Clinical Applications*, edited by S. F. Flaim and R. Zelis, pp. 245–264. Urban & Schwarzenberg, Baltimore.

81. Spedding, M. (1982): *Br. J. Pharmacol.*, 75:25c (abstract).

82. Stone, P. H., Antman, E. M., Muller, J. E., and Braunwald, E. (1980): *Ann. Int. Med.*, 93:886–904.

83. Surprenant, A. (1980): *Pfluegers Arch.*, 386:85–91.

84. Suzuki, H., Itoh, T., and Kuriyama, H. (1982): *Am. J. Physiol.*, 242:H325–H336.

85. Tanaka, K., Gotoh, F., Muramatsu, F., Fukuuchi, Y., Amano, T., Okayasu, H., and Suzuki, N. (1980): *Arzneim. Forsch.* (*Drug Res.*), 9:1494–1497.

86. Taylor, D. G., and Kowalski, T. E. (1983): In: *Calcium Entry Blockers, Adenosine and Neurohumors*, edited by G. F. Merrill and H. R. Weiss pp. 137–153. Urban & Schwarzenberg, Baltimore.

87. Taylor, D. G., and Kowalski, T. E. (1982): *Fed. Proc.*, 41:1588.

88. Tomita, T. (1981): In: *Smooth Muscle: An Assessment of Current Knowledge*, edited by E. Bülbring, A. W. Jones, and T. Tomita, pp. 127–156. University of Texas Press, Austin.

89. Towart, R. (1981): *Circ. Res.*, 48:650–657.

90. Triggle, D. J. (1981): In: *New Perspectives on Calcium Antagonists*, edited by G. B. Weiss, pp. 1–18. American Physiological Society, Bethesda.

91. Tsien, R. W. (1983): *Annu. Rev. Physiol.*, 45:341–358.

92. Vághy, P. L., Johnson, J. D., Matlib, M. A., Wang, T., and Schwartz, A. (1982): *J. Biol. Chem.*, 257:6000–6002.

93. van Breemen, C., Aaranson, P. I., Cauvin, C. A., Loutzenhiser, R. D., Mangel, A. W., and Saida, K. (1982). In: *Calcium Blockers—Mechanisms of Action and Clinical Applications*, edited by S. Flaim and R. Zelis, pp. 121–134. Urban & Schwarzenberg, Baltimore.

94. van Breemen, C., Hwang, O., and Meisheri, K. D. (1981): *J. Pharmacol. Exp. Ther.*, 218:459–463.

95. Vanhoutte, P. M. (1982): *Circulation*, 65 (Suppl. I):I11–I19.

96. Van Nueten, J. M., and Vanhoutee, P. M. (1981): *Fed. Proc.*, 40:2862–2865.
97. Van Zwieten, P. A., Van Meel, J. C. A., and Timmermans, P. B. M. W. M. (1981): *Pharmaceutisch Weekblad*, 3:237–247.
98. Vater, W., Kroneberg, G., and Hoffmeister, F., Saller, H., Meng, K., Oberdorf, A., Puls, W., Schlossmann, K., and Stoepel, K. (1972): *Arzneim. Forsch.*, 22:1–14.
99. Vater, W., and Schlossmann, K. (1976): In: *3rd International Adalat Symposium*, edited by A. D. Jatene and P. R. Lichtlen, pp. 33–41. Excerpta Medica, Amsterdam.
100. Walus, K. M., Fondacaro, J. D., and Jacobson, E. D. (1981): *Circ. Res.*, 48:692–700.
101. Weiss, B., Prozialeck, W. C., and Wallace, T. G. (1982): *Biochem. Pharmacol.*, 31:2217–2230.
102. Weiss, G. B. (1982): In: *Calcium Blockers—Mechanisms of Action and Clinical Applications*, edited by S. F. Flaim and R. Zelis, p. 135–153. Urban & Schwarzenberg, Baltimore.
103. Wiggins, J. R., and Bassett, A. L. (1976): *Eur. J. Pharmacol.*, 37:217–220.
104. Williams, L. T., and Tremble, P. (1982): *J. Clin. Invest.*, 70:209–212.
105. Williams, L. T., and Jones, L. R. (1983): *J. Biol. Chem.* 258:5344–5347.

Calcium Antagonists and Cardiovascular Disease, edited by L. H. Opie.
Raven Press, New York © 1984.

Chapter 15

Structural/Activity Relationships in Calcium Antagonists

H. Meyer

Chemical Research Laboratories, Pharmaceutical Division, Bayer AG Wuppertal-Elberfeld, Federal Republic of Germany

Fifteen years have now passed since A. Fleckenstein published his pioneering work in which he described Ca^{2+} antagonism as the fundamental mode of action of the coronary therapeutics, prenylamine and verapamil (7). Meanwhile, numerous drugs with completely different pharmacological qualities have been designated as Ca^{2+} antagonists (35,36,47). The majority of these agents, however, only exert a weak, nonspecific inhibitory action upon the influx of extracellular Ca^{2+} through the slow Ca^{2+} channel in the cell membrane. Inorganic cations such as Mn^{2+}, Co^{2+}, La^{3+}, on the other hand, must be regarded as general, unspecific Ca^{2+} antagonists which can replace Ca^{2+} at the latter's binding sites (38).

"Specific" Ca^{2+} antagonists, according to Fleckenstein's definition, are therapeutic agents with a vasodilatory action in which the Ca^{2+} antagonistic effect predominates both qualitatively and quantitatively. Vasodilators of the aralkylamine type, such as prenylamine, fendiline, cinnarizine, diltiazem, bencyclan, verapamil, gallopamil, and tiapamil, come particularly to mind (Fig. 1).

These Ca^{2+} antagonists are structurally related in that they all have an aryl ring, frequently alkoxy substituted, which is connected to an alkylamino or aralkylamino group. This analogy suggests similar, if not the same, binding sites for this group of drugs. Binding studies with ³H-cinnarizine support this hypothesis. A saturable binding site in smooth muscle can be blocked by the verapamil analog, gallopamil (8).

Ca^{2+} antagonistic structures without an essential basic structure have been found in the form of 4-aryl-1,4-dihydropyridinedicarboxylates (4,5,15,23)—the standard agent is nifedipine—and, latterly, in the benzthiazolylbenzylphosphonates of the KB-944 type (32) (Fig. 2).

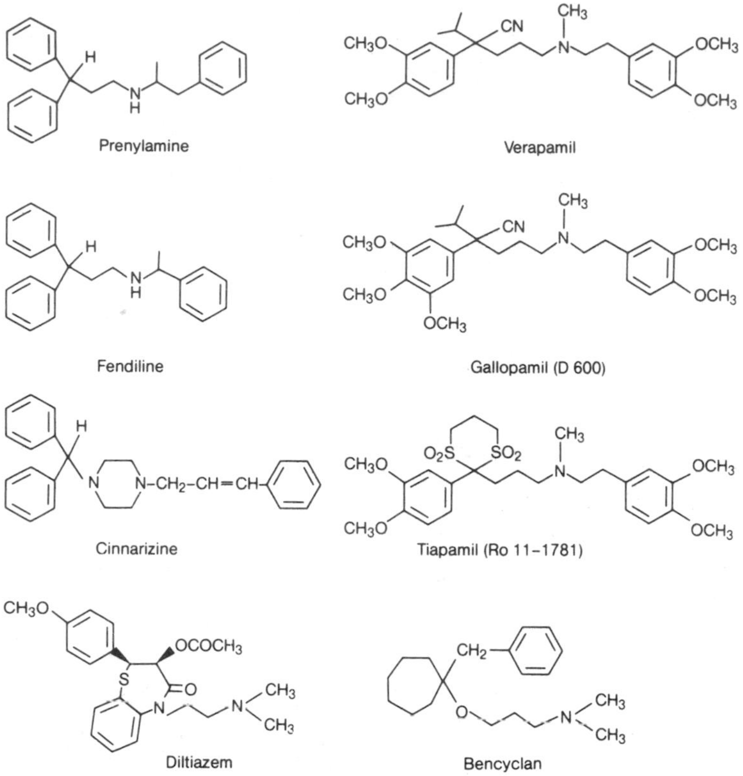

FIG. 1. The aralkylamine group of Ca²⁺ antagonists.

The 1,4-dihydropyridine, nimodipine, is only displaced from its binding sites (cerebral membranes) by a more than a thousandfold greater concentration of aralkylamine-type Ca²⁺ antagonists such as verapamil or fendiline; diltiazem does not bind at all (2). These observations confirm the postulate, based on the completely different structural features, that the 1,4-dihydropyridines represent a class of Ca²⁺ antagonists in their own right.

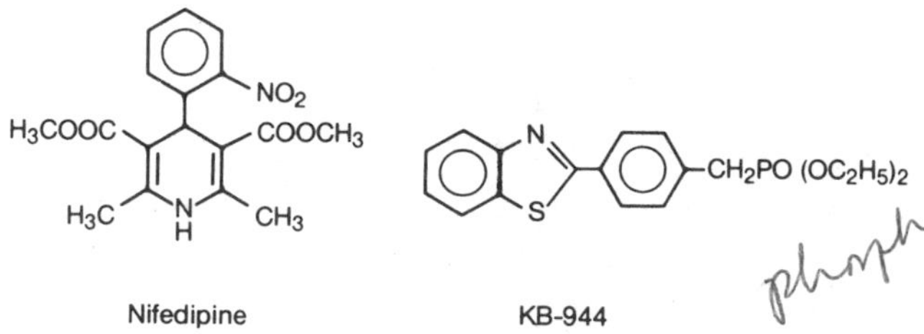

FIG. 2. Nonbasic Ca²⁺-antagonistic structures.

VERAPAMIL

Qualitative structure-activity studies in the verapamil series (coronary blood flow in the dog) have indicated 3,4-dimethoxy and 3,4,5-trimethoxy (gallopamil, D 600) to be the optimal substitution pattern in the left-hand benzene ring. Of the other substituents investigated only a *meta*-trifluoromethyl group was tolerated without loss of activity when the aromatic substituent R^1 was varied, the remaining functionality being held constant (9,17).

Quantitative structure-activity correlations were found with a similar collection of compounds studied for negative inotropic activity on cat papillary muscle (18,19). According to this work, the substitution of the phenyl ring neighboring the chiral center had the greatest influence on activity. Good correlations of activity with the electronic parameter σ and the steric parameter mv (molar volume) show that activity decreases with diminishing electron density of the substituted phenyl ring and, simultaneously, is also dependent upon the steric requirement of the substitution. Interestingly, lipophilic parameters provided no useful correlations.

Replacement of the isopropyl group in verapamil by ethyl, or of the methoxy group by hydroxy, led to compounds of weaker activity, as did dealkylation of the nitrogen atom.

The chiral center at the benzylic carbon atom is of significance with regard to the quality of activity, but not critical. In general the S(−)-enantiomers of verapamil and gallopamil are more active than the R (+)-antipodes in various experimental models (1,12,16). Starting with the knowledge that the quaternary benzylic carbon atom of verapamil is an essential structural element, but that the replacement of the nitrile function and the isopropyl group (which can be advantageously replaced by long-chain aliphatic substituents) is tolerated within certain limits, a non-chiral verapamil analog with comparable qualities was found in tiapamil (Ro 11–1781). The main metabolites are the products resulting from dealkylation at nitrogen (37) (Fig. 3).

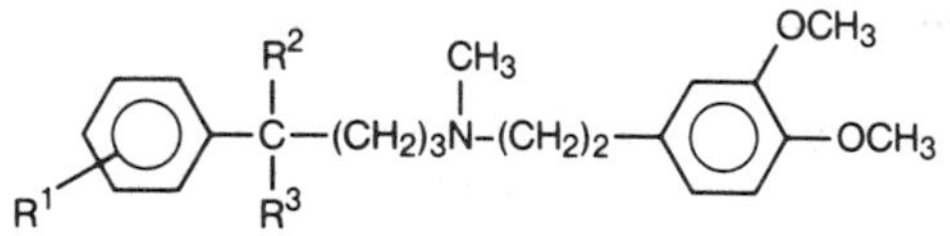

Verapamil	$R^1 = 3,4\text{-}(OCH_3)_2$	$R^2 = CH(CH_3)_2$	$R^3 = CN$
Gallopamil	$R^1 = 3,4,5\text{-}(OCH_3)_3$	$R^2 = CH(CH_3)_2$	$R^3 = CN$
Tiapamil	$R^1 = 3,4\text{-}(OCH_3)_2$	$R^2, R^3 = SO_2(CH_2)_3SO_2$	

FIG. 3. The verapamil group.

Metabolic studies on ^{14}C-verapamil in rats and dogs pinpointed the ether cleavage of the methoxy groups in both benzene rings as a major step in the biotransformation, in addition to the dealkylation at nitrogen (20).

DILTIAZEM

Stereoselectivity in the pharmacological activity has been observed in the diltiazem series just as in the verapamil group (Fig. 4).

Apart from having two chiral centers (C_2 and C_3), the diltiazem molecule is also capable of *cis-trans* isomerism at these two carbon atoms. In general, the *trans* compounds are devoid of vasodilating properties. The laevorotatory *cis*-enantiomer of diltiazem has a 10-fold longer duration of activity than its dextrorotatory antipode (i.e., diltiazem itself) in increasing blood flow in the canine coronary sinus.

The scope for variation of the substitution in the noncondensed aromatic ring is limited. Introduction of further alkoxy substituents or replacement of a methoxy group by hydroxy are accompanied by a drop in activity. Only the replacement of methoxy by *para*-methyl is tolerated without any marked loss of activity (33). In the condensed aromatic ring, substitution with chlorine in the 7-position is possible; other substitution patterns lead to a weakening of activity.

The alkylaminoalkyl substitution at the N_5 atom is essential for activity. Dealkylation or quaternization at the terminal nitrogen lead to almost inactive products. The possibilities for replacement of the acetoxy function at C_3 are more flexible. Substitution by hydroxy, alkoxy, or aralkoxy provides products with comparable activity to diltiazem, as does the replacement of the acetoxy group by longer-chain aliphatic or aromatic acyloxy groups. The 3-hydroxy compound, itself active, is one of the major metabolites of diltiazem (22), thus making the broad variability of substitution at this O atom plausible. Other primary steps in the biotransformation of diltiazem are demethylation at the terminal nitrogen, ether cleavage of the *para*-methoxy group and oxidative hy-

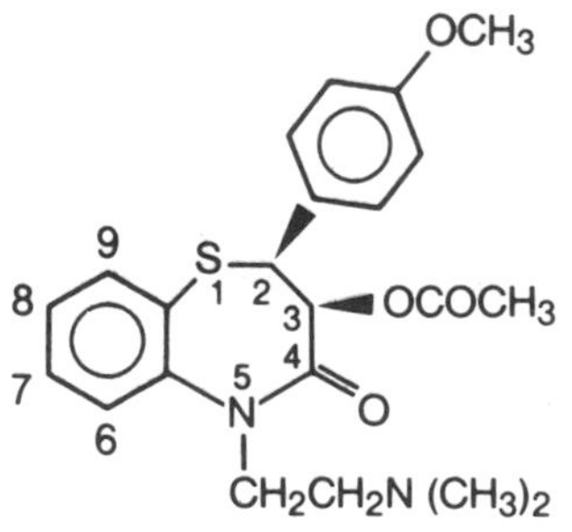

FIG. 4. Diltiazem.

? The bippyridene milrenone
is the metapsil

droxylation in one of the two aromatic rings. The secondary metabolites exhibit combinations of these primary steps.

NIFEDIPINE

4-Aryl-1,4-dihydropyridine-3,5-dicarboxylates of the nifedipine type represent a completely new group of Ca^{2+} antagonists not having an essential basic function (Fig. 5).

Numerous studies on the elucidation of structure-activity relationships have been carried out in this class owing to the wide variability of the active structure and its superior intensity of activity. Good vasodilatory activity is to be expected under the following conditions (4,15): (a) No substitution at nitrogen ($R^1 =$ H); (b) substitution at C_2 and C_6 (R^2,R^6) by a lower alkyl group, preferably methyl [replacement of an alkyl group by amino (24,28), cyano, or formyl is tolerated, but hydrogen or aryl weaken the activity]; (c) carboxylic ester functions are optimal substituents at C_3 and C_5 (R^3,R^5). One of these can be replaced by acyl, nitrile, or sulphonyl with some loss of activity. The aliphatic or araliphatic alcohol component of the ester functions is variable in terms of chain length, branching, degree of saturation, and heterosubstitution (3,11). The ester groups mainly affect vascular selectivity and duration of activity. (d) The degree of activity is mainly determined by the substituent in the 4-position (R^4); substitution by an aromatic or heteroaromatic ring here is essential for optimal activity. For monosubstitution of a 4-phenyl residue the following, simplified rules are valid: *Ortho*-substitution is superior to *meta*. In the *meta* series, only the nitro group provides activity comparable to that of *ortho*-substituted compounds. *Para*-substituted compounds are practically inactive. Acceptor substituents such as NO_2, CN, CF_3, SO_2 alkyl, Cl, etc., intensify the activity in comparison to donor substituents. Hydrophilic substituents such as amino or hydroxy lead to a drop, if not total loss, in activity. Disubstitution is acceptable when in the *ortho* and/or *meta* positions, making 2,3-, 2,5-, and 2,6-disubstitutions of particular interest.

With the aid of Hansch analysis, certain physicochemical substituent properties have been related quantitatively to the negative inotropic effect on cat papil-

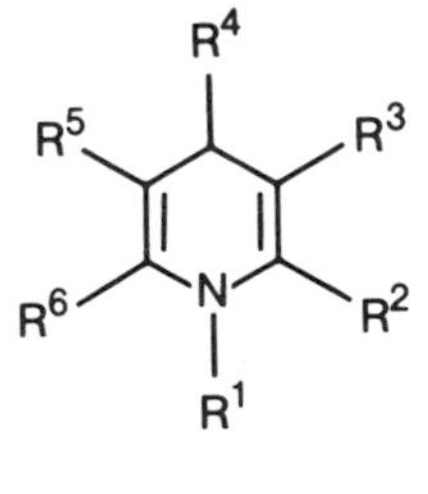

FIG. 5. General structure of dihydropyridine Ca^{2+} antagonists.

lary muscle, for a small selection of dihydropyridine derivatives (39). In this test model, the steric influence of the substituents in the 4-phenyl group was much more significant than their lipophilic and electronic properties. To a certain extent, this finding disagreed with qualitatively assessed relationships (e.g., antihypertensive effect in spontaneously hypertensive rats). In a series of 4-(3-nitrophenyl)-1,4-dihydropyridines with varied ester groups, increasing lipophilicity and/or an increasing volume caused a decrease in negative inotropic effect. A quantitative relationship between Ca^{2+} antagonistic properties of substituted 4-phenyldihydropyridines and the torsion angle at C_4 of the dihydropyridine core has been demonstrated in a small series (46).

The most active Ca^{2+}-antagonistic nifedipine analogs—nicardipine (43), nitrendipine (25), nimodipine (27), nisoldipine (13), felodipine (6), FR 34235 (48), PN 200–110 (10)—conform structurally to all the qualitative and quantitative structure-activity relationships just described (Fig. 6). One important characteristic of all these products is the nonidentity of the carboxylate groups in the 3- and 5-positions. Dihydropyridine Ca^{2+} antagonists with nonidentical ester groups have, in most cases, a higher vasodilatory or antihypertensive activity than their symmetrically substituted counterparts (25).

Nonidentical substituents in the 3- and 5-positions make the 1,4-dihydropyridine molecule chiral (Fig. 7). It can thus exist in two enantiomeric forms which differ in their absolute configuration at the C_4 carbon atom and in their direction of optical rotation. It has been shown for a series of products that the enantiomers exhibit significantly different *in vitro* and *in vivo* activities in several test models (41,42,45).

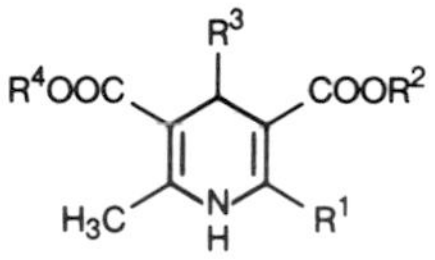

	R^1	R^2	R^3	R^4
Nifedipine	CH_3	CH_3	$2-NO_2-C_6H_4$	CH_3
Nicardipine	CH_3	$CH_2CH_2N\overset{CH_2C_6H_5}{\underset{CH_3}{}}$	$3-NO_2-C_6H_4$	CH_3
Nitrendipine	CH_3	C_2H_5	$3-NO_2-C_6H_4$	CH_3
Nimodipine	CH_3	$CH_2CH_2OCH_3$	$3-NO_2-C_6H_4$	$CH(CH_3)_2$
Nisoldipine	CH_3	CH_3	$2-NO_2-C_6H_4$	$CH_2CH(CH_3)_2$
Felodipine	CH_3	C_2H_5	$2,3-Cl_2-C_6H_3$	CH_3
FR 34235	CN	CH_3	$3-NO_2-C_6H_4$	$CH(CH_3)_2$
PN 200–110	CH_3	CH_3	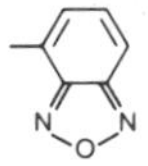	$CH(CH_3)_2$

FIG. 6. The nifedipine group.

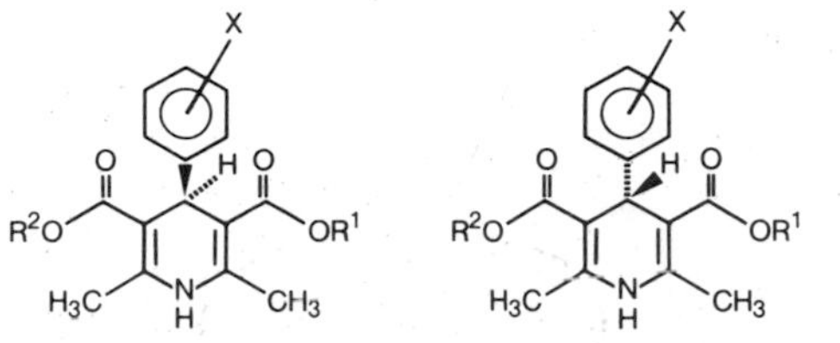

FIG. 7. Chirality of unsymmetrical 1,4-dihydropyridines.

The metabolic breakdown of dihydropyridine Ca²⁺ antagonists follows the principle of increasing hydrophilicity starting from the comparably lipophilic primary structure (14,21,27,34,44). The biotransformation of nitrendipine is a good example of this (40) (Fig. 8).

The first step is oxidation to the pyridine derivative, practically devoid of vasodilatory activity, which is followed by saponification of one of the two ester functions to give the pyridine-monocarboxylic acid. The final products of biotransformation are the hydroxymethyl-pyridine-carboxylic acids resulting from oxidative hydroxylation of the methyl group neighboring the carboxylic acid function. These are characterized as their corresponding γ-lactones after acidification.

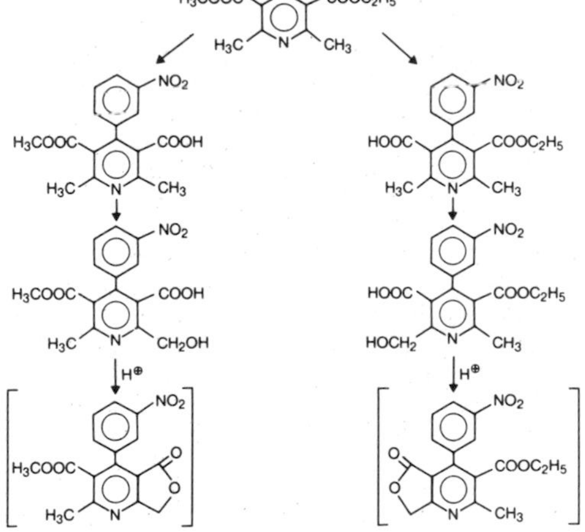

FIG. 8. Metabolic pathway of nitrendipine.

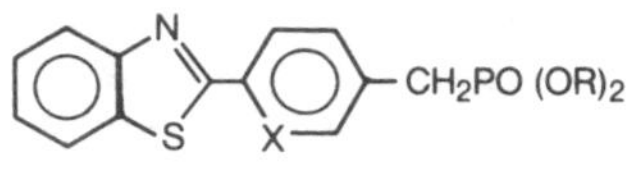

FIG. 9. Arakyl phosphonate Ca^{2+} antagonists.

KB-944   X=CH   R=C_2H_5

KB-944

The new Ca^{2+}-antagonistic structure of the (benzothiazol-2-yl)-dialkoxy-phosphinylmethylbenzenes and pyridines of the KB-944 type also has no essential basic structure (Fig. 9).

KB-944 is similar to diltiazem both in terms of pharmacological profile and of level of activity. That is, the dosages used in animal experiments are 10-to-50-fold higher than the limiting doses attainable with nifedipine (3,26,29,32). According to the activity data available, the introduction of a pyridine nitrogen ($X = N$) and variations in the alkoxy substitution at the phosphorus atom (OR) are possible without loss of activity.

SUMMARY

Ca^{2+} antagonists can be divided into several groups with regard to their essential active structure. In the case of verapamil, diltiazem, nifedipine, and their analogs, some qualitative and quantitative structure/activity relationship can be deduced. The metabolic pathways are discussed with this background.

REFERENCES

1. Bayer, R., Kalusche, D., Kaufmann, R., and Mannhold, R. (1975): *Naunyn Schmiedebergs Arch. Pharmacol.*, 290:81–97.
2. Bellemann, P., and Schade A. (1983): In: *Proceedings of "Cell Surface Receptors,"* edited by P. G. Strange. Ellis Horwood Publishing, Chichester, United Kingdom (*in press*).
3. Bossert, F., Horstmann, H., Meyer, H., and Vater, W. (1979): *Arzneim. Forsch.*, 29:226–229.
4. Bossert, F., Meyer, H., and Wehinger, E. (1981): *Angew. Chem. (Engl.),* 20:762–769.
5. Bossert, F., and Vater, W. (1971): *Naturwissenschaften,* 58:578.
6. Ek, B., Ahnoff, M., Hallbäck-Nordlander, M., and Ljung, B. (1980): *Arch. Pharmacol.,* 313: Suppl. R 37.
7. Fleckenstein, A., Kammermeier, H., Döring, H. J., and Freund, H. J. (1967): *Z. Kreislauff.,* 56:716–744, 839–858.
8. Godfraind, T., and Morel, N. (1977): *Eur. J. Pharmacol.* 41:245–246.
9. Haas, H., and Busch, E. (1967): *Arzneim. Forsch.,* 17:257–272.
10. Hof, R. B., Vuorela, H. J., Hof, A., and Neumann, B. (1982): *International Symposium on Calcium Modulators,* Venice, (Abstracts, p. 103).
11. Iwanami, M., Shibanuma, T., Fujimoto, M., Kawai, R., Tamazawa, K., Takenaka, T., Takahashi, K., and Murakami, M. (1979): *Chem. Pharm. Bull. (Tokyo),* 27:1426–1440.
12. Jim, K., Harris, A., Rosenberger, L. B., and Triggle, D. J. (1981): *Eur. J. Pharmacol.,* 76:67–72.

13. Kazda, S., Garthoff, B., Meyer, H., Scholssmann, K., Stoepel, K., Towart, R., Vater, W., and Wehinger, E. (1980): *Arzneim. Forsch.,* 30:2144–2162.
14. Kondo, S., Kuchiki, A., Yamamoto, K., Akimoto, K., Takahashi, K., Awata, N., and Sugimoto, I. (1980): *Chem. Pharm. Bull (Tokyo),* 28:1–7.
15. Loev, B., Goodman, M. M., Snader, K. M., Tedeschi, R., and Macko, E. (1974): *J. Med. Chem.,* 17:956–965.
16. Ludwig, C., and Nawrath, H. (1977): *Br. J. Pharmacol.,* 59:411–417.
17. Mannhold, R., and Bayer, R. (1976): *Arch. Pharmacol.,* 293: Suppl. R21.
18. Mannhold, R., Steiner, R., Haas, W., and Kaufmann, R. (1978): *Naunyn Schmiedebergs Arch. Pharmacol.,* 302:217–226.
19. Mannhold, R., Zierden, P., Bayer, R., Rodenkirchen, R., and Steiner, R. (1981): *Arzneim. Forsch.,* 31:773–780.
20. McIlhenny, H. M. (1971): *J. Med. Chem.,* 14:1178–1184.
21. Medenwald, H., Schlossmann, K., and Wünsche, C. (1972): *Arzneim. Forsch.,* 22:53–56.
22. Meshi, T., Sugihara, J., and Sato, Y. (1971): *Chem. Pharm. Bull. (Tokyo),* 19:1546–1556.
23. Meyer, H. (1982): In: *Annual Reports in Medicinal Chemistry,* edited by H.-J. Hess, pp. 71–77. Academic Press, New York.
24. Meyer, H., Bossert, F., and Horstmann, H. (1977): *Liebigs Ann. Chem.,* 1977:1895–1908.
25. Meyer, H., Bossert, F., Wehinger, E., Stoepel, K., and Vater, W. (1981): *Arzneim. Forsch.,* 31:407–409.
26. Meyer, H., Scherling, D., and Kah, W. (1983): *Arzneim. Forsch. (in press).*
27. Meyer, H., Wehinger, E., Bossert, F., and Scherling, D. (1983): *Arzneim. Forsch.,* 33: 106–112.
28. Meyer, H., Wehinger, E., Bossert, F., Stoepel, K., and Vater, W. (1981): *Arzneim. Forsch.,* 31:1173–1177.
29. Morita, T., Fukuda, T., Sukamoto, T., Tajima, S., Sato, I., Ikeda, Y., Kanazawa, T., Hamada, Y., Morimoto, Y., Kitamura, H., Kawakami, K., Ito, K., and Nose, T. (1982): *Arzneim. Forsch.,* 32:1060–1068.
30. Morita, T., Ito, K., and Nose, T. (1982): *Arzneim. Forsch.,* 32: 1053–1056.
31. Morita, T., Kanazawa, T., Ito, K., and Nose, T. (1982): *Arzneim. Forsch.,* 32:1043–1046.
32. Morita, T., Yoshino, K., Kanazawa, T., Ito, K., and Nose, T. (1982): *Arzneim. Forsch.,* 32:1037–1042.
33. Nagao, T., Sato, M., Nakajima, H., and Kiyomoto, A. (1973): *Chem. Pharm. Bull. (Tokyo),* 21:92–97.
34. Parker, S. E., and Weinstock, J. (1973): *J. Med. Chem.,* 16:34–37.
35. Rahwan, R. G., Piascik, M. F., and Witiak, D. T. (1979): *Can. J. Physiol. Pharmacol.,* 57: 443–460.
36. Rahwan, R. G., Witiak, D. T., and Muir, W. W. (1981): In: *Annual Reports in Medicinal Chemistry,* edited by H.-J. Hess, pp. 257–268. Academic Press, New York.
37. Ramuz, H. (1978): *Arzneim. Forsch.,* 28:2048–2051.
38. Reuter, H. (1973): *Prog. Biophys. Mol. Biol.,* 26:3–43.
39. Rodenkirchen, R., Bayer, R., Steiner, R., Bossert., F., Meyer, H., and Möllcr, E. (1978): *Naunyn-Schmiedebergs Arch. Pharmacol.,* 310:69–78.
40. Shibanuma, T., Iwanami, M., Fujimoto, M., Takenaka, T., and Murakami, M. (1980): *Chem. Pharm. Bull. (Tokyo),* 28:2609–2613.
41. Shibanuma, T., Iwanami, M., Okuda, K., Takenaka, T., and Murakami, M. (1980): *Chem. Pharm. Bull. (Tokyo),* 28:2809–2812.
42. Takenaka, T., Miyazaki, I., Asano, M., Higuchi, S., and Maeno, H. (1982): *Jpn. J. Pharmacol.,* 32:665–670.
43. Takenaka, T., Usuda, S., Nomura, T., Maeno, H., and Sado, T. (1976): *Arzneim. Forsch.,* 26:2172–2178.
44. Towart, R., Wehinger, E., and Meyer, H. (1981): *Naunyn-Schmiedebergs Arch. Pharmacol.,* 317:183–185.
45. Towart, R., Wehinger, E., Meyer, H., and Kazda, S. (1982): *Arzneim. Forsch.,* 32:338–346.
46. Triggle, A. M., Shefter, E., and Triggle, D. J. (1980): *J. Med. Chem.,* 23:1442–1445.
47. Triggle, D. J., and Swamy, V. C. (1980): *Chest,* 78(*Suppl.*):174–179.
48. Warltier, D. C., Zyvoloski, Brooks, H. L., and Gross, G. J. (1982): *Eur. J. Pharmacol.,* 80:149–153.

Calcium Antagonists and Cardiovascular
Disease, edited by L. H. Opie.
Raven Press, New York © 1984.

Chapter 16

Binding Sites for Dihydropyridine Calcium Antagonists

W. U. Dompert and J. Traber

Neurobiology Department, Troponwerke, D5000 Köln 80, Federal Republic of Germany

Among the Ca^{2+} antagonists, the dihydropyridines belong to the most potent compounds known at present. Because of the high pharmacological potency, their structure and stereospecificity already known from animal experiments, it was proposed that dihydropyridines may act via distinct receptor sites in a way similar to many neurotransmitters and hormones. The search for specific recognition sites, which may mediate the pharmacological action of dihydropyridines, became feasible when the synthesis of radioactively labeled nitrendipine and nimodipine of high specific activity was successful. Using these tracers, it was, in fact, possible to detect specific binding sites for dihydropyridines in heart muscle and brain (1,2). By this breakthrough, many researchers who are interested in Ca^{2+} channel function have come to use radiolabeled dihydropyridines as a tool. Future work will show if these binding sites represent pharmacologically relevant receptors.

METHODS AND RESULTS

To study the organ and structure specificity of dihydropyridine-binding sites in the pig, pig tissues were minced with scissors and homogenized 1:10 (w/v) in ice-cold buffer (25 mM Tris HCl, containing 300 mM sucrose and 0.5 mM $CaCl_2$, pH 7.4 at 37°C). Homogenization, centrifugation, and incubation for the binding assay was performed essentially as described in the literature (2). Protein was measured using the Bradford method (4). The radioligand nimodipine [isopropyl-^{3}H], custom synthesized by New England Nuclear with a specific radioactivity of 160 Ci/mmoles, was checked for radiochemical purity by thin-layer chromatography (> 95%) every few weeks. Substances were supplied by Bayer AG, Wuppertal.

The binding of nimodipine [isopropyl-^{3}H] (1.2 nM) to pig cerebral cortical membranes was reversible with a half-life time for association and dissociation of about 1 and 5 min, respectively.

Saturation of membranes with radioligand was reached at about 4 nM ligand. The nonspecific binding was as low as 10%. Scatchard transformation of the data revealed one class of noninteracting binding sites with a dissociation constant K_D of 1.4 ± 0.3 nM and a binding capacity B_{max} of 0.16 ± 0.07 pmoles/mg protein (mean and SD of 13 preparations). Binding of nimodipine [isopropyl-³H] to brain membranes required Ca^{2+} ions. The addition of 0.2 mM ethylenediamine tetraacetate decreased binding to 10% of the controls. Binding of nimodipine [isopropyl-³H] could be restored completely by the addition of 1 mM $CaCl_2$. Exposure of membranes to heat (70°C, 10 min) or pronase (1 μg/100 μg protein) resulted in a sharp decline of binding to 20 and 30% of the controls, respectively.

As shown in Table 1, cerebral cortex, adrenal gland, as well as heart and skeletal muscle, showed high specific binding (80–90% of total), cerebellum and blood vessels considerably less (65%). Other tissues studied (lung, thymus, ovary, thyroid, pancreas, kidney, and liver) showed poor specific binding (20–30%). The binding sites in the tissues with high specific binding seemed to be very similar to those in the brain with the remarkable exception of the skeletal muscle (binding affinity 5 times lower and binding capacity 5 times higher). These differences are in agreement with findings of other groups.

Dihydropyridine-binding is stereoselective. This is shown for the 4 S(−) enantiomer (Fig. 1, *open circles*) and R(+) enantiomer (Fig. 1, *solid circles*) of 2,6-dimethyl-3-isopropyl-5-methyl-4-(3-nitrophenyl)-1,4-dihydropyridine-3,5-dicarboxylate. The much more potent S(−) form determines the affinity of the racemic mixture (Fig. 1, *crosses*) as expected. Similar results were obtained with the isomers of nimodipine and nitrendipine. The inhibition constants K_i for these stereoisomers and for other selected dihydropyridines were also studied. In our hands, BAY E 6927 (K_i = 0.4 nM) and nisoldipine (0.5 nM) are the most potent dihydropyridines tested followed by nimodipine (2 nM), nitrendipine (3 nM), and nifedipine (10 nM). Oxidation of the dihydropyridine ring system resulted in loss of binding affinity. As an example of the phenylalkylamine series of Ca^{2+} antagonists, displacement characteristics of gallopamil are illus-

TABLE 1. *Specific binding of nimodipine isopropyl-³H to different organs and tissues of the pig*

Tissue	Specificity (% of total)	K_D (nM)	B_{max} (pmoles/mg protein)
Cerebral cortex	90	1.4	0.16
Adrenal gland	80	1.6	0.1
Heart muscle	80	1.4	0.18
Skeletal muscle	80	10.0	0.8
Cerebellum	65	1.2	0.04
Pia vessels	65	1.9	0.2
Coronary vessels	65	1.5	0.1

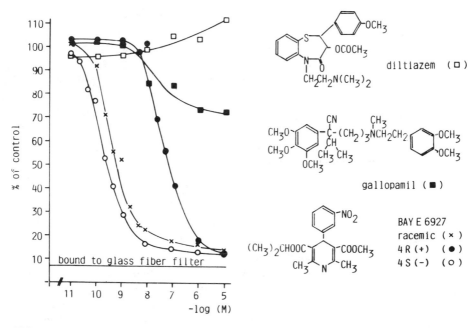

FIG. 1. Left: Effect of racemic BAY E 6927 (*crosses*), the 4R (+) isomer (*solid circles*), the 4S (−) isomer (*open circles*), of diltiazem (*open squares*) and gallopamil (*solid squares*) on binding of nimodipine [isopropyl-³H]. **Right:** Structures of BAY E 6927, diltiazem, and gallopamil.

trated in Fig. 1 (*solid squares*). This compound is only able to displace about 30% of the bound nimodipine even at very high concentrations. In contrast, diltiazem which belongs to the benzothiazepine series of Ca²⁺ antagonists, even increases the binding of nimodipine (*open squares*).

DISCUSSION

Three different types of dihydropyridine ligands have been used in the literature: nitrendipine [methyl-³H], nimodipine [isopropyl-³H], and nifedipine [³H] (11). Methods for membrane preparations and incubation conditions have been quite different, especially in the protein to ligand ratio and the assay volume. Nevertheless, in all published studies, the binding is reversible and saturable. The dissociation constants and binding capacities are in good agreement in many publications (K_D 0.1–2 nM and B_{max} 0.1–1 pmoles/mg protein, respectively). Structure specificity was shown in all cases. The uniqueness of the dihydropyridine-binding site is demonstrated by the fact that only dihydropyridine Ca²⁺ antagonists bind with high affinity, whereas structurally unrelated Ca²⁺ antagonists show only weak effects.

If one compares the inhibition for well known dihydropyridines from the literature, there are slight differences in the rank order of nifedipine, nitrendipine, nimodipine, and nisoldipine. Using pig cerebral cortical membranes, we found inhibition constants for dihydropyridines in the range from 0.1 nM (for (−) isomers) to 10 nM (nifedipine).

The absolute requirement of Ca^{2+} ions for dihydropyridine binding to membranes is generally accepted. Other ions also influence dihydropyridine-binding in an agonistic or antagonistic manner depending on their concentration used. At submaximal doses Ca^{2+}, Mn^{2+}, Sr^{2+}, and Ba^{2+} stimulate nitrendipine binding to carefully washed membranes in an additive way (10). For nimodipine-binding, the rank order in restoration is $Mn^{2+} > Ca^{2+} > Mg^{2+} > Sr^{2+}$. As a mechanism, the formation of a complex between Me^{2+}, Ca^{2+} channel, and dihydropyridines has been discussed (9). Inhibition of nitrendipine-binding is exerted by $Cd^{2+} > La^{3+} > Na^{+} > Co^{2+} = Mn^{2+} > Mg^{2+} \sim Ba^{2+} > Ca^{2+}$. Very low concentrations of La^{3+}, Cu^{2+} and Co^{2+} can stimulate nitrendipine-binding. These agonistic and antagonistic effects might depend on the different ion radii and motilities in the channel.

Besides the dihydropyridines themselves, there exist two other groups of Ca^{2+} antagonists acting at the dihydropyridine receptor. The phenylalkylamines, e.g., gallopamil, and the benzothiazepines, e.g., diltiazem, allosterically regulate dihydropyridine-binding. Verapamil and gallopamil show only partial displacement of labeled dihydropyridine in any case described so far. This may be due to a fast dissociation component for dihydropyridines, appearing in the presence of verapamil or gallopamil (5).

In contrast, diltiazem increases dihydropyridine-binding. For brain membranes, Ferry and Glossmann showed that this is due to an increased affinity and not to increased receptor density (6). Murphy et al. introduced a model in which only one recognition site for phenylalkylamines and benzothiazepines is present and allosterically linked to the dihydropyridine receptor site (13).

Sarmiento et al. (14) were able to localize nitrendipine-binding in the sarcolemma fraction of cardiac muscle. This is evidence for preferential dihydropyridine binding to cell surface membranes. An interesting new finding is the special type of binding sites for nimodipine and nitrendipine in skeletal muscle of guinea pig (7), rabbit (8), and pig (*this chapter*). Skeletal muscle binding is localized in membranes of transverse tubules which supply extracellular Ca^{2+} to the myofibrils. The physiological meaning of these results is an interesting subject for future research.

The characterization of specific binding sites for neurotransmitters, hormones, and drugs in biological material does not yet mean that one has found physiological relevant receptor sites. Evidence that this may be the case is provided by good correlation of binding data and physiological responses. In the case of dihydropyridines, inhibition constants correlate very well with their inhibitory potency on isolated contracting muscles like ileum (12) and aorta strips (3). The radiolabeled dihydropyridines provide a very valuable tool for studying the mechanism of action of Ca^{2+} antagonists which may give more insights in the molecular function of Ca^{2+} channels.

SUMMARY

High-affinity binding sites for dihydropyridine Ca^{2+} antagonists have been found in brain, heart, smooth muscle, and adrenal glands of various species. Dihydropyridine-binding seems to be allosterically modulated by two other types of Ca^{2+} antagonists, the phenylalkylamines (e.g., verapamil or gallopamil) and the benzothiazepines (e.g., diltiazem).

ACKNOWLEDGMENTS

We thank Drs. H. Meyer and E. Wehinger for kindly providing the drugs, and Drs. H. Glossmann, F. Hoffmeister, and H. Horstmann for helpful discussions.

The technical assistance of B. Häck, W. Scheip, and M. Wiertellorz is gratefully acknowledged.

REFERENCES

1. Bellemann, P., Ferry, D., Lübbecke, F., and Glossmann, H. (1981): *Arzneim. Forsch.*, 31:2064–2067.
2. Bellemann, P., Ferry, D., Lübbecke, F., and Glossmann, H. (1982): *Arzneim. Forsch.*, 32:361–363.
3. Bellemann, P., Schade, A., and Towart, R. (1983): *Proc. Natl. Acad. Sci.*, 80:2356–2360.
4. Bradford, M. M. (1976): *Anal. Biochem.*, 72:248–254.
5. Ehlert, F. J., Roeske, W. R., Itoga, E., and Yamamura, H. J. (1982): *Life Sci.*, 30:2191–2202.
6. Ferry, D., and Glossmann, H. (1982): *Naunyn-Schmiedebergs Arch. Pharmacol.*, 321:80–83.
7. Ferry, D. R., and Glossmann, H. (1982): *FEBS Lett.*, 148:331–337.
8. Fosset, M., Jaimovich, E., Delpont. E., and Lazdunski, M. (1983): *Eur. J. Pharmacol.*, 86:141–142.
9. Glossmann, H., and Ferry, D. (1983): In: *Drug Development and Evaluation 9: New Calcium Antagonists, Recent Developments and Prospects*, edited by A. Fleckenstein, K. Hashimoto, M. Herrmann, A. Schwartz, and L. Sipel. Gustav Fischer Verlag, Stuttgart.
10. Gould, R. J., Murphy, K. K., and Snyder, S. H. (1982): *Proc. Natl. Acad. Sci.*, 79:3656–3660.
11. Holck, M., Thomas, S., and Häussler, G. (1982): *Eur. J. Pharmacol.*, 85:305–315.
12. Janis, R. A., Maurer, S. C., Sarmiento, J. G., Bolger, G. T., and Triggle, D. J. (1982): *Eur. J. Pharmacol.*, 82:191–194.
13. Murphy, K. M. M., Gould, R. J., Largent, B. L., and Snyder, S. H. (1983): *Proc. Natl. Acad. Sci.*, 80:860–864.
14. Sarmiento, J. G., Janis, R. A., Colvin, D., Triggle, J., and Katz, A. M. (1983): *J. Mol. Cell. Cardiol.* (*in press*).

Calcium Antagonists and Cardiovascular
Disease, edited by L. H. Opie.
Raven Press, New York © 1984.

Chapter 17

Cellular Sites of Action of Calcium Antagonists and β-Adrenoceptor Blockers

Winifred G. Nayler, J. S. Dillon, and M. J. Daly

Department of Medicine, University of Melbourne, Austin Hospital, Heidelberg, Victoria, 3084 Australia

A useful way of starting this chapter might be to consider precisely what is meant by the term "Ca^{2+} antagonism." The substances which exhibit this property include verapamil, nifedipine, diltiazem, tiapamil, fendiline, niludipine, nimodipine, cinnarizine, and many more (5,6). These are the organic antagonists. In addition, there are the inorganic Ca^{2+} antagonists—including Ni^{2+}, Co^{2+}, Mn^{2+}, and La^{3+}. Clearly, therefore, when considered as a group, Ca^{2+} antagonists lack a common chemical structure; they also lack any β-adrenoceptor blocking activity (21). Nor is their Ca^{2+}-antagonistic activity widespread or lacking in specificity because, unless excessively high concentrations are used, this property appears to be largely restricted to an inhibitory effect on the processes which are involved in the voltage-activated displacement of Ca^{2+}. Thus, in the case of cardiac muscle, smooth muscle, or nodal and conducting tissues, for example, where Ca^{2+} can enter in a variety of ways—including in exchange for Na^+, by passive diffusion, through voltage-activated slow channels (27), and in exchange for K^+, the inhibitory effect of these substances on Ca^{2+} transport is limited to their effect on the movement of Ca^{2+} through the voltage-activated slow channels (Fig. 1).

OTHER ACTIONS OF THE CALCIUM ANTAGONISTS

The original classification of substances such as verapamil, nifedipine, and diltiazem as Ca^{2+} antagonists (5) was based on two requirements: (a) the predominant characteristic of inhibiting the voltage-activated inward movement of Ca^{2+} through voltage-sensitive channels, and (b) the ability of an increased extracellular Ca^{2+} to overcome this inhibition.

These criteria still apply, but with the passage of time, the development of

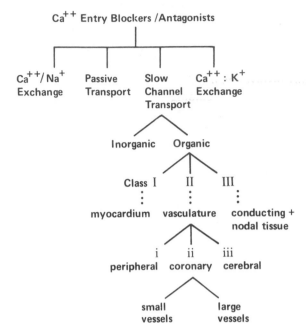

FIG. 1. Schematic representation of the possible routes of Ca^{2+} entry into excitable cells, and the subdivision of the Ca^{2+} antagonists determined with regard to their tissue specificity.

new and highly potent compounds, and with increasing experience, it has become clear that the pharmacology of these substances is far more complex than was at first appreciated. For example, some Ca^{2+} antagonists interact with α_1- and α_2-adrenoceptors (4), some inhibit the fast Na^+ current particularly when used in high concentrations (29), and some interact with muscarinic receptors (18). Even their inhibitory effect on the voltage-activated inward displacement of ions through the slow channels is no longer regarded as being specific for Ca^{2+}, because some of these substances have been found to inhibit the Na^+-dependent component of the slow current (10). At the outset, therefore, we can assume that the mode of action of the Ca^{2+} antagonists contrasts with that of the β-adrenergic blockers, the antagonistic activity of which can be accounted for simply in terms of the classical concepts of receptor occupancy and inactivation.

ARE THERE "RECEPTORS" FOR THE CALCIUM ANTAGONISTS?

Because of their complex pharmacology and heterogeneous chemistry, it might have been concluded that specific receptors for the Ca^{2+} antagonists do not exist. On the contrary, the dose-dependency of their electrophysiological and pharmacological actions implies that specific membrane-located binding sites should occur—and, indeed, specific high-affinity binding sites for ^3H-nitrendipine and other closely related dihydropyridine derivatives (1) have now been identified. However, since not all of the substances which are currently classed as Ca^{2+} antagonists appear to be capable of displacing ^3H-labeled nitrendipine from these newly identified binding sites, we must assume that Ca^{2+} antagonism does not simply involve the interaction of a heterogeneous group of compounds with a single population of binding sites. Instead, we may be dealing with a multiplicity of binding sites; some may even be located intracellularly, in structures which are not necessarily part of, or attached to, the cell surface. Even at the cell surface there appears to be a multiplicity of actions, with the various Ca^{2+} antagonists exerting slightly different inhibitory actions on the functioning of the slow channels. Thus, for example, whereas nifedipine inhibits slow-channel activity without altering the kinetics of slow-channel transport (12), verapamil and its methoxyderivative, D600, alter the kinetics of slow-channel transport, slowing down the rate of recovery after a period of activation (10).

β-BLOCKERS AND SLOW-CHANNEL TRANSPORT

The currently available Ca^{2+} antagonists lack any appreciable β-adrenoceptor blocking activity (21). Likewise, when used in therapeutic concentrations, the β-blockers have no *direct* inhibitory effect on the slow channels. However, the β-blockers do exert an *indirect* inhibitory effect which is evident when catecholamines are present. This can be explained as follows: Some, but not necessarily all, of the channels which are concerned with the inward movement of Ca^{2+} appear to be under phosphorylation control (33,36). This phosphorylation control may be mediated by way of a sarcolemmal protein, the phosphorylation of which is dependent on cyclic $3'5'AMP$. Since the interaction of a β-agonist with its receptor triggers a raised tissue level of cyclic $3'5'AMP$, we can surmise that β-adrenoceptor stimulation will facilitate the phosphorylation of the sarcolemmal protein. There are at least three different ways in which this process might alter the ion-carrying capacity of the channels: (a) Phosphorylation of the protein may cause a conformational change in the geometry of the slow channels; (b) there may be a conformational change in the supporting plasmalemma resulting indirectly in an altered channel geometry; or (c) an altered chemistry of the channel may directly affect its ion carrying capacity.

The end result is that more of the existing channels are open at any one time, without the formation of *de novo* channels (28), and under these conditions Ca^{2+} influx is enhanced. Against this background, the inhibitory effect of β-blockers on the influx of Ca^{2+} through the slow channels can be explained in terms of the occupancy of the β-receptors by the β-blockers—an occupancy which renders the β-receptors inaccessible to the β-agonists, but which leaves the α-adrenoceptors available for activation.

We can conclude, therefore, that whereas the Ca^{2+} antagonists and β-adrenoceptor antagonists may both reduce the amount of Ca^{2+} which enters through the slow channels per unit of time, their mode of action is entirely different.

∴ Ca ant don't block Ca influx due to Catamines whereas BB do.∴ best in infarctn & Isch...n also Caunns are involved

my Beautiful theinking

The Ca^{2+} antagonists have a *direct* inhibitory effect. By contrast the β-adrenoceptor antagonists act *indirectly*, by inhibiting the catecholamine-induced production of cyclic 3′5′AMP. It follows, therefore, that whereas the inhibitory effect of β-adrenoceptors on slow-channel transport is expressed only in the presence of catecholamine-induced stimulation, the slow-channel blockers (Ca^{2+} antagonists) exert their inhibitory effect irrespective of whether catecholamines, including the neurotransmitters, are present. As a corollary, we should perhaps question whether there are not two populations of myocardial Ca^{2+} channels, some under phosphorylation (and, hence, hormonal) and others under voltage control, as proposed for vascular smooth muscle. *There are (2)*

EVIDENCE FOR A DIRECT EFFECT OF THE CALCIUM ANTAGONISTS ON THE CALCIUM TRANSPORTING ACTIVITY OF CARDIAC SARCOLEMMAL PREPARATIONS

One of the major unresolved problems relating to the pharmacology of the Ca^{2+} antagonists is that of identifying their membrane-located receptor binding sites. Evidence for a direct interaction with sites in the sarcolemma comes not only from radioligand-binding (1), enzymatic degradation (17), and electrophysiological studies (33). It also comes from experiments in which the Ca^{2+}-transporting activity of isolated sarcolemmal preparations has been monitored (17). These studies have consistently shown a dose-dependent inhibitory action which, at least in the case of verapamil, is now known to be pH-sensitive—its inhibitory effect on Ca^{2+} binding being greater at pH 6.8 than at 7.4. The significance of this pH effect is still being investigated, but it is tempting to assume that it may contribute to the enhanced sensitivity which ischemic (and, hence, acidotic) heart muscle displays towards this compound (32).

At first sight, it is difficult to explain how such an inhibitory effect on Ca^{2+} transport in the absence of voltage activation could contribute to the pharmacology of these compounds. One possibility is, however, that what is being monitored in these experiments is the translocation of Ca^{2+} to the superficially located storage sites for future mobilization and inward displacement through the voltage-activated channels. Such a concept is compatible with the earlier observation that verapamil decreases the size of the lanthanum-displaceable and, hence, superficially located pool of Ca^{2+} (22).

IS THERE AN INTRACELLULAR SITE OF ACTION FOR THE CALCIUM ANTAGONISTS?

The vast majority of the organic Ca^{2+} antagonists are lipophilic and it is not unreasonable, therefore, to ask if they interfere with intracellular Ca^{2+}-mediated processes. Possible sites of action include the sarcoplasmic reticulum, the myofibrillar apparatus, the mitochondia, and the Ca^{2+}-regulator protein, calmodulin.

Sarcoplasmic Reticulum

At dose-levels which might be encountered therapeutically, none of the Ca^{2+} antagonists seem to affect the Ca^{2+}-accumulating activity of the sarcoplasmic reticulum (22). Also, for those substances which have been tested under carefully controlled conditions, there is no evidence of an effect on the Ca^{2+}-induced release of Ca^{2+} from this organelle (3).

Myofibrillar Apparatus

Even when used in relatively high concentrations, verapamil has been shown not to inhibit either the direct Ca^{2+}-induced activation of chemically skinned cardiac myofibrils (19) or the Ca^{2+}-binding activity of troponin.

Mitochondria

Again, although pretreatment of the myocardium with Ca^{2+} antagonists prevents the mitochondria from becoming overloaded with Ca^{2+} upon postischemic reperfusion (20), these drugs have no direct inhibitory effect on the Ca^{2+}-accumulating activity of the mitochondria.

Calmodulin—the Calcium Regulator Protein

Although some investigators (9) have shown that high doses of some of the relatively potent Ca^{2+} antagonists may interact with calmodulin, this does not seem to be relevant to the clinical situation. When clinically applicable doses are used and the Ca^{2+}-binding activity of calmodulin is assayed in terms of its effect on Ca^{2+}-induced stimulation of phosphodiesterase activity, evidence of an interaction between the Ca^{2+} antagonists and the Ca^{2+}-binding activity of calmodulin has not been obtained.

Therefore, the major site of action of the Ca^{2+} antagonists is located within the sarcolemmal complex, where at least two quite distinct effects on Ca^{2+}-mediated processes have been observed. These are: (a) an inhibition of the entry of Ca^{2+} through the voltage-activated channels, and (b) a slowed rate of Ca^{2+} binding.

TISSUE SPECIFICITY

As already stated, the Ca^{2+} antagonists lack a common chemical structure. They also exhibit marked differences in tissue specificity. For example, all of the Ca^{2+} blockers which have been developed so far are relatively ineffective in blocking slow-channel transport in bronchiolar and tracheal smooth muscle cells (8). Hence, in doses which can be achieved in clinical practice, they do not relieve asthma. Contrasting with this low specificity for bronchiolar and tracheal smooth muscle is their relatively high specificity for other smooth muscle cells (6). An extreme example of this is provided by cinnarizine and its difluorinated derivative, flunarizine (7,35), because these substances are 1,000 times more potent as blockers of slow-channel transport in vascular smooth muscle cells than for the myocardium. Even within the vasculature there are preferred sites of action, with nimodipine, for example, acting preferentially on cerebral blood vessels (34), whereas diltiazem is more selective for the coronary vasculature (14). Differences in tissue specificity are not limited to differences between myocardial, bronchiolar, and vascular smooth muscle muscle cells. Thus, verapamil, for example, is a highly potent inhibitor of the slow Ca^{2+} current in nodal and conducting tissue (37), whereas nifedipine is relatively ineffective (25). On the myocardium, the Ca^{2+} antagonists all exhibit a dose-dependent spectrum of negative inotropy. In terms of their "direct" cardiac depressant activity, nifedipine and verapamil are more potent than diltiazem.

Why the Ca^{2+} antagonists are tissue specific is not known for certain. Various factors may be involved:

1. There are differences in the relative importance of the Ca^{2+} which enters through the slow channels. Thus, vascular smooth muscle, which derives almost all of the Ca^{2+} it requires for contraction from extracellular sources (7) is generally more sensitive to the Ca^{2+} antagonists than is other smooth muscle which derives some of its Ca^{2+} from intracellular stores.

2. Differences in the surface chemistry of the cells may be involved (16).

3. The slow channels themselves may be heterogenous, with some channels being under receptor control as discussed previously, and others under voltage-activation control. If only the voltage-activated channels were affected by the Ca^{2+} antagonists, the differences in the tissue distribution of the receptor and voltage-activated channels could contribute to this tissue specificity.

4. A further possibility is that, as with the β-receptors, there may be different types of Ca^{2+} receptors with the distribution of these receptors being tissue specific.

5. Yet another possibility is that the tissue specificity of these substances reflects, in part at least, their other properties. For example, is the potent antiarrhythmic activity of verapamil (37) and its potency in slowing atrioventricular conduction (30) due entirely to its Ca^{2+} antagonist activity? The effect of verapamil on the fast Na^+ current could also possibly be involved.

Whereas the precise cause of this tissue specificity is unknown, its effect on the clinical usage of these drugs is profound. Thus, in man, the preferred site of action of verapamil is the atrioventricular node (13). This does not mean that verapamil does not have an effect on slow-channel activity in vascular smooth muscle (15) or myocardial cells (22). It does mean, however, that relatively higher concentrations are required to achieve an effect. This same argument applies to the *relative* insensitivity of the atrioventricular node to the direct inhibitory effect of nifedipine (30). When added to isolated nodal tissue, nifedipine can slow atrioventricular conduction (11). However, in man, such an effect is concealed, presumably because of the reflex-induced activation of the sympathetic system that occurs in response to nifedipine's profound vasodilator effect. The same problem does not occur with verapamil, because its relatively high specificity for nodal and conducting tissues ensures that any reflex-induced increase in sympathetic activity that may be triggered by a vasodilator response does not speed up atrioventricular conduction.

SPECIES SPECIFICITY

In view of the described marked tissue specificity, it is not altogether surprising to find that the Ca^{2+} antagonists also exhibit evidence of species specificity. This has been most thoroughly documented for verapamil where the order of potency based on affinity constants is for the myocardium (rat > cat > rabbit) and for arterial smooth muscle (rat = rabbit > cat) (24). Why such pronounced species specificity should occur is not known. As far as the myocardium is concerned, the presence or absence of T-tubules cannot be the main determinant because rat atrial and rat papillary muscle are equisensitive. Possibly it is the species-dependent differences in the Ca^{2+} handling properties of the individual tissues that determines their responsiveness. Species-dependent differences in the responsiveness of heart muscle to inotropically active drugs is not peculiar to the Ca^{2+} antagonists. Other examples include caffeine and the cardiac glycosides.

Thus, when compared with the β-adrenoceptor antagonists, the Ca^{2+} antagonists are an exceedingly heterogeneous and complex group of drugs. Their heterogeneity is expresssed not only in terms of their chemical composition, but also in terms of their differing tissue specificities and potencies, their interaction with other receptors, and even, for some of them, an interaction with other ion conducting channels. Nevertheless, and despite their different modes of action, the Ca^{2+} antagonists and the β-blockers are often used in the treatment of similar diseased states.

CLINICAL CONSIDERATIONS

Vasculature

Irrespective of whether we are dealing with peripheral, coronary, or cerebral blood vessels, the addition of a Ca^{2+} antagonist can be expected to cause vasodilation. In the case of the coronary vasculature (Fig. 2), this will result in an enhanced blood flow and O_2 supply provided the myocardium does not become underperfused as the result of a massive decline in perfusion pressure. In many ways, this effect of the Ca^{2+} antagonists contrasts with that of the β-blockers, where vasoconstriction may be intensified because (a) the β-adrenoceptors in the coronary vasculature mediate dilation; and (b) by blocking off the β-adrenoceptors, excess neurotransmitter will remain available for interaction with the α-receptors to mediate constriction.

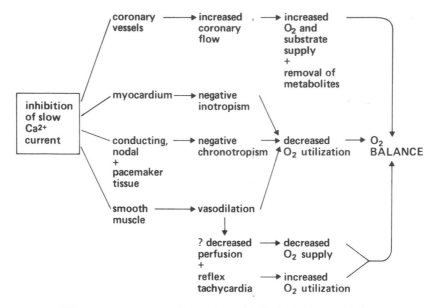

FIG. 2. Consequences of slow-channel inhibition in the circulation.

This does not mean that the β-adrenoceptor antagonists cannot be used in the management of angina pectoris. It only means that their effective use is restricted to those conditions which depend upon reducing the O_2 requirement of the myocardium—rather than increasing coronary flow.

There are at least two ways whereby the β-blockers can cause a rapid reduction in the myocardial O_2 requirement: (a) by reducing heart rate via their inhibition of catecholamine-induced stimulation of slow-channel activity in the pacemaker tissue (23), and (b) by interfering with the direct stimulant effect of β-adrenoceptor stimulation on the inotropic state of the heart, an effect (Fig. 3) which is indirectly mediated by the slow Ca^{2+} channels.

ISCHEMIC-REPERFUSION DAMAGE

Whereas the efficacy of using β-blockers to protect the ischemic myocardium against the deleterious effects of ischemia and reperfusion is now well founded (23a,31) the use of the Ca^{2+} antagonist is still in its infancy. Nevertheless, there is evidence that they can be effective, particularly when used prophylatically (2,20,26).

Like the β-adrenoceptor antagonists, the Ca^{2+} antagonists also reduce the energy requirements of the myocardium, causing a slowed rate of ATP depletion during conditions of inadequate oxygenation and flow (20). The β-adrenoceptor antagonists probably achieve their effect by reducing excessive cardiac work

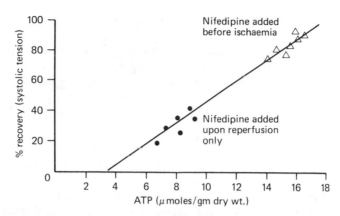

FIG. 3. Effect of 50 μg/liter (1.4 × 10⁻⁷M) nifedipine on the percentage recovery of isolated rabbit hearts made ischemic for 60 min at 37°C and then reperfused, plotted as a function of their ATP content at the end of the reperfusion period. (From Nayler et al., ref. 22a.)

due to the entry of Ca^{2+} through the phosphorylation-controlled slow channels. As described previously, the Ca^{2+} antagonists probably interact *directly* with the channels; the end result, however, is the same—that of energy conservation. Thus, whereas neither the β-adrenoceptor antagonists nor the β-blockers have a direct effect on the energy-dependent pumps which are responsible for maintaining intracellular ionic homeostasis, they both indirectly ensure that ionic homeostasis is maintained (at least for some time) under conditions of poor oxygenation and flow. Evidence of this energy-sparing effect following the prophylactic use of nifedipine is shown by the data (Fig. 3) which come from experiments in which the ATP content of hearts, reperfused after 60 min ischemia at 37°C, was measured. Since the hearts were isolated, this must represent a direct energy-sparing effect.

ARRHYTHMIAS

By far the most difficult thing to account for in terms of the Ca^{2+} antagonists is why only some of them are effective in slowing conduction at the atrioventricular node, when the ion-carrying currents in these tissues are known to involve Ca^{2+} (23). There is no easy explanation for this—unless it is assumed, as in the case of nifedipine, for example, that it is so highly potent an inhibitor of the slow Ca^{2+} channels in the peripheral vasculature that a concentration which might be effective in blocking the slow channels in the atrioventricular node in man cannot be achieved. Or is it that the "Ca^{2+} receptors are tissue-specific," and that verapamil, for example, has a high affinity for these receptors in nodal tissue?

PERIPHERAL CIRCULATION

With regard to peripheral circulation, there is again marked evidence of tissue specificity, with the nifedipine-type drugs being far more potent than verapamil and D600. Hence, in the intact circulation, the main energy-sparing effect of nifedipine may be derived from its ability to "unload" the peripheral circulation.

SUMMARY

The hypothesis is proposed that although the β-adrenoceptor and Ca^{2+}-antagonist drugs do not share a common pharmacology, their use has one common endpoint—that of controlling myocardial slow-channel activity. This they do in entirely different ways: The β-blockers indirectly prevent the activation of phosphorylation-dependent channels; and the Ca^{2+} antagonists prevent Ca^{2+} entry through the voltage-activated channels. In neither instance, however, is the entry of Ca^{2+} via other routes affected.

REFERENCES

1. Bellemann, P., Ferry, D., Lubbecke, F., and Glossmann, H. (1981): *Arzneim. Forsch.* 31:2064.
2. Christlieb, I. Y., Clark, R. E., Nora, J. D., Henry, P. D., Fischer, A. E., Williamson, J. R., and Sobel, B. E. (1979): *Am. J. Cardiol.,* 44:825–831.
3. Dunnett, J., and Nayler, W. G. (1979): *Biochem. Biophys. Acta,* 198:434–438.
4. Fairhurst, A. S., Whittaker, M. L., and Ehlert, F. J. (1980): *Biochem. Pharmacol.,* 29:155–162.
5. Fleckenstein, A. (1971): In: *Calcium and the Heart,* edited by P. Harris and L. Opie, pp. 135–188. Academic Press, London.
6. Fleckenstein, A. (1977): *Annu. Rev. Pharmacol. Toxicol.,* 17:149–166.
7. Godfraind, T., and Kaba, A. (1972): *Arch. Int. Pharmacodyn. Ther.,* 196:35–49.
8. Himori, N., and Taira, N. (1980): *Br. J. Pharmacol.,* 68:595–598.
9. Johnson, J. D., Vaghy, P. L., Crouch, T. H., Potter, J. D., and Schwartz, A. (1981): In: *Advances in Pharmacology and Therapeutics,* Vol. 3, edited by H. Yoshida, T. Hagihara, and S. Ebashi, pp. 121–138. Pergamon, London.
10. Kass, R. S., and Tsien, R. W. (1975): *J. Gen. Physiol.,* 6:169–192.
11. Kawai, C., Konishi, T., Matsuyama, E., and Okazaki, H. (1981): *Circulation,* 63:1034–1042.
12. Kohlhardt, M., and Fleckenstein, A. (1977): *Naunyn Schmiedebergs Arch. Pharmacol.,* 298:267–272.
13. Krikler, D. M., and Spurrell, R. A. J. (1974): *Postgrad. Med. J.,* 50:47–453.
14. Kusukawa, R., Kinoshita, M., Shimoto, Y., Tomonaga, G., and Hoshina, T. (1977): *Arzneim. Forsch.,* 21:878–883.
15. Lewis, G. R. J., Morley, K. D., Lewis, B. M., and Bones, P. J. (1978): *New Zealand Med. J.,* 612:351–354.
16. Martinez-Polomo, A. (1970): *Int. Rev. Cytol.,* 29:29–75.
17. Mas-Oliva, J., and Nayler, W. G. (1980): *Br. J. Pharmacol.,* 70:612–624.
18. McGee, R., Jr., and Schneider, J. E. (1979): *Mol. Pharmacol.,* 16:877.
19. Nayler, W. G. (1980): *Eur. Heart J.,* 1:225–237.
20. Nayler, W. G., Ferrari, R., and Williams, A. (1980): *Am. J. Cardiol.,* 46:242–248.
21. Nayler, W. G., McInnes, I., Swann, J. B., Price, J. M., Carson, V., Race, D., and Lowe, T. E. (1968): *J. Pharmacol. Exp. Ther.,* 161:83–96.
22. Nayler, W. G., and Szeto, J. (1972): *Cardiovasc. Res.,* 6:120–128.
22a. Nayler et al. (1982): *J. Thorac. Cardiovasc. Surg.,* 84:897–905.
23. Noble, D. (1975): *The Initiation of the Heart Beat.* Clarendon Press, Oxford.

23a. Norwegian Multicenter Study Group (1981): *N. Engl. J. Med.,* 304:801–807.
24. Quinn, P., Briscoe, M. G., Nuttall, A., and Smith, H. J. (1981): *J. Cardiovasc. Res.,* 15:398–403.
25. Raschack, M. (1976): *Arzneim. Forsch.,* 26:1330–1333.
26. Reimer, K. A., Lowe, J. W., and Jennings, R. B. (1977): *Circulation,* 55:581–587.
27. Reuter, H. (1979): *Annu. Rev. Physiol.,* 41:413–424.
28. Reuter, H., and Scholz, H. (1977): *J. Physiol.,* 264:49–62.
29. Rosenberger, L., and Triggle, D. J. (1978): In: *Calcium in Drug Action,* edited by G. B. Weiss, pp. 3–31. Plenum Press, New York.
30. Rowland, E., Evans, T., and Krikler, D. (1979): *Br. Heart J.,* 42:124–12.
31. Sleight, P. (1981): *N. Engl. J. Med.,* 304:837–838.
32. Smith, H. J., Goldstein, R. A., Griffith, J. M., Kent, K. M., and Epstein, S. E. (1976): *Circulation,* 54:629–635.
33. Sperelakis, N., and Schneider, J. A. (1978): *Am. J. Cardiol.,* 37:1079–1085.
34. Towart, R., and Perzborn, E. (1981): *Eur. J. Pharmacol.,* 69:213–215.
35. Van Nueten, J. M., Van Beek, J., and Janssen, P. A. J. (1978): *Arch. Int. Pharmacodyn. Ther.,* 233:42–49.
36. Watanabe, A. M., and Besch, H. R. (1974): *Circ. Res.,* 35:316–324.
37. Zipes, D. P., and Fischer, J. C. (1974): *Circ. Res.,* 34:184–192.

Calcium Antagonists and Cardiovascular Disease, edited by L. H. Opie.
Raven Press, New York © 1984.

Chapter 18

α-Adrenergic-Mediated Effects on Myocardial Calcium

Peter B. Corr and Arjun D. Sharma

*Cardiovascular Division, Washington University School of Medicine,
St. Louis, Missouri 63110*

Recent evidence suggests that α-adrenergic mechanisms may modulate the movement of Ca^{2+} during both myocardial ischemia as well as reperfusion. This increased Ca^{2+} movement across the sarcolemma may not only be of significance in the development of malignant dysrhythmias, but also in the ultimate extent of ischemic injury. In reviewing the potential mechanisms involved in the movement of Ca^{2+} across the sarcolemma, the data available at present have been derived primarily from *in vitro* studies, and the application of these findings to myocardial ischemia *in vivo* must be done with caution. During ischemia *in vivo,* increases in the extracellular concentration of H^+ and K^+ ions, the intracellular concentration of Na^+, and the presence of amphiphilic metabolites such as lysophosphatides and long-chain acyl carnitines may alter the normal homeostatic mechanisms controlling the influx and efflux of cellular Ca^{2+}.

Although there is considerable evidence to suggest that catecholamine modulation of Ca^{2+} movement in the myocardium is mediated through stimulation of β-adrenergic receptors, more recent evidence indicates an important role of the myocardial α-adrenergic receptor.

MYOCARDIAL CALCIUM FLUX

The potential mechanisms of Ca^{2+} flux in the myocyte are reviewed by E. Carafoli (Chapter 3, *this volume*), and we will only briefly consider mechanisms of Ca^{2+} accumulation in ischemic and reperfused tissue. Although during physiological conditions, the free intracellular Ca^{2+} concentration remains within narrow limits, during myocardial ischemia and reperfusion, intracellular Ca^{2+} increases. Myocardial ischemia activates sympathetic reflexes and also results in local release of catecholamines which could stimulate Ca^{2+} uptake via the slow inward current (I_{si}), particularly in depolarized tissue. Recent observations indicate that infarcted myocardium possesses a greatly increased capacity to metabolize arachidonic acid to prostaglandin products (21). During ischemia or evolving infarction, Ca^{2+} influx may be augmented by the presence of agents such as prostaglandins which can experimentally act as Ca^{2+} ionophores (43). Furthermore, Ca^{2+} efflux would be expected to be depressed during myocardial ischemia, Na^+-Ca^{2+} exchange by the increased intracellular Na^+ and loss of membrane potential, and active Ca^{2+} transport out of the cell due to the fall in cellular ATP. These mechanisms may contribute to the increase in tissue Ca^{2+} that has been determined to occur *in vivo*. In the rat, even brief intervals of ischemia result in increased intracellular Ca^{2+} assessed with X-ray microanalysis (28). Reperfusion of ischemic tissue results in dramatic increases in tissue Ca^{2+}, which appear to be a function of the preceding ischemic interval (37). This increase in intracellular Ca^{2+} may increase resting tension of the tissue, and may activate enzymes such as sarcolemmal Ca^{2+}-dependent phospholipases (15). This may increase the concentrations of lysophosphoglycerides, compounds which have been implicated not only in arrhythmogenesis, but also in the extension of cellular damage (6). Thus, enhanced Ca^{2+} influx during ischemia and reperfusion has significance not only in arrhythmogenesis, but also in myocardial preservation.

INFLUENCE OF α-ADRENERGIC RECEPTOR STIMULATION IN THE MYOCARDIUM UNDER PHYSIOLOGICAL CONDITIONS

The presence of myocardial α-adrenergic receptors was first obtained from pharmacological investigations demonstrating a prolongation of the effective refractory period by norepinephrine mediated through α- rather than β-adrenergic mechanisms (17). Subsequently, additional effects mediated through α-adrenergic mechanisms have included positive inotropy (34), prolongation of action potential duration (16), and a reduction in automaticity in isolated Purkinje fibers (33) and the sinus node *in situ* (19). More recently, radioligand-binding studies have revealed the presence of myocardial α-adrenergic receptors and confirmed the subclassification of these receptors into both α_1 and α_2 (42). Originally, α_1-adrenergic receptors were categorized as postsynaptic, and α_2-receptors as presynaptic. However, it is now clear that α_2-receptors may also mediate postsynaptic events in vasculature tissue (10). The α_1-adrenergic receptor site has a high affinity for prazosin, whereas the α_2-receptor site has a high affinity for either clonidine or yohimbine (42). α_2-Receptors are also modulated by guanine nucleotides and are coupled to adenylate cyclase in an inhibitory manner. In the myocardium, both α_1- and α_2-adrenergic receptors are present, and, for this reason, a number of previous experiments using nonspecific α-adrenergic agonists and antagonists are open to multiple interpretations. Our interest has focused on the α_1-adrenergic receptor, as this appears to be the predominant receptor in the myocardium, particularly at the postsynaptic site

(42). The cellular events resulting from α_1-adrenergic stimulation in the myocardium are unknown, since the augmentation of contractility produced by α_1-adrenergic stimulation occurs without increases in cellular cyclic AMP (46), unlike β-adrenergic stimulation. However, this augmentation of contractility and prolongation of the plateau phase of the action potential by α_1-adrenergic stimulation suggests that the effects may be mediated through modulation of intracellular Ca^{2+}. The recent purification of the α_1-adrenergic receptor may aid in identifying the second messengers involved in mediating these effects (18). Our findings relative to α_1-adrenergic stimulation during ischemia, discussed in the following sections, also implicate enhanced influx of Ca^{2+}.

α-ADRENERGIC STIMULATION AND CALCIUM FLUX IN NONMYOCARDIAL TISSUE

In a number of other tissues, including vascular smooth muscle, liver, nerve, and parotid gland, there is strong evidence that α_1-adrenergic stimulation produces an increase in cytosolic Ca^{2+}. In vascular smooth muscle, α_1-adrenergic stimulation releases Ca^{2+} from an intracellular source resulting in an early rapid phase of contraction followed by a late slow phase which is related to the influx of Ca^{2+} across the membrane (11). The combination of increased cytosolic Ca^{2+} and calmodulin, the Ca^{2+}-binding protein, activates myosin light-chain kinase resulting in phosphorylation of the myosin light chain and subsequent contraction. Studies using elevated $[K^+]_o$ and norepinephrine-induced contraction in vascular tissue suggest the presence of additional α-adrenergic receptor-operated Ca^{2+} channels independent of the voltage-dependent Ca^{2+} channel (45). The extent to which the receptor-operated channels are present in the myocyte is unknown.

Studies involving hepatic glycogenolysis have shown that α_1-adrenergic receptors act to modulate glycogenolysis via increases in cytosolic Ca^{2+} (13). This elevated cytosolic Ca^{2+} may be due to transsarcolemmal influx or release from intracellular stores, primarily mitochondria. The early phase of elevated cytosolic Ca^{2+} is associated with the metabolic effects of α_1-receptor stimulation, which is attributable to Ca^{2+}-mediated phosphorylation of phosphorylase, glycogen synthetase, and pyruvate kinase (13). Although α_1-adrenergic stimulation may directly elevate cytosolic Ca^{2+} in hepatic tissue, more recent evidence in vascular tissue suggests that hydrolysis of phosphatidylinositol (PI) is associated with α_1-receptor stimulation, and phosphate incorporation into PI is correlated with contraction (44). α-Receptor stimulation may also increase phosphate incorporation into phosphatidic acid, an agent which stimulates the breakdown of PI (44).

α-Adrenergic receptors have also been demonstrated in brain tissue. Interestingly, in neuroblastoma-glioma cells, either α_1-adrenergic blockade or Ca^{2+} channel blockade with D-600 prevented Ca^{2+} spikes recorded by intracellular microelectrodes in the presence of tetrodotoxin (1), suggesting that α-receptor stimulation can modulate Ca^{2+} influx in brain tissue as well. Likewise, α_1-adrenergic receptor stimulation in parotid gland tissue produces a biphasic elevation in cytosolic Ca^{2+} similar to the effect seen in vascular smooth muscle (31). This increased Ca^{2+} results in increased membrane permeability to K^+ with a secondary osmotic secretion of water. Thus, while the functional consequences of α_1-receptor stimulation varies in different tissues, several common features emerge. α_1-Adrenergic receptor stimulation at the plasma membrane results in increased cytosolic Ca^{2+}, resulting in phosphorylation of a number of cell proteins producing an intracellular response. These effects appear to be independent of cyclic AMP, but may be mediated by alteration in phospholipids, particularly PI. Although the biochemical events responsible for α_1-adrenergic receptor stimulation in the heart are unknown, evidence to suggest that these receptors may modulate the transsarcolemmal movement of Ca^{2+} is now emerging.

α-ADRENERGIC-MEDIATED EFFECTS ON DYSRHYTHMIA DURING ISCHEMIA AND REPERFUSION

The electrophysiologic mechanisms responsible for the dysrhythmias induced by occlusion alone appear to differ from those due to reperfusion (29). Dysrhythmia induced by reperfusion of the ischemic myocardium is characterized by improved conduction, a rapid idioventricular rate, and both shortening and lengthening of refractory periods. In our initial studies in the cat, α-adrenergic blockade with either phentolamine or the specific α_1-adrenergic blocking agent, prazosin, significantly reduced the number of premature ventricular complexes and abolished the occurrence of ventricular fibrillation during both coronary occlusion and reperfusion (38). Several findings suggest that the protective effect of α-adrenergic blockade during ischemia is mediated through interaction with α_1-adrenergic receptor, rather than any other nonspecific action of the drugs (38). First, depletion of myocardial catecholamines with 6-hydroxydopamine also abolishes ventricular fibrillation, whereas β-adrenergic blockade with propranolol failed to alter the incidence of ventricular fibrillation. Second, the increase in idioventricular rate during reperfusion from 50 to 180 beats/min was responsive to modulation by sympathetic nerve stimulation through activation of α-adrenergic receptors, a phenomenon which was mediated through β-adrenergic receptors prior to reperfusion. Thus, the increase in idioventricular rate produced by left stellate ganglion stimulation was blocked by phentolamine, but not propranolol, suggesting α-adrenergic mediation of the response. Likewise, intracoronary administration of the α-agonist, methoxamine, increased the idioventricular rate only on reperfusion. In contrast, prior to coronary occlusion, the increased idioventricular rate during stellate stimulation was blocked by propranolol suggesting a β-adrenergic mechanism. Third, the beneficial effects of α-adrenergic blockade were independent of alterations in heart rate, mean arterial pressure, left ventricular end-diastolic pressure, cardiac output, peak left ventricular dP/dt, stroke work, or regional coronary blood flow. Fourth, the antiarrhythmic effect of α-adrenergic blockade was confirmed in a subsequent randomized study utilizing the combined α- and β-adrenergic blocking agent, labetalol (30). Labetalol produces shifts in the dose-response curves for phenylephrine-induced arterial pressure elevation (α) and isoproterenol-induced heart rate increases (β). From the shifts in the dose-response curves, the dose ratio 10 (DR_{10}) was calculated for α- and β-adrenergic blockade. Labetalol is 11.5 times less potent as an α-adrenergic blocking agent than as a β-adrenergic blocking agent. A dose of labetalol (1 mg/kg) that produces predominantly β-adrenergic blocking effects had little antiarrhythmic efficacy. In contrast, a dose of labetalol (5 mg/kg) that produces significant α-adrenergic blocking effects, abolished ventricular fibrillation on reperfusion (30). Thus, α_1-adrenergic blockade produces significant antiarrhythmic effects during both coronary occlusion and reperfusion, which appears to be mediated through specific blockade of the α_1-adrenergic receptor.

The antiarrhythmic effects of prazosin in the cat at low doses (50 μg/kg) have been confirmed recently (9). In dogs, phentolamine virtually obliterates dysrhythmia induced by reperfusion, and blocks the increase in effective refractory period (41). Intracoronary phentolamine in the dog also attenuates reperfusion-induced ventricular fibrillation (47). Although prazosin or phentolamine did not alter the incidence of ventricular fibrillation induced by reperfusion in one report (2), the disparity may be due to inappropriately high doses of α-adrenergic blockade employed for dogs in that study.

To examine if this enhanced, yet reversible, α_1-adrenergic responsivity during ischemia and the early reperfusion interval was mediated through changes in the α_1-adrenergic receptor, radioligand-binding procedures were performed. ^{3}H-Prazosin-binding was specific, rapid, saturable, reversible, stereoselective, and demonstrated an affinity in the nanomolar range indicating that it represented binding to the α_1-adrenergic receptor site. The number of α_1-adrenergic receptor sites in the ischemic tissue increased twofold to 28 fmoles/mg protein within 30 min of ischemia and remained significantly increased after 2 min of reperfusion, before returning to control levels after 15 min of reperfusion (7), a time course that paralleled the enhanced α_1-adrenergic responsivity. Similar studies have also demonstrated an increase in α_1-adrenergic receptors in the canine heart during ischemia (23). Thus, the reversible increase in α_1-adrenergic receptors in the ischemic heart may explain the augmented electrophysiological effects of α_1-adrenergic stimulation.

POTENTIAL MECHANISMS INVOLVED IN THE INCREASE IN α_1-ADRENERGIC RECEPTORS

Although the mechanisms responsible for the increase in α_1-adrenergic receptors in ischemic myocardium are unknown, several potential mechanisms may apply based on findings in nonmyocardial tissue. The role of membrane phospholipids, such as phosphatidylinositol, in mediating α-adrenergic effects has been alluded to previously (44). There is also evidence, although inconclusive, to suggest that membrane phospholipids may be associated with the α_1-adrenergic receptor. ^{14}C-Dibenamine (an irreversible α-antagonist) bound to aortic tissue can be extracted with organic solvents which extract phospholipids. Also ^{3}H-norepinephrine extracted from tissue tends to be partitioned to the phase containing phospholipids (14). However, these findings may represent nonspecific interactions between lipid and the α_1-adrenergic agents. A more convincing finding implicating the phospholipid interaction was that a proteolipid extracted from bovine spleen binds ^{3}H-norepinephrine, and when this proteolipid was added to an artificial membrane, norepinephrine induced a transient increase in membrane conductance, a response which was stereospecific and blocked by phentolamine (27). The role of phospholipids in receptor site recognition may be particularly important during ischemia, since alterations in phospholipids are prominent in ischemic myocardium with increases in lysophosphoglycerides, amphiphilic metabolites of phospholipids (6,8). Considerable evidence suggests that the accumulation of these lysophosphoglycerides may mediate, at least in part, the electrophysiologic derangements characteristic of ischemic tissue *in vivo*. In addition, lysophosphoglycerides can increase the size of the exchangeable pool of intracellular Ca^{2+} in isolated myocytes assessed using [45]Ca^{2+} (35). Thus, the accumulation of lysophosphoglycerides in ischemic myocardium may be responsible for the apparent increase in α_1-adrenergic receptors, as well as increased responsivity to α-adrenergic stimulation. Lysophosphoglycerides may alter receptor density through changes in membrane fluidity, resulting in uncovering of cryptic receptors; or lysophosphoglycerides may increase the nonspecific binding of α-adrenergic agents to the sarcolemma, thereby enhancing the binding of specific α-agonists. Alternatively, lysophosphoglycerides may modulate α-adrenergic responses through changes in phosphotidylinositol turnover. The role of lysophosphoglycerides in the alteration of α_1-adrenergic receptor density is particularly attractive, since the reduction in pH which occurs during ischemia *in vivo* has been shown to potentiate the electrophysiological effects of these compounds (40), as well as inhibit their degradation by lysophospholipase (6). Since reperfusion results in a rapid reversal of the acidosis, with concomitant removal of accumulating metabolites such as lysophosphoglycerides, these changes may explain the reversal of the increase in α_1-adrenergic receptors in reperfused myocardium (7). Thus, there is circumstantial evidence to link membrane phospholipids with α-adrenergic receptors in nonmyocardial tissue, and the accumulation of lysophosphoglycerides in ischemic myocardium with the associated electrophysiologic derangements, alteration in density of α_1-adrenergic receptors, and augmentation of Ca^{2+} uptake into the myocyte.

α-ADRENERGIC MODULATION OF MYOCARDIAL CALCIUM DURING REPERFUSION

Based on the previous discussion, it is evident that α-adrenergic stimulation alters cytosolic Ca^{2+} in a number of different tissues. Reperfusion of ischemic tissue results in a large increase in total tissue Ca^{2+} with increased mitochondrial Ca^{2+}, malignant dysrhythmia, and the potential extension of ischemic damage. Since α_1-adrenergic blockade is antiarrhythmic during the reperfusion interval, the influence of this intervention on the accumulation of Ca^{2+} was recently assessed (36). Regional ischemia for 35 min in the cat resulted in no measurable increase in tissue Ca^{2+}. However, when ischemia was followed by 10 min reperfusion, total tissue Ca^{2+} doubled and continued to do so for the next 30 min. In contrast, in animals pretreated with either phentolamine, prazosin, or labetalol, no significant increase in tissue Ca^{2+} content was evident during reperfusion. The increase in both the extracellular space (^{3}H-inulin) and calculated intracellular Ca^{2+} was prevented by pretreatment with the α-adrenergic blocking agents, suggesting a site of action at both the endothelial cell as well as at the myocyte. Electron microscopy of tissue that had been rendered ischemic for 35 min and reperfused contained striking precipitates in the mitochondria which were verified as Ca^{2+} antimonate by X-ray microanalysis (36). There was also evidence of ischemia, including glycogen depletion. In contrast, animals treated with α-adrenergic blocking agents failed to demonstrate deposition of Ca^{2+} in the mitochondria after reperfusion, although evidence of ischemia including glycogen depletion was apparent. Thus, α-adrenergic blockade specifically prevents the increase in intracellular Ca^{2+} and mitochondrial Ca^{2+} deposition induced by reperfusion.

Previous studies in isolated perfused tissues have concluded that Ca^{2+} influx during ischemia and reperfusion can be attenuated by agents that reduce the work performed during the ischemic interval (3,24,25). Thus, the Ca^{2+} entry blockers, verapamil and nifedipine, and the β-adrenergic blocking agent, propranolol, were each shown to prevent cellular accumulation of Ca^{2+} only when administered prior to ischemia, but not prior to reperfusion (3,25). In these studies using isolated tissue perfused with artificial media at 32°C, the authors have concluded that mitochondrial Ca^{2+} uptake occurs independent of any alterations in the sarcolemma (3,24). However, in these isolated preparations there is a very large extracellular space and the conditions of ischemia in vivo were not reproduced—in particular, the accumulation of metabolites. Accordingly, when isolated, blood-perfused, septal preparations are utilized at 37°C, altered sarcolemmal permeability to Ca^{2+} appears to be prominent (39), consistent with our observations in vivo. In our studies in vivo, either phentolamine, or the water soluble α_1-specific adrenergic blocking agent, BE 2254, given even 33 min after ischemia and 2 min prior to reperfusion also prevented the increase in tissue Ca^{2+} (36). Thus, α-adrenergic blockade specifically prevents the uptake of Ca^{2+} during reperfusion. It is likely that the protection conferred by α-adrenergic blockade occurs only in tissues that are functionally deranged but structurally intact. This conclusion is suggested by the finding that, in contrast to ischemia for only 35 min, when the ischemic interval was extended to 70 min followed by 10 min of reperfusion, light microscopy of the tissue showed hemorrhage and contraction-banding with thin, wavy fibers suggesting necrosis, and there was a fourfold increase in tissue Ca^{2+}. With 70 min of ischemia prior to reperfusion, α-adrenergic blockade with phentolamine produced only a partial reduction in tissue Ca^{2+}, presumably reflecting protection only in intact cells.

CALCIUM ANTAGONISTS AND THE α-ADRENERGIC RECEPTOR

Since previous studies have indicated that verapamil may attenuate the increase in tissue Ca^{2+} during reperfusion, the potential interaction of several Ca^{2+} antagonists with the myocardial α_1-adrenergic receptor was recently examined. ^{3}H-Prazosin-binding was used to define the α_1-adrenergic receptor based on specific displacement by agonists and antagonists in rat myocardial membrane preparations. Verapamil, nifedipine, and diltiazem displaced prazosin from α_1-adrenergic receptor sites, but the potency varied, being greatest for verapamil and less for nifedipine and diltiazem (Fig. 1). The K_I for verapamil was 4.8×10^{-7} M; based on recent plasma and myocardial tissue concentrations, verapamil is the only one of these Ca^{2+} antagonists that would be expected to have potent α-adrenergic blocking properties at doses used clinically. These findings may explain why verapamil, but not nifedipine, attenuates dysrhythmia induced by reperfusion in the dog. Similar results demonstrating the relative α_1-adrenergic blocking activity of several Ca^{2+} antagonists has recently been reported by Nayler and colleagues (26). These findings further suggest that Ca^{2+} influx secondary to α_1-adrenergic stimulation is not likely to be mediated through activation of the voltage-dependent Ca^{2+} channel, since the potency for blockade of the voltage-dependent channel is greatest for ^{3}H-nitrendipine and nifedipine, and least for verapamil (12). Rather, it appears that Ca^{2+} entry blockers have multiple sites of action, one of which is the α_1-adrenergic receptor. It remains to be determined if the α_1-adrenergic receptor controls specific Ca^{2+} channels, or if it modulates the degree of Na^+–Ca^{2+} exchange. Whereas there is evidence that the antiarrhythmic potency of verapamil, nifedipine, and diltiazem parallels their affinity for the α_1-adrenergic receptor, there is contradictory evidence regarding the effectiveness of verapamil in preventing Ca^{2+} uptake following reperfusion. With prolonged ischemia of 60 min or more, verapamil was relatively ineffective *in vivo* in preventing dysrhythmias (32), which is likely to be related to the presence of irreversible cell damage.

POTENTIAL MECHANISMS RESPONSIBLE FOR THE ELECTROPHYSIOLOGIC EFFECTS OF α-ADRENERGIC STIMULATION

α-Adrenergic stimulation under physiological conditions results in a decrease in Purkinje fiber automaticity, with an increase in action potential duration (16) and refractoriness *in vitro*, and a slowing in sinus node rate *in situ* (19). In contrast, in tissue depressed *in vitro* by high $[K^+]_o$, to simulate conditions during ischemia *in vivo*, α- rather than β-adrenergic mechanisms appear to

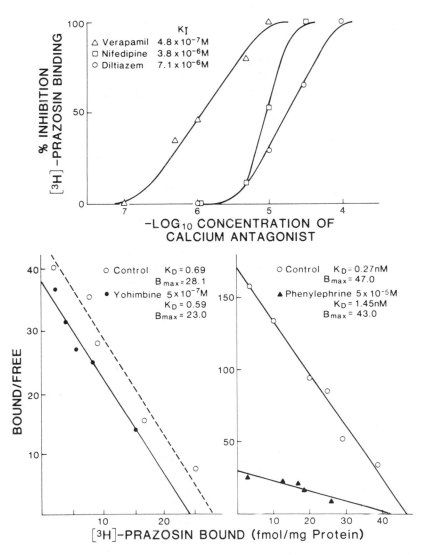

FIG. 1. The displacement of ^{3}H-prazosin by increasing concentrations of 3 different Ca^{2+} antagonists (**upper**). The K_I was calculated as IC$_{50}$/(1 + [ligand]/K$_D$). The IC$_{50}$ was calculated as the concentration of antagonist required to produce a 50% displacement of the specific binding of the radioligand. Scatchard analysis with verapamil (10 μM) as the displacing agent for ^{3}H-prazosin-binding (**lower**) in the presence of yohimbine (**lower left**) or phenylephrine (**lower right**).

augment the I_{si} in rabbit papillary muscle (22). Analogous findings have been reported in bovine ventricular tissue (4). *In vivo* during ischemia, the augmentation in contractility induced by stellate nerve stimulation is also mediated by α-adrenergic mechanisms in the ischemic, but not normal, regions (20). Thus, responses to catecholamines in ventricular muscle that are normally mediated by β-adrenergic receptors appear to be controlled by α-adrenergic mechanisms during ischemia. The production of slow-response action potentials with concomitant slowing of conduction, and the presence of postrepolarization refractoriness, may predispose to the development of dysrhythmia due to reentry.

An alternative mechanism for mediation of electrophysiologic effects of α-adrenergic stimulation during ischemia relates to the finding that an inward current channel can be activated by elevation of the cytosolic Ca^{2+} concentration (5). Using microelectrodes and membrane patches derived from cultured neonatal myocytes, an inward current channel has been characterized which is activated by increased cytosolic Ca^{2+}, but was only slightly voltage-dependent and discriminated poorly between Na^+ and K^+ (5). In depolarized tissue, which is prominent during ischemia *in vivo,* an elevated intracellular Ca^{2+} concentration may activate these channels and could result in oscillatory activity that could reach threshold and produce multiple ectopic depolarizations *in vivo.* α-Adrenergic stimulation may indirectly activate such channels through its effects on increasing cytosolic Ca^{2+}. Thus, $α_1$-adrenergic stimulation may result in malignant dysrhythmia in the setting of ischemia and reperfusion through increases in both sarcolemmal permeability to Ca^{2+} and accumulation of cytosolic Ca^{2+}.

SUMMARY

There is considerable evidence from the study of nonmyocardial tissues to suggest that α-adrenergic stimulation mediates Ca^{2+} uptake and that the functional consequences of this varies between organs. In the myocardium, α-adrenergic receptors also appear to modulate Ca^{2+} influx and may thereby result in electrophysiologic alterations which predispose to ventricular fibrillation. The interaction between the $α_1$-adrenergic receptor and Ca^{2+} antagonists suggests that, of the major Ca^{2+} antagonists, only verapamil is likely to have significant α-adrenergic blocking effects at doses used clinically, and that the site of action of the α-blocking agents is not the voltage-dependent Ca^{2+} channel.

ACKNOWLEDGMENTS

Research from the authors' laboratory was supported by National Institutes of Health Grants HL-17646, SCOR in Ischemic Heart Disease, and by grant RROO396 from the Division of Research Resources, National Institutes of Health. For Dr. Peter B. Corr, this work was done during the tenure of an Established Investigatorship of the American Heart Association and with funds contributed in part by the Missouri Heart Affiliate.

REFERENCES

1. Atlas, D., and Adler, M. (1981): *Proc. Natl. Acad. Sci. USA,* 78:1237–1241.
2. Bolli, R., Brandon, T. A., Fisher, D. J., Taylor, A. A., and Miller, R. R. (1982): *Clin. Res.,* 30:173A (Abstract).

3. Bourdillon, P. D., and Poole-Wilson, P. A. (1982): *Circ. Res.,* 50:360–368.
4. Brüchner, R., and Scholz, H. (1980): *Naunyn-Schmiedebergs Arch. Pharmacol.,* 311:R37 (Abstract).
5. Colquhoun, D., Neher, E., Reuter, H., and Stevens, C. F. (1981): *Nature,* 294:752–724.
6. Corr, P. B., Lee, B. I., and Sobel, B. E. (1981): *Acta Medica Scand.,* 210 (Suppl. 651):59–69.
7. Corr, P. B., Shayman, J. A., Kramer, J. B., and Kipnis, R. J. (1981): *J. Clin. Invest.,* 67:1232–1236.
8. Corr, P. B., Snyder, D. W., Lee, B. I., Gross, R. W., Keim, C. R., and Sobel, B. E. (1982): *Am. J. Physiol.,* 243(12):H187–H195.
9. Davey, M. J. (1980): *J. Cardiovasc. Pharmacol.,* 2:S287–S301.
10. Deth, R., and Lynch, C. (1981): *Eur. J. Pharmacol.,* 71:1–11.
11. Deth, R., and van Breemen, C. (1974): *Pfluegers Arch.,* 348:13–22.
12. Ehlert, E. J., Roeske, W. R., Hoga, E., and Yamamura, H. I. (1982): *Life Sci.,* 30:2191–2202.
13. Exton, J. H. (1981): *Mol. Cell Endocrinol.,* 23:233–264.
14. Formby, B. (1968): *Mol. Pharmacol.,* 4:288–292.
15. Franson, R. (1981): In: *Liposomes: From Physical Structure to Therapeutic Applications,* edited by G. Knight, pp. 349–380. Elsevier/North-Holland, New York.
16. Giotti, A., Ledda, F., and Mannaioni, P. F. (1973): *J. Physiol. (Lond.),* 229:99–113.
17. Govier, W. C. (1967): *Life Sci.,* 6:1367–1371.
18. Graham, R. M., Hess, H.-J., and Homcy, C. J. (1982): *Clin. Res.,* 30:190A (Abstract).
19. James, T. N., Bear, E. S., Lang, K. F., and Green, E. W. (1968): *Am. J. Physiol.,* 215:1366–1375.
20. Juhasz-Nagy, A., and Aviado, D. M. (1976): *Physiologist,* 19:245 (Abstract).
21. McCluskey, E. R., Corr, P. B., Lee, B. I., Saffitz, J. E., and Needleman, P. (1982): *Circ. Res.,* 51:743–750.
22. Miura, Y., Inui, J., and Imamura, H. (1978): *Naunyn-Schmiedebergs Arch. Pharmacol.,* 301:201–205.
23. Mukherjee, A., Hogan, M., McCoy, K., Buja, L. M., and Willerson, J. T. (1980): *Circulation,* 64(Suppl. III):III–149 (Abstract).
24. Nakanishi, T., Nishioka, K., and Jarmakani, J. M. (1982): *Am. J. Physiol.,* 242(11):H437–H449.
25. Nayler, W. G., Ferrari, R., and Williams, A. (1980): *Am. J. Cardiol.,* 46:242–248.
26. Nayler, W. G., Thompson, J. E., and Jarrott, B. (1982): *J. Mol. Cell. Cardiol.,* 14:185–188.
27. Ochoa, E., De Plazas, S. F., and De Robertis, E. (1972): *Mol. Pharmacol.,* 8:215–221.
28. Osornio-Vargas, A. R., Berezesky, I. K., and Trump, B. F. (1981): *Scan. Electron Microsc.,* II:463–472.
29. Penkoske, P. A., Sobel, B. E., and Corr, P. B. (1978): *Circulation,* 58:1023–1035.
30. Pogwizd, S. M., Sharma, A. D., and Corr, P. B. (1982): *Cardiovasc. Res.,* 16:398.
31. Putney, J. W. (1979): *Pharmacol. Rev.,* 30:209–245.
32. Reimer, K. A., Lowe, J. E., and Jennings, R. B. (1977): *Circulation,* 55:581–587.
33. Rosen, M. R., Hordof, A. J., Ilvento, J. P., and Danilo, P., Jr. (1977): *Circ. Res.,* 40:390–400.
34. Schumann, H. J., Wagner, J., Knorr, A., Reidemeister, J. C., Sadony, V., and Schramm, G. (1978): *Naunyn Schmiedebergs Arch. Pharmacol.,* 302:333–336.
35. Sedlis, S. P., Corr, P. B., Sobel, B. E., and Ahumada, G. G. (1983): *Am. J. Physiol.:* 244(13):H32–H38.
36. Sharma, A. D., Saffitz, J. E., Lee, B. I., Sobel, B. E., and Corr, P. B. (1983): *J. Clin. Invest. (in press).*
37. Shen, A. C., and Jennings, R. B. (1972): *Am. J. Pathol.,* 67:417–440.
38. Sheridan, D. J., Penkoske, P. A., Sobel, B. E., and Corr, P. B. (1980): *J. Clin. Invest.,* 65:161–171.
39. Shine, K. I., Douglas, A. M., and Ricchiuti, N. V. (1978): *Circ. Res.,* 43:712–720.
40. Snyder, D. W., Crafford, W. A., Glashow, J. L., Rankin, D., Sobel, B. E., and Corr, P. B. (1981): *Am. J. Physiol.,* 241(10):H700–707.
41. Stewart, J. R., Burmeister, W. E., Burmeister, J., and Lucchesi, B. R. (1980): *J. Cardiovasc. Pharmacol.,* 2:77–91.
42. Story, D. D., Briley, M. S., and Langer, S. Z. (1979): *Eur. J. Pharmacol.,* 57:423–426.

43. Sugiyama, S., Norimatsu, I., and Takayuki, O. (1979): *J. Appl. Biochem.*, 1:402–409.
44. Villalobos-Molina, R., Mirna, U. C., Hong, E., and Garcia-Sainz, J. A. (1982): *J. Pharmacol. Exp. Ther.*, 222:258–261.
45. van Breemen, C., Aaronson, P., Loutzenhiser, R., and Meisheri, K. (1980): *Chest*, 78:157–165.
46. Watanabe, A. M., Hathaway, D. R., Besch, H. R., Jr., Farmer, B. B., and Harris, R. A. (1977): *Circ. Res.*, 40:596–602.
47. Williams, L. T., Guerrero, J. L., and Leinbach, R. C. (1982): *Am. J. Cardiol.*, 49:1046 (Abstract).

Calcium Antagonists and Cardiovascular Disease, edited by L. H. Opie.
Raven Press, New York © 1984.

Chapter 19

Angina and Myocardial Infarction—Introduction

G. Kroneberg

*Pharmaceutical Research Development, Bayer AG, D-5600 Wuppertal 1,
Federal Republic of Germany*

The subject of this volume, the field of the Ca^{2+} antagonists, has had to
pass through several developmental stages to reach the present one (Fig. 1).

Today, the vascular smooth muscle with its mechanism of Ca^{2+} fluxes, Ca^{2+}
movements, and cellular Ca^{2+} distribution is the focus of the theoretical interest.
With regard to the pathogenesis of disease, our knowledge of the metabolic
situation in the hypoxic myocardial fiber, and the interrelationship with Ca^{2+}
and Ca^{2+} antagonists is incomplete. With regard to the clinical side, the importance of spasm—functional narrowings or increased wall tension of the coronary
arteries in the pathogenesis of different forms of angina pectoris—is under continuing investigation.

In 1969, Fleckenstein and co-workers published studies showing that verapamil and D 600 inhibited the mechanical contraction of the cardiac papillary
muscle without inhibiting the action potential, and that this was due to a selective
inhibition of the transmembrane Ca^{2+} influx. The conclusion seemed to be justified that the beneficial effect of verapamil in myocardial ischemia might be
related to its negative inotropic activity.

After having seen the results with verapamil, I asked Prof. Fleckenstein if
a new compound, later to become nifedipine, then under pharmacological investigation and having both a strong negative inotropic effect in the isolated heart
and strong coronary dilatory effects, could also be a Ca^{2+}-antagonist agent.

Later in 1969, he enthusiastically told me that this substance was the most
potent Ca^{2+} antagonist he had ever investigated.

Due to its strong dilatation of the coronary vessels, nifedipine was tried in
cases of angina pectoris; and in some double-blind studies, a significant antianginal effect was demonstrated.

It became clear that the Ca^{2+}-antagonistic property was also the reason for

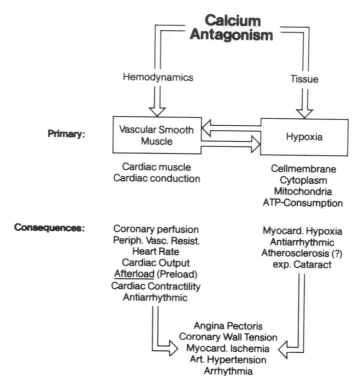

FIG. 1. A condensed summary of present knowledge.

the relaxation of the vessels, but it remained an open question as to how far the *negative inotropic action* was of clinical significance. Neither in the conscious awake animal, nor in man, could such an effect of nifedipine be demonstrated because peripheral vasodilatation activated baroreceptor reflexes which abolished the negative inotropism by a compensatory regulation.

Then more attention was drawn to the *afterload reduction* after nifedipine, which is a consequence of the vasodilatation and which discharges the O_2-consuming resistance work of the heart.

A further step towards a better understanding of the antianginal effect was made by Lichtlen in Hannover who showed, with nifedipine, a significant increase in the retrograde perfusion of underperfused, hypoxic myocardial areas in patients with coronary artery obstruction. Another important, if not decisive, step in the understanding of the Ca^{2+}-antagonist action was the demonstration of a convincing nifedipine effect in Prinzmetal's angina, obviously the result of its strong smooth muscle relaxant property in coronary vessels. And, finally, it was to the credit of Professor Maseri who provided evidence—in fact, against the general opinion—that spasm and increased wall tension of the coronary arteries are involved in the pathogenesis of angina pectoris. To complete the rational basis of the application of Ca^{2+} antagonists, Hugenholtz and his group could show that, not only in Prinzmetal's angina but also in unstable angina, functional narrowings and vasoconstriction of the coronary arteries are involved.

Calcium Antagonists and Cardiovascular Disease, edited by L. H. Opie. Raven Press, New York © 1984.

Chapter 20

Calcium Antagonists as Antiatherogenic Agents

Philip D. Henry

Department of Medicine, Baylor College of Medicine, Houston, Texas 77030

Blumenthal et al. (2) were among the first to suggest that Ca^{2+} may play an important role in the pathogenesis of atherosclerotic vascular injury. They concluded from their anatomic studies of human aortas that disease of the media, more specifically medial calcification, was a constant precursor of intimal lesions. Experimental support for this concept was first provided by Wartman et al. (17) who demonstrated that parenteral administration of magnesium edetic acid suppressed atherosclerosis in rabbits maintained on a high cholesterol diet. In subsequent years, anionic compounds that chelate Ca^{2+}, such as the diphosphonates, were shown to exert antiatherogenic effects in cholesterol-fed rabbits (12). More recently, Kramsch and collaborators (10) showed that trivalent lanthanum, a cation that nonselectively displaces Ca^{2+} from its extracellular binding sites, inhibits atherosclerotic plaque formation in rabbits and monkeys given high-fat diets.

The concept that Ca^{2+} may play an important role as a mediator of cell injury derives primarily from studies in skeletal and cardiac muscle. Pathological conditions in which Ca^{2+} accumulation may act as a pathogenic mechanism include catecholamine-induced cardiac necrosis, myocardial hypoxia, regional and global myocardial ischemia, various myopathies, and malignant hyperthermia (8). In these various forms of muscle injury, Ca^{2+} antagonists have been reported to reduce the accumulation of intracellular Ca^{2+}, and at the same time to prevent cell necrosis.

In view of these findings, we have become interested in the question whether Ca^{2+} antagonists might exert protective effects on vessels undergoing atherosclerotic injury (9). In this chapter, we show that nifedipine suppresses atherogenesis in cholesterol-fed rabbits. This finding supports the hypothesis that Ca^{2+} contributes to vascular injury in atherosclerosis, and that Ca^{2+} antagonists may protect arteries exposed to an atherogenic environment.

RESULTS

Response of the Rabbits to the Diet and Drug Regimens

Details of methods are given in ref. 9. Two cholesterol-fed rabbits, one receiving placebo, the other nifedipine, died of unknown causes during the diet period. The diet and drug regimens were well tolerated, and weight gain during the 8-week period was similar in the different groups. High-dose nifedipine (30 mg/kg/day) has been previously shown to be well tolerated in rats (6).

Peak effects on mean arterial pressure and heart rate after each dose of nifedipine were -11 ± 3 mm Hg and $+44 \pm 18$ beats/min during the first week of treatment. These effects were transient, values returning to baseline within 2 hr or less. Hemodynamic effects of nifedipine did not differ significantly between the dietary groups, nor was there a difference in each group between values during the first and last weeks of treatment, indicating that tolerance to the dihydropyridine did not develop.

Blood Chemistry

Nifedipine treatment had no effect on plasma cholesterol levels of rabbits maintained on standard diet or 2% cholesterol diet (9).

Structural Changes in Aorta

In cholesterol-fed rabbits, the percentage of the intimal surface covered by Sudan-positive lesions averaged $40 \pm 5\%$ (SEM) in placebo-treated rabbits ($n = 13$), and $17 \pm 3\%$ in nifedipine-treated rabbits ($n = 13$; $p < 0.001$) (Fig. 1).

Microscopic evaluation of aortic tissue revealed qualitatively similar lesions in the two cholesterol-fed groups, but a quantitative structural analysis was not performed.

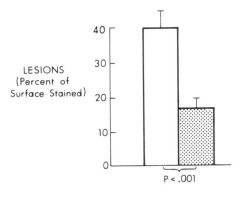

LESIONS (Percent of Surface Stained)

FIG. 1. Effect of nifedipine on the extent of aortic lesions (planimetry of sudan-ophilic lesions) induced by cholesterol feeding. Key ($n = 13$): □, placebo; ▨, nifedipine.

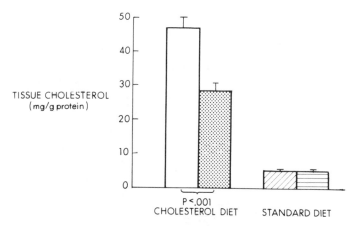

FIG. 2. Effect of nifedipine on aortic cholesterol content following cholesterol feeding. Key ($n = 13$): □, placebo and cholesterol; ⊞, nifedipine and cholesterol; ($n = 14$): ▨, placebo and control diet; ⊟, nifedipine and control diet.

Biochemical Changes in Aorta

The cholesterol concentrations in aortas from rabbits given standard pellets were 6.1 ± 0.3 mg/g protein for the placebo group, and 6.3 ± 0.4 mg/g protein for the nifedipine group (Fig. 2). In cholesterol-fed rabbits, values for the placebo and nifedipine groups differed significantly ($p < 0.001$), averaging 47 ± 5 and 29 ± 1 mg/g protein (Fig. 2). Treatment with nifedipine altered the relationship between the formation of Sudan-positive lesions and the accumulation of aortic cholesterol. The ratio relating planimetered lesions (percent) to tissue cholesterol (mg/g protein) averaged 0.85 ± 0.05 and $0.58 \pm 0.04\%$ ($\% \cdot$ g protein/mg) in untreated and treated rabbits, respectively ($p < 0.001$).

In rabbits given the standard diet, Ca^{2+} concentrations in aortic tissue for the placebo and nifedipine groups were 190 ± 11 and 194 ± 14 μg/g protein. In cholesterol-fed rabbits, aortic Ca^{2+} for the nifedipine groups was significantly lower than that for the placebo group, values averaging 202 ± 14 and 297 ± 18 μg/g protein ($p < 0.005$).

DISCUSSION

Results of this study demonstrate that nifedipine suppresses structural and biochemical changes of atherosclerosis in rabbits fed a high cholesterol diet. Cholesterol-fed rabbits have been used for many years as a model of experimental atherosclerosis, and the arterial disease produced in these animals has been extensively characterized. Unfortunately, rapidly developed lesions are of the foam-cell variety, and do not resemble the usual atherosclerotic plaques in man. However, cholesterol-fed rabbits kept alive for longer intervals (2 years) developed lesions similar to those in man (4). Therefore, foam-cell lesions may reflect predominantly the briefness of the atherogenic insult, rather than a special property of rabbit arteries. Foam-cell lesions are observed in most species susceptible to dietary cholesterol, including monkeys (5). Recently, Rouleau et al. (13) reported that verapamil, like nifedipine, suppressed atherogenesis in cholesterol-fed rabbits. Therefore, it appears that Ca^{2+} antagonists, in general, might exert antiatherogenic effects in rabbits. It will be very important to ascertain if Ca^{2+} antagonists suppress atherogenesis in other models of atherosclerosis.

The present experiments provide little information regarding the mechanisms by which nifedipine exerts its antiatherogenic effects. Nifedipine had no apparent effect on the induced hypercholesterolemia, and study on the lipoprotein pattern of cholesterol-fed rabbits treated with nifedipine has thus far failed to reveal significant quantitative changes (P. Henry, 1983, *unpublished observations*). A decreased lipid overload of arterial cells in the absence of a hypolipidemic effect might occur, if Ca^{2+} antagonists inhibited Ca^{2+}-dependent lipoprotein uptake by arterial cells. However, experiments in our laboratory with smooth muscle cells in culture have thus far failed to demonstrate that Ca^{2+} antagonists influence the endocytosis of lipoproteins (R. Ostlund and P. Henry, 1983, *unpublished observations*). The antiatherogenic effects of Ca^{2+} antagonists might be related to the mechanism of action invoked in various syndromes associated with membrane injury, Ca^{2+} overload, and cell necrosis. Atherogenesis is accompanied by a proliferation of smooth muscle cells, a key process of lesion formation that goes hand-in-hand with cell necrosis (14,15). Necrosis of foam cells releasing membrane-active lipids and catabolic enzymes might affect neighboring cells and accelerate cell necrosis and turnover. Therefore, if Ca^{2+} antagonists were capable of retarding cell necrosis, they might slow down cellular turnover and atherosclerotic lesion formation.

Vasodilators and hypotensive agents may conceivably influence atherogenesis by reducing arterial pressure. It has been generally recognized that arterial pressure is an important determinant of atherosclerosis, and elevated pressure has been shown to aggravate atherosclerosis in cholesterol-fed rabbits (3). Therefore, vasodilator-induced hypotension might exert protective effects, although hypotensive responses to nifedipine were modest and not sustained in our rabbits. Moreover, potent vasodilators such as nifedipine might influence arteries by increasing vasa vasorum flow (7).

Recently, Garthoff and Kazda (6) have demonstrated that dihydropyridines may be effective in lowering blood pressure and preventing hypertensive vascular injury in spontaneously hypertensive rats. In addition, Fleckenstein and collaborators (Chapter 2, *this volume*) have reported that vascular injury induced in rats by the administration of large doses of vitamin D can be prevented by verapamil. It would be of interest to determine if verapamil lowered blood pressure and hypercalcemia in these vitamin D-treated rats.

Platelets may play an important role in atherogenesis, and recent reports indicate that Ca^{2+} antagonists may affect platelet functions. However, antiaggregating effects of verapamil and diltiazem occur only at high drug concentrations known to exert multiple nonspecific actions, including local anesthetic and antiadrenergic blocking effects (1,8,11). On the other hand, dihydropyridines, such as nifedipine, are virtually devoid of local anesthetic effects and have not been noted to affect the aggregation of human platelets *in vitro* (11,16). Nevertheless, the possibility that Ca^{2+} antagonists affect atherogenesis by modifying platelets cannot be ruled out on the basis of the present evidence. It is important to recognize that platelets exposed to hyperlipidemic environments may exhibit altered reactivity to aggregating stimuli.

CONCLUSIONS

Since Ca^{2+} antagonists are used extensively for the treatment of coronary disease, this study appears to have potential clinical implications. Obviously, it would be important to determine if Ca^{2+} antagonists retard the progression of atherosclerosis in man. Unfortunately, clinical trials aimed at assessing antiatherogenic interventions have proved difficult in the past.

REFERENCES

1. Blackmore, P. F., El-Refai, M., and Exton, J. H. (1979): *Mol. Pharmacol.,* 15:598–606.
2. Blumenthal, H. T., Lansing, A. I., and Wheeler, P. A. (1944): *Am. J. Pathol.,* 20:665–679.
3. Bretherton, K. N., Day, A. J. and Skinner, S. L. (1977): *Atherosclerosis,* 27:79–87.
4. Constantinides, P., Booth, J., and Carlson, G. (1960): *Arch. Pathol.,* 70:712–724.
5. Fowler, S., Berberian, P. A., Shio, H., Goldfischer, S., and Wolinsky, H. (1980): *Circ. Res.,* 46:520–530.
6. Garthoff, B., and Kazda, S. (1981): *Eur. J. Pharmacol.,* 74:111–112.
7. Heistad, D. D., Armstrong, M. L., and Marcus, M. L. (1981): *Circ. Res.,* 48:669–675.
8. Henry, P. (1982): In: *Calcium Blockers—Mechanisms of Action and Clinical Applications,* edited by S. E. Flaim and R. Zelis, pp. 135–153. Urban & Schwarzenberg, Baltimore.
9. Henry, P. D., and Bentley, K. I. (1981): *J. Clin. Invest.,* 1366–1369.
10. Kramsch, D. G., Aspen, A. J., and Rozler, L. J. (1981): *Science,* 213:1511–1512.
11. Margolis, B., Lucas, C., and Henry, P. D. (1980): *Circulation,* (Suppl. III) 62:191 (Abstract).
12. Rosenblum, I. Y., Flora, L., and Fisenstein, R. (1975): *Atherosclerosis,* 22:411–424.
13. Rouleau, J. L., Parmley, W. W., Stevens, J., Wikman-Coffelt, J., Sievers, R., Mahley, R. S., and Havel, R. J. (1982): *Am. J. Cardiol.,* 46:889.
14. Stary, H. C. (1977): *Prog. Biochem. Pharmacol.,* 14:241–247.
15. Thomas, W. A., Imai, H., Florentin, R. A., Reiner, J. M., and Scott, R. F. (1977): *Prog. Biochem. Pharmacol.,* 14L:234–240.
16. Vater, W., Kroneberg, G., Hoffmeister, F., Kaller, H., Meng, K., Oberdorf, A., Puls, W., Schlossmann, K., and Stoepel, K. (1972): *Drug Res.,* 22:1–14.
17. Wartman, A., Lampe, T. L., McCann, D. S., and Boyle, A. J. (1967): *J. Atheroscler. Res.,* 7:331–341.

Calcium Antagonists and Cardiovascular Disease, edited by L. H. Opie.
Raven Press, New York © 1984.

Chapter 21

Clinical Experience With Calcium Antagonists in Angina: What We Have Learned; What We Should Know

Attilio Maseri and Peter A. Crean

Cardiovascular Unit, Royal Postgraduate Medical School, Hammersmith Hospital, London W12 OHS, United Kingdom

Interest in the heterogeneous class of drugs called Ca^{2+} antagonists derives largely from their remarkable efficacy in preventing coronary spasm, now well established by a number of studies.

However, it is remarkable that the discovery of their efficacy has been rather empirical: They can often prevent a syndrome, of which we do not know the causes, by mechanisms which are only speculative. They are also found efficacious in other forms of angina, both spontaneous and exertional. For these reasons and because, in general, their side-effects are fewer and less severe than those of β-blockers, their use is gaining widespread acceptance. Therefore, before they enter the cooking books of therapy in a definitive way, it seems appropriate to review the available clinical information in the light of our personal experience.

METHODS OF CLINICAL TRIALS

A simple and wise means of assessing the results of treatment is by the daily records of patients who can often easily tell the changes in their condition with treatment. Although in practice this subjective approach remains the final yardstick, when confronted with a changing understanding of the disease (9,10), and with novel forms of treatment, carefully controlled clinical trials are desirable.

For trials of the initial clinical phase, a double-blind, double-cross-over design with placebo is necessary. Only this design allows (a) assessment of the stability of symptoms during the trial (hence the separation of the effects of the drug from a possible changing course of the disease), and (b) assessment of the consistency of the response in each patient (hence the identification of responders and nonresponders). For the trials of the second phase, simpler double-blind studies can be performed on larger, but selected, groups of patients who appear reasonably homogeneous on the basis of characteristics identified in phase 1 studies.

EVIDENCE OF EFFICACY IN ANGINA

Variant Angina

In the mid-1970s we became convinced of the role of spasm in variant angina and, having been unimpressed by the results with propranolol and practolol, we began to try verapamil which was made available to us in 1974. We decided to design a double cross-over trial because we were intrigued by our very favorable clinical impression, and the result fully confirmed this impression (11). Similar findings were obtained subsequently with nifedipine (13). Other nondouble cross-over studies with nifedipine and diltiazem yielded a comparable degree of success (7,14). A double cross-over trial with verapamil/propranolol/placebo, initiated in 1978 in Pisa and recently completed, confirmed the remarkable superiority of Ca^{2+} antagonists over propranolol in variant angina and unstable angina at rest (12).

Summarizing the present experience, it can be stated that these drugs are remarkably effective in over 80% of patients with variant angina.

Angina at Rest

The anticipated efficacy of Ca^{2+} antagonists in the treatment of rest angina, requiring admission to the Coronary Care Unit, depends on the composition of this subset of patients and thus is largely determined by the local referral policy. If referral is predominantly patients with a long history of exertional angina followed by a progressive reduction in exercise tolerance to only a few yards, associated with rest pain, then it is unlikely that any form of medical treatment will produce good results. Conversely, in patients with angina of recent onset, or with increasing frequency of rest pain, the results of treatment with Ca^{2+} antagonists is similar to those of variant angina, as shown in our previous studies (11,12) and by our general clinical impression.

Exertional Angina

Exertional angina that may be reproducibly induced by stress testing has shown an improvement following treatment with verapamil, nifedipine, and diltiazem in numerous well conducted trials. These drugs prolong the time to ST-segment depression, onset of angina, and total duration of exercise during short- and long-term treatment (2,6,8). The mechanism of improvement in exercise-induced angina may be mediated by a reduction in myocardial O_2 demand during exertion due to the blunting of the rate/pressure product rise similar to that seen with β-blockade. This mechanism has been suggested by the data obtained in a placebo-controlled trial using diltiazem (6). However, in a similarly constructed trial using the same drug and dosage, no consistent alteration in the rate/pressure product was seen between treatment and placebo periods (3a,16).

These conflicting data suggest that the fundamental action by which improvement in exercise performance is achieved has not yet been elucidated. In general, the improvement that may be expected in the treatment of exercise-induced angina has been shown to be similar to that with β-blocker therapy (1).

Mechanisms of Action

As with all systemically distributed drugs, multiple rather than single sites of action may be expected. Among their diverse effects, Ca^{2+} antagonists have been shown to cause relaxation of smooth muscle and to abolish experimentally induced arterial spasm (5). In unstable angina, due to documented coronary artery spasm, the smooth muscle relaxant action offers a ready explanation for their efficacy, but does not necessarily provide the whole picture. Despite adequate treatment with nitrates and Ca^{2+} antagonists, some 10 to 15% of patients failed to respond to medical therapy, and a proportion of patients required cardiac denervation and autotransplantation for relief of continuing symptoms (3). This lack of a homogenous response in patients with coronary spasm leaves in our minds doubts regarding the possible mechanisms through which Ca^{2+} antagonists achieve their improvement in individual patients.

Another pathway by which Ca^{2+} antagonists are postulated to improve angina is via a reduction in myocardial oxygen demand (MVO_2) during therapy. This fall in MVO_2 is suggested by experimental studies demonstrating reduced myocardial contractility, the finding in certain clinical trials of a reduction in heart rate or blood pressure during treatment, and the observation that nifedipine reduces preload by its potent vasodilatory action. It remains difficult, however, to assess the relative importance of reduction in MVO_2 compared with relaxation of the epicardial coronary arteries in patients with exercise-induced angina. It is reasonable to assume that in exertional angina, the mechanism of action responsible for symptomatic improvement differs from that responsible for the beneficial effect seen in variant angina, as the pathogenesis also differs.

It is obvious that the mechanisms of action of these drugs can only be appreciated when we have achieved a clearer understanding of the causes responsible for spasm and for angina occurring in the absence of an increase of myocardial demand in patients with stable angina (4,15).

PERSPECTIVES

Looking to the future, a number of problems remain to be defined. It is important that we establish the mode of action of these agents in the various types of angina, and, in particular, that we obtain knowledge of the pharmacological characteristics responsible for the relative potency of different agents within this group on different sites of action. With this knowledge of relative potency, it should be possible to subselect patients who will achieve the maximum therapeutic benefit in a particular type of angina with avoidance of side-effects using the appropriate drug.

In angina, as in other conditions, combination therapy with drugs possessing different modalities of action, but similar end-points, is often necessary to control moderate to severe symptoms. These combinations allow reduction in individual drug dosages, and thus lessens side-effects while attaining a cumulative effect on the target organ. The potential use of Ca^{2+} antagonists in this way is multiple. Nifedipine, with its lack of negative inotropism and peripheral vasodilatory properties, would appear ideal for combination with a β-blocker and, indeed, initial studies support this concept (8). Verapamil and diltiazem, on the other hand, would probably be best used combined with nitrates. Further trials of various combinations of Ca^{2+} antagonists with long-acting nitrates and β-blockers should be performed to assess this potential.

Following myocardial infarction, coronary artery spasm, angina at rest, and reinfarction are common events. Theoretically, at least, it should be possible to reduce these postinfarction ischemic events by the use of Ca^{2+} antagonists alone, or in combination, in the early period. It may be that improvement in morbidity and mortality would be maximized by the identification of the subset of patients at risk for ischemic events from a subset in whom arrhythmias may be the major risk factor. In the latter group, the use of β-blockers may be more relevant because of their antiarrhythmic properties.

As we extend our research into the mechanism of action of these agents in unstable, rest and exercise-induced angina, we may obtain valuable clues on the pathogenesis of these forms of angina. The discovery of Ca^{2+} antagonists should not be the only fortunate accident which we encounter during this process.

REFERENCES

1. Balasubramanian, V., Bowles, M. J., Khurmi, N. S., and Raftery, E. B. (1982): *Circulation,* 66(II):18 (Abstract).
2. Balasubramanian, V., Lahiri, A., Paramaswan, R., Raftery, E. B. (1980): *Lancet,* 1:841–4.
3. Bertrand, M. E., Lablanche, J. M., Rousseau, M., Waremburg, H. H., Stankowtax, C., and Soot, G. (1980): *Circulation,* 61:877–882.
3a. Crean, P. A., Riebeiro, P. A., Wright, C. W., Shapiro, L., and Fox, K. M. (1983): *Ir. Med. J.,* 76:179–180.
4. Deanfield, J. E., Fox, K. M., Ribeiro, P., Crean, P. A., Chierchia, S., and Maseri, A. (1982): *Circulation,* 66(II):17 (Abstract).
5. Fleckenstein-Grun, G., and Fleckenstein, A. (1980): In: *Calcium Antagonismus,* edited by A. Fleckenstein and H. Roskamm, pp. 191–207. Springer Verlag, Berlin.

6. Hossack, K. F., and Bruce, R. A. (1981): *Am. J. Cardiol.*, 47:95–101.
7. Hugenholtz, P., Michels, H. R., Serruys, P., and Brower, R. (1981): *Am. J. Cardiol.*, 47:163–74.
8. Lynch, P., Dargie, H. J., Krikler, S., and Krikler, D. M. (1980): *Br. Med. J.*, 281:184–7.
9. Maseri, A. (1980): *Br. Heart J.*, 43:648–60.
10. Maseri, A., and Chierchia, S. (1981): *Am. J. Med.*, 71:639–44.
11. Parodi, O., Maseri, A., and Simonetti, I. (1979): *Br. Heart J.*, 41:167–74.
12. Parodi, O., Simonetti, I., L'Abbate, A., Maseri, A. (1982): *Am. J. Cardiol.*, 50:923–8.
13. Previtali, M., Salerno, J., Tavazzi, L., Ray, M., Medici, A., Chimienti, M., Specchia, G., and Bobba, P. (1980): *Am. J. Cardiol.*, 45:825–30.
14. Rosenthal, S. J., Ginsburg, R., Lamb, I. H., Baim, D. S., and Schroeder, J. S. (1980): *Am. J. Cardiol.*, 46:1027–32.
15. Schang, J. J., and Pepine, C. J. (1977): *Am. J. Cardiol.*, 39:396–402.
16. Starling, M. R., Crawford, M. H., and O'Rourke, R. (1982): *Int. J. Cardiol.*, 1:229–37.

Calcium Antagonists and Cardiovascular Disease, edited by L. H. Opie.
Raven Press, New York © 1984.

Chapter 22

Calcium Entry Blockers, Especially Nifedipine, in Angina of Effort: Possible Mechanisms and Clinical Implications

Paul R. Lichtlen, Hans-Jürgen Engel, and Wolfgang Rafflenbeul

Department of Medicine, Division of Cardiology, Hannover Medical School, Hannover, Federal Republic of Germany

MYOCARDIAL OXYGEN SUPPLY VERSUS DEMAND

In preventive drug treatment in angina of effort, a number of physiological, pathophysiological, and anatomical factors of the normal and abnormal coronary system play an important role. Some of these factors are summarized in Table 1.

Prevention of ischemia provoked by increased O_2 demand, for instance, through exercise or rapid atrial pacing raising heart rate, contractility, and wall tension (i.e., increase of blood pressure and heart size), basically is achieved by maintaining the balance between the increased O_2 demand and the ensuing rise of O_2 supply. This mainly concerns the endocardium, the first myocardial zone to be deficient in O_2 and become ischemic. Exercise-induced ischemia is thus defined as a situation in which O_2 supply to the endocardium becomes deficient to the extent where aerobic metabolism cannot be maintained any longer and anaerobic energy supply is installed; this results in a massive drop of myocardial cell function, affecting mainly the possibility to develop and maintain contractility and wall tension, as well as relaxation. At this time the arteriolar bed is maximally dilated, its resistance has reached its minimum, whereas coronary flow is at its possible maximum which, however, is far too low to maintain O_2 supply. This balance between energy demand and supply can be improved either by decreasing O_2 consumption and demand for the entire myocardium, and thus especially for the poststenotic ischemic area, or by increasing O_2 supply, mainly in the ischemic zone, or, finally, by a combination of both manoeuvers. So far, most of the drugs have been mainly concerned with a decrease in the parameters responsible for O_2 consumption (heart rate, contractility, wall tension,

TABLE 1. *Pathophysiological concepts of angina pectoris important for the understanding of antianginal drug treatment*

Autoregulation of coronary system
Epi- to endocardial flow gradient
Relation between coronary flow and degree of fixed coronary obstructions at rest and under maximal flow (coronary reserve)
Collateral flow versus antegrade flow
Eccentric versus concentric obstructions, the normal wall segment within obstructions
Vascular smooth muscle tone (coronary spasm)
Stable versus unstable angina
Intravascular and extravascular coronary resistance
Coronary steal phenomenon

heart size) by reducing either heart rate and force of contraction (β-blocking agents) or wall tension, i.e., blood pressure (afterload reduction) (nitrates, Ca^{2+}-entry blockers), or heart size, i.e., end-diastolic volume and pressure (preload reduction) (nitrates). The other way, the restoration of O_2 supply to the ischemic area, was felt to be impossible as the arteriolar bed during ischemia was assumed to be already maximally dilated. Indeed, drugs like dipyridamole, resulting mainly in maximal coronary arteriolar dilatation and inhibition of autoregulation, were not only unable to further increase exercise flow (17) but even provoked angina through a steal phenomenon (18,19). This is based on the observation that dipyridamole acts only on the arteriolar level and completely blocks autoregulation, increasing the resting flow to the level of exercise, and at the same time decreasing blood pressure and thus coronary flow in critically perfused regions (18,19). Recent pharmacological studies, performed both in animals and in man, demonstrated that coronary flow to the ischemic zone could be increased through a number of ways without critically affecting autoregulation.

Poststenotic Flow

In recent years, the behavior of regional myocardial blood flow during ischemia has been analyzed in detail, especially in animals. It was shown that during ischemia flow in the endocardial layers is minimal or even abolished, and a considerable flow gradient exists from epi- to endocardium (26). Hence, zones of low or minimal, medium, and high ischemic flow have to be distinguished in the myocardium, especially in presence of myocardial infarctions (14), but also (in man) during angina of effort. These differences in flow throughout the myocardium occur in spite of the presence of maximal arteriolar dilatation in all these areas, resistance to flow being increased through augmented wall stiffness due to the absence of local contractility. In man, we substantiated this concept by observations made with the precordial xenon-clearance technique (see later sections for details) in 45 patients with single-vessel disease; this technique distinguishes between flow in a poststenotic, eventually ischemic region from a normally perfused region of the heart in the individual patient. It was observed that the increase in transmural flow in the poststenotic zone during pacing-induced ischemia (rapid atrial pacing up to angina and ST depression > 0.1 mV) reached significantly lower levels ($p < 0.001$) than in the normally perfused area where coronary blood flow corresponded to the level of O_2 demand, i.e., the increase in rate-pressure product (Fig. 1). Furthermore, in 3 patients with severe angina and ST depressions > 0.2 mV, poststenotic flow during atrial pacing even decreased when compared to the resting level. As the xenon-133 clearance technique records transmural flow only, one has to assume that in these few cases myocardial blood flow in the endocardial zone was extremely low or even had stopped so that the flow increase in the epicardial zone remained unnoticed. Therefore, it seems justified to assume that not only in animals (26,27)

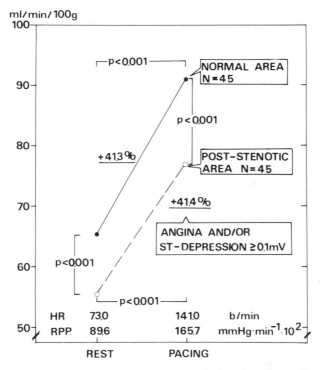

FIG. 1. Myocardial blood flow in poststenotic (*dotted line*) and corresponding normal areas (*solid line*) at rest and during rapid atrial pacing in 45 patients with severe single-vessel coronary artery disease (obstructions >70%). *Ordinate:* myocardial blood flow in ml/min/100 g myocardium; *abscissa:* flow at rest and during rapid atrial pacing (average 141 beats/min). HR, heart rate, RPP, rate-pressure product. (For details see text.)

but also in man, it is primarily endocardial flow which is severely jeopardized during ischemia.

EFFECTS OF NIFEDIPINE

An improvement of coronary flow can be achieved in various ways, for example, by a decrease in extravascular resistance through a reduction in myocardial stiffness with improved compliance brought about by a decrease in pre- and afterload, through additional arteriolar dilatation in the endocardial and middle layers of the myocardium concerning mainly arterioles which are compressed under the increased muscle stiffness and, finally, by functional dilatation of epicardial obstructions. It was found that all these mechanisms take place after administration of Ca^{2+} entry blockers (6,21). Nifedipine (Adalat®, Bayer), by partially inhibiting the entry of Ca^{2+} through the cell membrane, mainly impairs the contraction of vascular smooth muscle cells and the working myocardium; this results in vascular smooth muscle relaxation and—if nifedipine is applied directly into the coronary system—in a decrease in myocardial contractility (Fig. 2). Clinically, the more important effect, especially in angina of effort, is the one on smooth muscle vascular tone. This effect can be found on the arterioles of the peripheral and coronary circulation in man as well as on the large capacitance artery, especially the epicardial coronary arteries. The effect on the peripheral arteriolar system is mainly expressed by a decrease in blood pressure (afterload reduction), especially in the hypertensive patient (3), but also in the normotensive coronary patient especially during exercise (12) or rapid atrial pacing (7); this drop of blood pressure and peripheral vascular resistance (18) is associated with a significant increase in cardiac output (12,17). No direct changes on the venous system (preload, end-diastolic pressure and volume) have been observed by our group so far (1).

This chapter will concentrate mainly on the effect of nifedipine on the coronary system, both the arteriolar bed and the epicardial arteries, in preventing angina of effort.

CORONARY ARTERIOLAR DILATATION, CHANGES IN REGIONAL CORONARY BLOOD FLOW

Changes in regional myocardial blood flow in the normal and poststenotic area were assessed employing the precordial xenon-clearance technique, injecting 10 to 20 mCi xenon-133 directly into a major coronary artery. Details of the technique are described elsewhere (6,7,19).

Patients and Methods

Eleven patients with severe proximal obstructions (> 70%) of a single coronary artery and with a normally perfused control area, as shown by coronary angiogra-

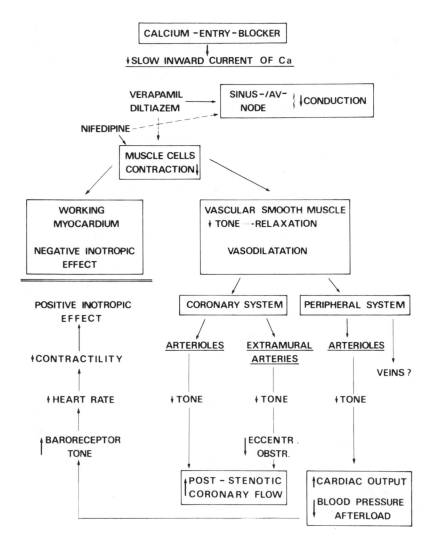

FIG. 2. Schematic drawing of the effects of nifedipine on muscle cells of the working myocardium as well as of coronary and peripheral arteries and arterioles. All changes indicated have been verified by our group. (For details see text.)

phy, were studied. Obstructions were quantitated by means of a vernier caliper (accuracy of 0.05 mm). Twenty minutes after angiography, a flow measurement was performed at rest. All flow studies were done in a LAO-40° projection in order to ensure optimal separation between the vascular distribution of the left anterior descending, the left circumflex, and the distal right coronary artery. Fifteen minutes later, rapid right atrial pacing was installed by increasing heart rate in steps of 20 beats/2 min until angina pectoris and/or ST depressions > 0.1 mV appeared in leads V_4 to V_6. The maximally tolerated heart rate was maintained for at least 2 min during the second flow measurement. After complete recovery from angina and normalization of the ST segment, 20 mg nifedipine were administered sublingually and, after a 10 min interval, right atrial pacing was repeated at the same heart rate and duration (i.e., under identical conditions); also, the xenon flow-recording during nifedipine was performed at the same moment, that is, after the same onset of pacing.

RESULTS

The effects of 20 mg nifedipine sublingually on regional myocardial blood flow during rapid atrial pacing are shown in Figs. 3 and 4. As described previously, during control pacing regional transmural myocardial blood flow increased both in poststenotic and normal areas in 10 of the 11 patients; in one case, a decrease in poststenotic flow was observed during pacing (Fig. 3). However, average flow in the poststenotic ischemic area was significantly lower than in the normal zone (78 ml/min/100 g versus 91 ml/min/100 g; $p < 0.0005$). After nifedipine, flow decreased slightly in the normal area (87 ml/min/100 g) and further increased mildly in the poststenotic zone (82 ml/min/100 g), both changes not being significant. Heart rate had increased from rest to pacing from 73 to 139 beats/min, the rate-pressure product from 97 to 182 mm Hg$\cdot$min$^{-1}\cdot10^2$ during control pacing and decreased to 142 mm Hg$\cdot$min$^{-1}\cdot10^2$ after nifedipine ($p < 0.005$). Hence, surprisingly, following nifedipine, regional myocardial blood flow in the poststenotic zone had further increased or had at least remained unchanged, in spite of a significant drop of O_2 demand. Based on the assumption that during control pacing (i.e., at the time of ischemia) mainly epicardial flow had increased and endocardial flow might even have decreased, and that after nifedipine transmural flow had further increased only in the ischemic zone, it has to be assumed that in the poststenotic area nifedipine led to an increase in regional myocardial blood flow throughout the myocardium, not only in the epi- but especially also in the endocardial layers.

The further increase in flow in the poststenotic area after administration of nifedipine can be attributed to several factors: First, nifedipine leads to a decrease in blood pressure (afterload), i.e., the rate-pressure product; this results in a decrease in wall tension (i.e., wall stiffness) and thus in extramural coronary resistance especially in the ischemic area; this also prevents a further increase in end-diastolic pressure. Second, during ischemia, the arteriolar system in the poststenotic area is maximally dilated; however, endocardial flow is low due to the increased extravascular resistance; after nifedipine the decrease of the latter leads to an increase of flow in the endocardial zone. Third, after nifedipine there is partial inhibition of autoregulation of flow, preventing an increase in arteriolar resistance in the poststenotic zone and, thus, a decrease in flow to the level corresponding to O_2 demand; hence, O_2 delivery remains slightly higher than demand. It is important to note that this does not lead to a steal phenomenon, as flow increases only mildly (by approximately 20%) at rest after nifedipine

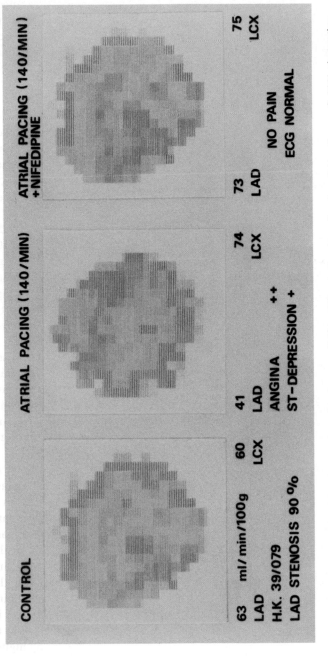

FIG. 3. Typical example of the changes in regional myocardial blood flow in the normal and poststenotic area (>90% obstruction of the left anterior descending branch) at rest (*left*), and during pacing-induced angina before (*middle*) and after nifedipine (20 mg sublingual) (*right*). Note the marked decrease of poststenotic flow from 63 ml/min/100 g at rest to 41 ml/min/100 g during control pacing up to 140 beats/min. At this time the patient suffered from severe angina. ST depression was >0.2 mV; at the same time flow in the normal area had increased from 60 to 74 ml/min/100 g. After nifedipine flow increased in the previously ischemic area from 41 to 73 ml/min/100 g and remained unchanged in the normal area; the patient was free of pain and the ECG was normalized. Coronary flow is represented through analog values, i.e., a "flow image" taken in a 40° LAO projection separating the myocardial area perfused by the left anterior descending branch (*left side of each panel*) from the area perfused by the normal left circumflex branch (*right side of each panel*). Each small quadrangle represents a matrix point, i.e., flow value for an area of 0.5 × 0.5 cm. The highest flow values (= 100%) are represented in *red*, the "flow scale" decreases by steps of 6.25% from *red* to *orange, yellow, green,* and *blue* as the lowest value.

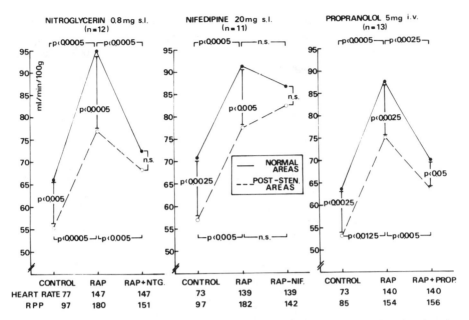

FIG. 4. Regional myocardial blood flow during rapid atrial pacing before and after nitroglycerin, propranolol, and nifedipine. *Ordinate:* myocardial blood flow in the normal (*solid line, closed circles*) and poststenotic zone (*broken line, open circles*) in ml/min/100 g. *Abscissa:* control flow at rest, flow during control pacing (RAP), and flow during pacing under drug administration. (For details see text.)

(6,17) and a further increase corresponding to the level of O_2 consumption is observed during exercise (17) or atrial pacing (6). This is a completely different behavior from the one observed after administration of dipyridamole where resting flow increases by approximately 100%, i.e., to the maximum of coronary reserve, and no further increase is seen during pacing or exercise (17,19). This raise in flow often results in angina due to a shift of blood from highly underperfused to normal zones, or a further drop in blood pressure and, consequently, in flow in areas of critical perfusion (18). Furthermore, it is interesting to note that the two other antiischemic drugs, nitrates and β-blockers, lead to a completely different behavior of regional myocardial blood flow under rapid atrial pacing (Fig. 4). In a study with an identical protocol, employing control pacing up to angina and ST depressions > 0.1 mV, and pacing after drug administration, we were able to demonstrate a significant decrease in flow both in the normal and poststenotic zone ($p < 0.0005$) after nitroglycerine (0.8 mg s.l.), as well as propranolol (5 mg i.v.) (6). This drop of flow was more pronounced in the normal than in the poststenotic zone, so that the difference between flow in both areas was almost abolished by drug administration. This autoregulatory decrease in flow corresponded to the drop in afterload, i.e., the rate-pressure product, from 180 to 151 mm Hg·min⁻¹·10² after nitroglycerin and, as we had to assume, in contractility following propranolol. Hence, nifedipine, in contrast to nitroglycerin and propranolol, which through a decrease in O_2 demand also prevented ischemia, increased O_2 supply to the ischemic area although O_2 demand was also considerably reduced.

CHANGES IN THE DEGREE OF THE PROXIMAL RESISTANCE AT THE LEVEL OF THE CORONARY OBSTRUCTION

Recent studies suggested that the further increase in transmural coronary flow in the poststenotic, previously ischemic, area in some patients might also be mediated through a decrease in resistance within critical obstructions, especially eccentric ones.

Technical Aspects

The most narrow diameters of coronary obstructions were measured from 35 mm angiograms on a Tage-Arno-projector applying at least four, often up to seven different projections. The measuring device was a vernier caliper with an accuracy of 0.05 mm, the tip of the SONES- or JUDKINS-catheter being used for calibration (measurements of 20 different catheter tips averaging 1.8 mm), the enlargement factor in the central beam of X-ray being approximately 1:3 (see ref. 25 for details). The intra- and interobserver variability was assessed in 82 double-measurements on different days in 12 diameters of obstructions; the average deviation between the first and second measurement amounted to 7.26 ± 3.33%. We, therefore, accepted only increases in diameter of more than 10% as biologically relevant.

Results

In 42 high-grade coronary obstructions with a most narrow diameter between 1.0 and 1.7 mm, 20 stenoses were found to be dilated by more than 10% (average 31%) 10 min after sublingual administration of 20 mg nifedipine; 22 obstructions remained unaffected (Fig. 5). A similar behavior was also found in 25 of 54 obstructions 10 min after sublingual administration of 0.8 mg nitroglycerin. Here, the average increase of the obstructions dilating by more than 10% was 28%; again, 29 of the stenoses (approximately half) did not react. Interestingly, the combined sublingual administration of 20 mg nifedipine and 0.8 mg nitroglycerin led to an additional effect (Fig. 6); 31 of 50 obstructions dilating more than 10% showed an average increase of 49%, and almost doubled their most narrow diameter from approximately 1.25 to more than 2.0 mm. A typical example is shown in Fig. 7 where the most narrow diameter was dilated from 1.4 to 1.96 mm (+ 38%). It is interesting to observe that pharmacological

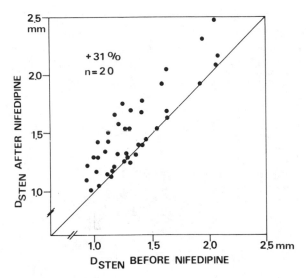

FIG. 5. Effect of nifedipine (20 mg sublingual) on the most narrow diameter (D_{sten}) in 42 high-grade coronary artery stenoses mainly of the left anterior descending branch. *Abscissa:* most narrow diameter before; *ordinate:* 10 min after drug administration. The average percent increase concerns only those obstructions with a biologically significant change (greater than intraobserver variability), i.e., an increase of more than 10% (see text).

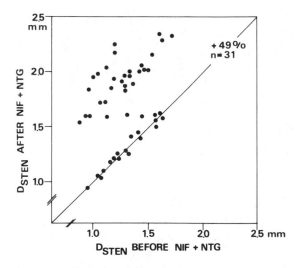

FIG. 6. Changes of the most narrow diameter (D_{sten}) in 50 coronary stenoses after combined sublingual administration of 0.8 mg nitroglycerin and 20 mg nifedipine; same arrangement as in Fig. 5.

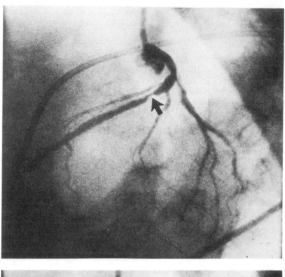

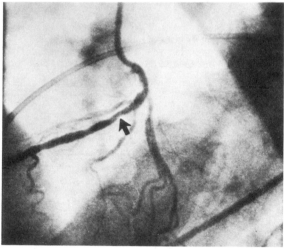

FIG. 7. Typical example of the effect of the combined sublingual administration of 0.8 mg nitroglycerin and 20 mg nifedipine on D_{sten} of an eccentric obstruction of the left anterior descending branch, half-axial LAO projection. There was an increase in D_{sten} from 1.4 mm (*top*) to 1.96 mm (*bottom*), i.e., by approximately 40%.

dilation of coronary obstructions mainly concerned *eccentric stenoses;* they were angiographically defined as obstructions in which the diameters measured in various projections 90° apart differed in length by more than 25%. In contrast, a stenosis was thought to be concentric in nature when the difference of various diameters was below 25%. Only three of the so-defined 32 eccentric obstructions did not dilate after the combined treatment of nifedipine and nitroglycerin, in contrast to 16 of 18 concentric obstructions. This leads to the assumption that in eccentric obstructions certain portions of the free wall are not yet diseased and are able to dilate considerably under Ca^{2+} entry blocking agents, in contrast to the concentric obstructions. In accordance, a postmortem analysis of 384 obstructions with narrowings of more than 50% (cross-sectional area at histology) performed in our laboratory (8) revealed the presence of a normal wall segment including at least one-quarter of the circumference in more than half of the obstructions studied.

DISCUSSION

Nifedipine Alone

Based on a host of studies performed in animals and in man, the preventive action of Ca^{2+} entry blockers, especially nifedipine, in ischemia and angina of effort can be described as follows:

The relaxing effect on vascular smooth muscle tone leads to arteriolar dilatation both in the peripheral and coronary system. On one hand, this results in a decrease in afterload, i.e., peripheral resistance and arterial pressure and—as venous pooling remains unaffected by Ca^{2+} entry blocking agents—in a mild increase in cardiac output. In spite of the slight increase in heart rate and dP/dt_{max} due to the decrease in blood pressure and increase in baroreceptor tone, the rate-pressure product, and thus probably also the average myocardial O_2 demand, decreases markedly. On the other hand, in the coronary bed, arteriolar dilatation maintained as autoregulation is partially abolished through the Ca^{2+} entry blocker; this leads to an improvement in perfusion especially in the jeopardized myocardium, i.e., in the poststenotic, previously ischemic area, mainly the endocardial region. Furthermore, in approximately 50% of the patients, nifedipine results in a considerable dilatation of proximal eccentric obstructions, resulting in a further decrease in total coronary resistance and increase in poststenotic flow. Hence, during increased O_2 demand due to exercise or rapid atrial pacing, O_2 delivery is increased to a level which is considerably higher than the reduced O_2 demand. To what extent the reduction in contractile force, observed after direct intracoronary injection of nifedipine (2), exerts an additional O_2-saving effect cannot be answered at the present time, as this effect with systemic administration is overridden by the increased sympathetic tone resulting in a mild rise in contractility.

The clinical efficacy of nifedipine in angina of effort has been confirmed in numerous exercise studies (15,22) demonstrating an improvement of ST-segment depression and of exercise tolerance in the majority of patients, as well as a decrease of anginal attacks. We believe that this is due to a combination of a decrease in afterload and an increase in poststenotic coronary blood flow due to dilatation of the arteriolar bed as well as of eccentric obstructions. The increased tone within proximal obstructions with crucially narrowed diameters (below 1.5 mm) seems to be a frequent phenomenon (Fig. 8). In 36 patients with high-grade proximal obstructions of the left anterior descending branch

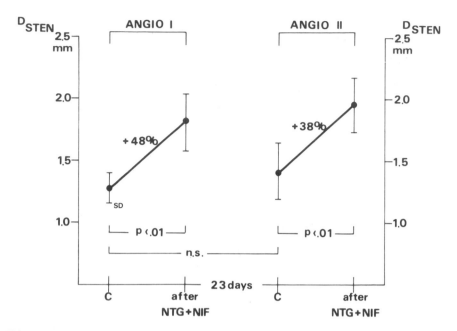

FIG. 8. Long-term course of residual vascular tone in 36 isolated coronary obstructions of the proximal left anterior descending branch, analyzed from angiograms performed in the same projection after an average interval of 23 days. In both instances, the combined administration of nitroglycerin (NTG) and nifedipine (NIF) led to a significant increase in the most narrow diameter (D_{sten}) by 48% and 38%, respectively (for details see text).

($> 70\%$), all being scheduled for balloon dilatation and, therefore, undergoing coronary angiography twice within an average of 23 days, we found a persistently increased tone of the remaining vascular smooth muscle within the obstruction; this could be relaxed in both instances. Hence, after the combined sublingual administration of nifedipine and nitroglycerin, a considerable increase of the most narrow diameters by 48% and 38%, respectively, was observed each time. We concluded that the increased tone indicated a lack of a feedback mechanism from the ischemic area to the epicardial artery, not leading to a maximal widening of the proximal obstruction. Treatment with Ca^{2+} antagonists in patients with severe angina of effort seems, therefore, especially of benefit in patients with high-grade eccentric obstructions, reducing the increased total coronary resistance.

Nifedipine Combined With Nitrates

Today the preventive treatment of angina of effort is based on three types of drugs, nitrates, β-blocking agents and, in addition, Ca^{2+} entry blockers. As already demonstrated, nifedipine can effectively be *combined with nitrates;* this results in a further relaxation of vascular smooth muscle tone, especially in

TABLE 2. Effects of nitrates versus calcium antagonists in vascular smooth muscle relaxation

Effect on:	Nitrites, nitrates	Ca^{2+} antagonists
Large extramural coronary arteries	+++	+++
Coronary arterioles	Only in high doses f.i. with intra-coronary, not s.l., administration	With low doses s.l., p.o., i.v.
Venous system	++++	None
	++	+++
Eccentric stenoses	Short (1 hr)	Long (3–4 hr)
Coronary spasm	++	++++
Mechanism	Intracellular sequestration of Ca^{2+} Induction of cGMP	Inhibition of Ca^{2+} influx into the cell No effect on Ca^{2+} efflux

Strong effect, ++++; moderate effect, +++; mild effect, ++.

the extramural eccentric obstructions and, in addition, in a reduction in pre- and afterload through combined arteriolar and venous dilatation. Some of the factors leading to an additional effect are summarized in Table 2. It is important to note that nitrates, when administered sublingually, exhibit only minimal effects on the coronary arteriolar level and act mainly on the peripheral venous bed by reducing preload: The different pharmacological actions of nifedipine and nitrates are explained by the way they influence Ca^{2+} fluxes across the membrane and within the vascular smooth muscle cell. Hence, a combination of nifedipine with nitrates is always desirable in the presence of eccentric obstructions with a markedly increased vasomotor tone, especially, of course, in the presence of coronary artery spasm, but also of an increased preload, i.e., end-diastolic volume and pressure.

The combination of Ca^{2+} entry blockers with β-blocking agents has become more popular recently, especially by using nifedipine, which in contrast to ver-apamil or diltiazem, exerts no inhibiting action on conductance both in the sinus- and atrioventricular node when clinical doses are used (4,5). A combination with β-blocking agents is advantageous in many patients, especially in the presence of a markedly elevated heart rate during exercise or insufficient control of blood pressure in hypertensive patients (3).

SUMMARY

Ca^{2+} entry blocking agents, and especially nifedipine, are not only useful in the presence of coronary spasm, Prinzmetal's angina, and unstable angina, but even more so in angina of effort, i.e., stable angina. This is of special importance for in most coronary patients a mixed form of angina is present including both angina of effort and angina at rest, where fixed anatomical obstructions as well as functional changes of vasomotor tone play a role. It should be mentioned that "fixed" obstructions completely unable to dilate are found rather rarely; in most patients some of the obstructions are eccentric in nature and still able to dilate to a certain extent. Ca^{2+} entry blocking agents are, therefore, beneficial in most patients with stable angina pectoris due to their action on the coronary arteriolar level, as well as on the proximal obstruction and the peripheral arteriolar system. For all these reasons, drug treatment of stable angina has become more successful during the last years, and it is conceivable that, for the first time, drug treatment might also have a significant prognostic impact.

REFERENCES

1. Amende, I., Simon, R., and Lichtlen, P. R. (1980): *Circulation,* 62:III-259.
2. Amende, I., Simon, R., Hood, W. P., Daniel, W., and Lichtlen, P. R. (1981): *Circulation,* 64:IV-293 (Abstract).
3. Bühler, F. (1984): In: *Calcium Antagonists and Cardiovascular Disease,* edited by L. H. Opie, pp. 313-322. Raven Press, New York.
4. Dargie, H. J., Lynch, P. G., Krikler, D. M., Harris, L., and Krikler, S. (1981): *Am. J. Med.,* 71:676.
5. Ekelund, L. G., and Orö, L. (1979): *Clin. Cardiol.,* 2:203.
6. Engel, H. J., and Lichtlen, P. R. (1981): *Am. J. Med.,* 71:658-666.
7. Engel, H. J., Lichtlen, P. R., and Hundeshagen, H. (1982): *Z. Kardiol.,* 71:326-333.
8. Freudenberg, H., and Lichtlen, P. (1981): *Z. Kardiol.,* 70:863-869.
9. Gould, K. L., Lipscomb, K., and Calvert, D. (1975): *Circulation,* 51:1085.
10. Gould, K. L. (1980): *Am. J. Cardiol.,* 45:286-292.
11. Gould, K. L., and Kelley, K. O. (1982): In: *Coronary Artery Disease,* edited by W. P. Santamore and A. A. Bove, pp. 173-198. Urban & Schwarzenberg, Baltimore.
12. Hanrath, P., Kremer, P., and Bleifeld, W. (1982): *Eur. Heart J.,* 3:325-330.
13. Hundeshagen, H., Geisler, S., Dittmann, P., Lichtlen, P., and Engel, H. J. (1976): *Eur. J. Nucl. Med.,* 1:107.
14. Jennings, R. (1984): In: *Calcium Antagonists and Cardiovascular Disease,* edited by L. H. Opie, pp. 85-95. Raven Press, New York.
15. Kaltenbach, M. (1974): In: *Proceedings of the 1st International Adalat Symposium,* Tokyo, p. 126. University of Tokyo Press, Tokyo.
16. Klein, W., Brand, D., Luch, N., and Maurer, E. (1982): *Z. Kardiol.,* 71:398-405.
17. Lichtlen, P. (1975): In: *Proceedings of the 2nd International Adalat Symposium,* edited by W. Lochner, W. Braasch, and G. Kroneberg, pp. 212-224. Springer, Heidelberg.
18. Lichtlen, P., Engel, H. J., Amende, I., Rafflenbeul, W., and Simon, R. (1976): In: *Proceedings of the 3rd International Adalat Symposium,* edited by A. D. Jatene and P. R. Lichtlen, pp. 14-29. Excerpta Medica, Amsterdam.
19. Lichtlen, P. R., and Engel, H. J. (1979): *Cardiovasc. Radiol.,* 2:203-216.
20. Lichtlen, P. R., and Engel, H. J. (1982): In: *Detection of Ischemic Myocardium with Exercise,* edited by F. Loogen and L. Seipel, pp. 98-110. Springer-Verlag, Heidelberg.
21. Lichtlen, P. R., Rafflenbeul, W., Amende, I., Simon, R., and Reil, G. (1983): In: *Angiology* (*in press*).
22. Mueller, H. S., and Chahine, R. A. (1981): *Am. J. Med.,* 71:645-657.
23. Rafflenbeul, W., Lichtlen, P. R., Kaltenbach, M., and Kober, G. (1982): *Z. Kardiol.,* 71:166 (Abstract).
24. Rafflenbeul, W., and Lichtlen, P. R. (1982): *Z. Kardiol.,* 71:439-444.
25. Rafflenbeul, W., Smith, L. R., Rogers, W. J., Mantle, J. A., Rackley, C. E., and Russel, R. O. (1979): *Am. J. Cardiol.,* 43:699-707.
26. Schaper, W. (1979): In: *The Pathophysiology of Myocardial Perfusion,* edited by W. Schaper, pp. 345-379. Elsevier/North-Holland, Amsterdam.
27. Winbury, M. M. (1974): In: *Pharmacologie Clinique des Médicaments Antiangineux,* p. 153. Edition Sandoz, Paris.

Calcium Antagonists and Cardiovascular Disease, edited by L. H. Opie.
Raven Press, New York © 1984.

Chapter 23

Nifedipine for Angina and Acute Myocardial Ischemia

P. G. Hugenholtz, P. D. Verdouw, J. W. de Jong, and
P. W. Serruys

Department of Cardiology, The Thoraxcenter, University Hospital Rotterdam, The Netherlands

Since their introduction in the early 1970s in Japan and Europe, Ca^{2+} antagonists have elicited great interest in the cardiological community. This is not only because one is dealing with an entirely new, although heterogeneous, group of compounds with a novel therapeutic principle, the manipulation of Ca^{2+} ion transport into and inside the cell, but also because they have proven to have great clinical efficacy in hitherto difficult to treat syndromes. Now that these compounds have been introduced in all parts of the world, it appears timely to review their profile in order to delineate their position in the therapeutic arsenal available to the practicing physician. Only the three main agents, nifedipine, verapamil, and diltiazem will be discussed, although several related or derived compounds are currently under development, and new compounds are imminent.

Combination therapy with nitrates, β-blockers, and Ca^{2+} antagonists has been recommended by several authors. This seems particularly advantageous when the dosages of the individual drugs in combination therapy are lower than with monotherapy, since side-effects can be reduced. For example, in a patient with angina pectoris who has hypertension and tachycardia, the combination of a β-blocker with nifedipine may be particularly advisable since the two main determinants of myocardial O_2 consumption, heart rate and afterload, can be reduced at the same time. Furthermore, the reflex-induced tachycardia after nifedipine will be blocked by the β-blocker. A schematic view of their overall (inter)action is provided in Fig. 1. Now let us return to reality and look at the evidence.

DETERMINANTS OF MYOCARDIAL OXYGEN CONSUMPTION

	HEART RATE	PRELOAD	AFTERLOAD	CONTRACTILITY	CORONARY VASCULAR TONE	CORONARY VASCULAR FLOW
A: NITRATES	↑	↓	↓	—	↧	↥
B: β-BLOCKERS	↓	↥	↑	↧	↑	—
C: CALCIUM ANTAGONISTS	↥	—	↓	↧	↓	↑
COMBINATION OF B AND C	↧	↓	↓	↧	↓	↑

FIG. 1. Schematic display of the principal effects of the nitrates, β-blocking agents, Ca^{2+} antagonists, and their combination. Aim of the therapy is to achieve oxygen demand–supply balance in the myocardium in angina pectoris. Note that when there is increased vasomotor tone, Ca^{2+} antagonists would seem to provide the best approach, since the combined effects of β-blocker and Ca^{2+} antagonists overcome increased vasomotor tone, while reducing cardiac work. *Upward arrow,* increase; *upward barred arrow,* lesser increase; *downward arrow,* decrease; *downward barred arrow,* lesser decrease; *bar,* effect undefined.

REPERFUSION IN THE PIG

Our reperfusion studies in the pig show that when coronary blood flow is reduced to 20 to 30% of control, mechanical action of the underperfused region of the heart all but ceases. Yet, if that area is reperfused soon enough, it will contract again normally. When reperfusion with blood is begun after 30 min of coronary artery occlusion, the contraction of the myocardial wall returns to only half the preocclusion level. However, when a nifedipine infusion (1 μg · kg⁻¹ min⁻¹, i.v.) is started just before reperfusion, myocardial contraction returns to 75% of the preocclusion level. This protective effect, presumably against reperfusion damage as detailed by Zimmerman et al. (72) and Hearse et al. (21), can also be shown in the same animal preparation after complete occlusion of the coronary artery near its origin. Most animals die of ventricular fibrillation within the first minutes after such ligation. In striking contrast, most animals in whom high doses of nifedipine or a combination of nifedipine and propanolol was administered in the coronary artery just before ligation, survived three consecutive 10 min periods of complete occlusion. Furthermore they did not show serious arrhythmias during reperfusion (68). In other words, nifedipine given immediately before reperfusion or, better, before ischemia is induced, preserves the heart's contractile properties much better than reoxygenation by itself can achieve (69). Nifedipine also increases capillary blood flow in non-ischemic tissue of animals in whom one of the coronary arteries has been partially occluded for 30 min. This is probably because overall resistance in the coronary vascular circuit is reduced further. However, even in the center of the ischemic area where little flow remains, perfusion increases, even favoring the endocardium (69). This augmentation of capillary flow, perhaps via collaterals that have opened, may well be an important factor in the suppression of reperfusion ventricular arrhythmias. In fact, in our patients submitted for percutaneous transluminal coronary angioplasty or streptokinase desobstruction, nifedipine is now given as a routine prophylaxis. In over 200 patients so treated, ventricular fibrillation occurred only twice. Many authors have observed that sudden reperfusion of ischemic myocardial tissue may cause an extension of myocardial damage, while Hearse (21), as well as others, found that such reperfusion damage, in fact, may be caused by sudden O_2-induced transmembrane Ca^{2+} fluxes. Fagbemi and Parratt (15) have also shown that under these circumstances reperfusion arrhythmias can be completely suppressed by nifedipine, as well as by some of its derivatives.

Though it is clear that reperfusion with O_2-rich blood may have a detrimental effect on the left ventricle, whether it is reperfused after a bout of vasoconstriction, such as after dissolving a platelet aggregate, or after coronary artery bypass grafting upon coming off the pump, our data provide direct evidence that during the acute ischemic conditions the addition of nifedipine preserves local mechanical function and increases capillary blood flow, even within the core of the ischemic area. Let us now see how these observations in the intact animal can be explained by measurements in the isolated heart, in which high-energy phosphate metabolism can be better studied in detail.

EFFECTS OF NIFEDIPINE ON HIGH-ENERGY PHOSPHATE COMPOUNDS

It has been shown by a number of authors that various Ca^{2+} antagonists can reduce high-energy phosphate breakdown during hypoxia. Although slow-channel blockers vary in their mode of action on the cardiac cells as shown by Opie (50), Henry (23) and, Fleckenstein et al. (16), nifedipine certainly acts by arresting mechanical activity, thus limiting phosphate utilization. However, there are only limited data supporting this view, mainly those published by Nayler et al. (48) and Higgins et al. (25), although Ichihara et al. (29) could not substantiate these. We decided, therefore, to study the effect of nifedipine on the myocardial release of the AMP catabolites adenosine, inosine, and (hypo)xanthine during ischemia. For that purpose we made isolated rat hearts ischemic. We showed that *breakdown of adenine nucleotides* was prevented by nifedipine (32). This evidence is based on measurements of purine nucleosides and oxypurines, of coronary flow and apex displacement, as well as of the adenylate energy charge (32). Nifedipine at 10 μg/liter concentration increased the control flow from 40 to 100 ml/min/g dry wt ($p < 0.001$). When the perfusion pressure was lowered from 72 to 17 mm Hg, coronary flow in the untreated hearts decreased by 60% ($p < 0.001$). During ischemia, flow in the presence and absence of nifedipine was comparable, about 15 ml/min/g dry wt, while during reperfusion, flow increased again to control levels. While nifedipine at a concentration of 10 μg/liter decreased apex displacement by 35% ($p < 0.01$), at 100 μg/liter, it diminished contractility during the preischemic perfusion to 10% of the control values observed with its solvent ($p < 0.001$). Since during ischemia, apex displacement was already reduced to about 25% of preperfusion values ($p < 0.001$) both in treated and untreated hearts, the heart could deliver a threefold *increase* ($p < 0.02$) in apex displacement, when the high dose of nifedipine (100 μg/liter) had been previously present in the perfusate. Purine release during the control period was 10 ± 5 nmoles/min/g dry wt. At the end of the ischemic period, purine release was 46 ± 17 nmoles/min/g dry wt ($p < 0.05$ versus control), while nifedipine in as low a dose as 10 μg/liter reduced this release by 75% ($p < 0.05$).

These relatively mild ischemic conditions resulted in a lactate release which was 2.6 times higher than the control value ($p < 0.02$). This, too, was completely abolished by 10 μg/liter nifedipine ($p < 0.05$). During reperfusion, purine and lactate production, after an initial sharp rise, decreased again, but the hearts released more of these compounds in the untreated group than in the treated group.

When ischemia was made more severe by reducing flow to a larger extent and by increasing heart rate, the highest dose of nifedipine, 100 μg/liter, *prevented adenosine release* during 10 min of ischemia by more than 90% ($p < 0.02$). This dose also decreased the release of inosine, hypoxanthine, and xanthine during ischemia by 85% ($p < 0.002$), 75% ($p < 0.05$), and 64% ($p < 0.05$). In these experiments, the solvent itself also had an effect on purine production during the control period as the release of adenosine rose from levels 1 nmoles/10 min to 7 to 11 nmoles/10 min. Differences in lactate release during the control period were only observed with 3 μg/liter nifedipine: This induced a 42% decrease ($p < 0.05$). The nifedipine dose had to be increased to levels ten times as high to prevent lactate release ($p < 0.001$). The best results, in terms of restricting adenosine release, were obtained when nifedipine (30 μg/liter) was combined with propanolol (30 μg/liter) (Fig. 2).

We were unable to measure a significant decrease in *myocardial ATP content* when flow was restricted to as little as 2.5 ml/min with a heart rate of 360 beats/min. However, adenylate energy charge decreased by about 15% due to ischemia ($p < 0.02$). This decrease was prevented by 100 μg/liter nifedipine ($p < 0.05$ versus solvent). Although we found that the release of lactate, a marker of myocardial ischemia (e.g., see ref. 31), was reduced by nifedipine, Ichihara et al. (29) were unable to detect an effect of nifedipine on myocardial lactate release during ischemia in the dog. Perhaps species differences exist to explain this.

These protective effects found in our experiments are not primarily due to the negative inotropic action of nifedipine, because we found that the drug did not affect contractility further when, as a result of ischemia, mechanical action had been reduced. Similarly, Perez et al. (52) found, at these doses, no

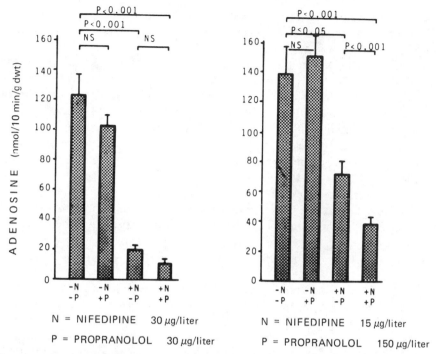

FIG. 2. The release of adenosine was studied in the efflux of the isolated rat heart driven at 360 beats/min and with coronary flow reduced to 25% of control. The prior administration of 30 μg/liter of nifedipine with a similar concentration of propranolol virtually eliminated the loss of this high-energy phosphate metabolite during ischemia; propranolol by itself was much less cardioprotective. (From ref. 33.)

nifedipine- or diltiazem-induced depression of the mechanical activity of ischemic canine heart but, instead, as in our experiments, observed a significant enhancement of its performance. In fact, with the highest dose of nifedipine we found an actual increase in apex displacement (32) concomitant with the decrease in purine release.

Atkinson (3) has reviewed the activities of important regulatory enzymes *in vitro* as a function of *energy charge*. With an increase in energy charge from 0 to 1, the regulatory enzymes in ATP-using sequences increase in activity, and those which regenerate ATP decrease in activity. Nifedipine appears capable of increasing the energy charge to the levels necessary for the proper functioning of the heart even when, under ischemic conditions, less O_2 is available. Perhaps its beneficial intracellular action is related to this regulatory function (12,34,41).

It is of interest that rat heart produces relatively large amounts of *xanthine* during ischemia (34). Xanthine oxidase, which converts hypoxanthine to xanthine (and xanthine to urate) is reported to be absent or to be present in low amounts (41). On the other hand, the extent to which xanthine oxidase in heart and blood vessels is present has been implicated as a causative factor in atherosclerosis by Carr et al. (12); further studies are clearly needed in this area. Could nifedipine be a primary antiatherosclerotic agent by this mechanism as suggested by the data of Fleckenstein and Henry (Chapters 2 and 20, *this volume*)?

Nayler et al. (48) were among the first to show that hearts from rabbits treated with nifedipine, verapamil, or propranolol were protected against the ischemia-induced decline in the ATP-generating and O_2-utilizing capacity of the mitochondria. According to Nayler and Poole-Wilson (49), at that time no simple explanation for the protection afforded by Ca^{2+} antagonists to hypoxic and ischemic heart muscle could be given. However, from our experiments we conclude that nifedipine prevents myocardial adenine nucleotide breakdown in ischemic rat heart, and presumably in the ischemic intact pig heart, by an energy regulatory action over and above its negative inotropic action. The precise mechanism remains to be solved, but little doubt can remain of its beneficial action, and further investigation in the human heart appears in order.

OBSERVATIONS IN PATIENTS: EFFECTS ON HEMODYNAMICS

To demonstrate the direct effect of nifedipine on the human heart, the intra-coronary route of administration was used by Kaltenbach and co-workers in 1979 (36). While 0.1 mg intravenously administered nifedipine had no effects on systemic hemodynamics or coronary sinus O_2 saturation, intracoronary injection of the same dose caused a significant increase of coronary sinus O_2 saturation, which terminated 5 min after infusion. During exercise, 15 min after 0.1 mg nifedipine i.c., an antiischemic effect, documented by a reduction in exercise-induced increase in left ventricular end-diastolic pressure and exercise-induced ST-T-segment depression, was apparent. The authors stated that this effect could not be entirely explained by the effects on the coronary arteriolar reserve, because it persisted after coronary flow had returned to normal. A central effect of the drug on cardic metabolism and/or contractility was considered as an alternative explanation. The effects of intracoronary nifedipine on left ventricular contractility were further studied by Serruys and co-workers (60,61). Epicardial wall motion was shown to be decreased and delayed by measuring the distances between metal markers which had been sutured on the epicardium during prior surgery in regions directly supplied by bypasses. An impaired left ventricular relaxation pattern after intracoronary injection of 0.1 mg nifedipine was also demonstrated by Rousseau et al. (57), both in patients and normal subjects. In addition, several authors have shown a powerful spasmolytic and vasodilating effect after intracoronary nifedipine (6,7,26,62).

The duration of the effect of intracoronary nifedipine on *cardiac metabolism* was also studied by Serruys et al. (62) during atrial pacing with heart rates up to 140 beats/min. Pacing-induced angina pectoris threshold was not affected 25 min after 0.1 mg intracoronary nifedipine, but at that time the efflux of hypoxanthine and lactate became significantly reduced although a lesser degree of efflux of these catabolites was also seen after injection of the solvent, which acted as a placebo. This indicates an O_2-sparing effect and also that the cause of induced anginal pain is not only the release of high-energy phosphate catabolites. This action may reflect increased efficiency of O_2 utilization.

Lydtin et al. (40) studied the hemodynamic effect of intravenous nifedipine (0.0075 mg/kg body wt) in *healthy volunteers*. There was an increase in heart rate by 25 beats/min, while systolic and diastolic blood pressures decreased. The cardiac output increased from 8.3 to 12 liters/min. From the observed shortening of the preejection period, these authors concluded that an increase in contractility takes place after intravenous nifedipine which can be explained by β-sympathomimetic stimulation related to the decrease in peripheral resistance.

The differences between the intrinsic negative inotropic effect of nifedipine, shown after direct intracoronary injection of the drug in humans and its absence after intravenous administration of nifedipine, can be explained by the reflex sympathetic drive, due to baroreceptor stimulation after the reduction in peripheral vascular resistance. Joshi et al. (35), at a constant atrial-paced rate, administered 10 mg nifedipine sublingually to 10 patients with coronary artery disease already pretreated with atenolol (400 mg/day). They observed a significant decrease of peak dP/dt and peak $dP/dt/P$, which suggested the negative inotropic effect of the drug was more evident after β-blockade. In their experiments, cardiac output, however, remained unchanged. Koch (37) gave 10 mg nifedipine sublingually to patients with coronary artery disease pretreated with metoprolol. An increase of epinephrine and norepinephrine plasma levels was observed after nifedipine. Stroke volume increased and the left ventricular filling pressure, which had increased after metoprolol alone, was reduced. These studies indicate that the stimulation of the sympathetic nervous system after nifedipine administration can be blocked by β-receptor antagonists. Although the intrinsic negative inotropic effect of the drug, thereby, may become more apparent after β-blockade, the vasodilatory effect of nifedipine appears to predominate.

There is now considerable evidence from the literature (63,66) to show that major coronary arteries can approximately double their luminal diameter from their most constricted to their most dilated state. When partial vasoconstriction takes place around an already preexisting, fixed, often eccentric, obstruction, critical reduction in flow may occur much earlier. In fact, when such increased vasomotor tone of the coronary vascular wall is invoked by a variety of stimuli, sudden reduction in flow may lead to irreversible ischemia. This is the current understanding of the mechanisms lying behind unstable angina and, often the next step, impending infarction.

Clinical experience has convinced all but perpetual skeptics of the *spasm-relieving properties of nifedipine*. Treating 127 patients with symptoms of myocardial ischemia associated with electrocardiographic or angiographic evidence of coronary artery spasm, Antman et al. (2) demonstrated complete control of anginal attacks in 63% of all patients and marked relief in 89%. They considered the drug highly effective for coronary artery spasm. Similar positive results were obtained by other authors in patients with coronary artery spasm produced by ergonovine (20,24,53) or by α-adrenergic stimulation such as by the cold pressor test (20,63). Coronary resistance is usually elevated during hand-grip isometric exercise and also decreases after nifedipine (63). With the xenon-133 clearance technique at rest, Engel et al. (14) and Heeger et al. (22) observed an increase in coronary blood flow after nifedipine. According to Lichtlen's group (14), this increase is present in normal as well as in poststenotic areas of coronary arteries. This increase in regional myocardial blood flow in poststenotic areas was confirmed by Malacoff et al. (42), although they observed a decrease in flow in regions with normal coronary arteries. During angina pectoris induced by atrial pacing, Engel et al. (14) also observed a tendency towards an increase in blood flow in poststenotic and a decrease in normal areas after nifedipine. Thus blood (re)distribution during atrial pacing appeared to become more homogeneous. As the xenon washout technique cannot differentiate between flow of subendocardial, medial, or subepicardial layers and only measures transmural flow, there remains the possibility that flow after nifedipine is only increased in the nonischemic subepicardium, but the animal data from our laboratory shown earlier would mitigate against this.

The effects of nifedipine on *coronary sinus blood flow* have been investigated by other authors. Kohler (38) observed in 6 patients with mitral stenosis, a rise in coronary sinus blood flow by 40% after 15 min, while a maximal increase of 70% was present after one-half hour. Merillon et al. (45) observed an increase in coronary sinus blood flow and a decrease in coronary vascular resistance in 20 patients with coronary artery disease. Almost identical changes in coronary sinus blood flow (+ 16%) and coronary vascular resistance (− 18%) were seen by Simonsen et al. (65) 15 min after administration of nifedipine. Neither Merillon et al. (45), Simonsen et al. (65), or Schaefer et al. (58) could, however, demonstrate a significant increase in flow during atrial pacing-induced tachycardia. The latter authors suggested that coronary artery disease in their patients was too severe and that the vessels were already maximally dilated, preventing an additional effect of nifedipine. Such an explanation would also fit some of our clinical observations in (un)stable angina pectoris described in the next section. Experimental data from our laboratory confirm that low doses of intracoronary nifedipine, while having no effect on myocardial, global, and regional function, will significantly lower the O_2 consumption of the myocardium (67). It has lead to the hypothesis of a *metabolic effect* of the drug. Could nifedipine reduce the O_2-wasting effect of free fatty acids by blocking intramyocardial lipolysis without affecting the overall dynamic state? Only further studies at the cellular level will tell.

EFFECTS ON ANGINA AND ISCHEMIA

At first sight, these differing (64) and perhaps complementary actions of Ca^{2+} antagonists and β-blockers would make it seem advisable to combine both in the clinical treatment of unstable angina and other acute ischemic states of the myocardium. This part of the chapter deals with the clinical evidence that is in favor of such concerted action while, in addition, available reports on unwanted effects with this combination of drugs will be reviewed.

The possible clinical beneficial actions of β-blockers in coronary artery disease can be summarized as follows: They may reduce or improve the ischemic state by a reduction of cardiac work, mainly through bradycardia, and by suppression of ventricular arrhythmias which improves the efficiency of cardiac function. In addition, there could be a selective cardioprotective action on subcellular systems which reduce myocardial metabolism further, while with hypertensive patients a reduction of afterload can be expected in particular with compounds with intrinsic sympathomimetic activity.

The principal clinical benefits of Ca^{2+} antagonists have been detailed in previous pages. Could they act in concert with β-blockade? Our own observations support the concept of concerted action of Ca^{2+} antagonists and β-blockers. During a one-year period, out of 1,263 admissions to our coronary care unit, 73 patients were identified with unstable angina (26) (Fig. 3). Each of these individuals had persistent pain during bedrest, coincident with intermittent changes in the electrocardiogram with elevation or depression of the ST segment, and changes in the T waves without any evidence of myocardial necrosis such as the development of Q waves or an elevation of the various cardiac enzymes. Of these 73 patients, 21 became asymptomatic within 8 hr on β-blockers with nitrates alone. In the 52 remaining patients, nifedipine in a dose of 60 mg, in divided doses of 10 mg, was added to the treatment. Forty-two out of the 52 then became asymptomatic, usually after the second dose. Ten patients remained symptomatic, 9 of whom required urgent bypass grafting. Two patients with persistent pain received intraaortic balloon pumping with immediate relief of their symptoms. One year later all are alive, as are all patients who were placed on nifedipine.

The extent of coronary artery obstructive disease as seen at cardiac catheterization has been detailed (26). Of the total group of 73 patients, 55 (75%) underwent coronary angiography during the initial hospital stay. The severity of coronary artery disease was not unlike that found in stable angina, but the incidence of advanced obstructive coronary artery disease was clearly higher in the group that remained symptomatic, despite all pharmacological interventions. On the other hand, there was a slight predominance of single- and two-vessel disease in those that responded to nifedipine.

The hemodynamic response to nifedipine was also studied in 18 of the 73 patients in whom invasive baseline data were available, from indwelling catheters, before therapy was given. No significant peripheral hemodynamic changes could be demonstrated, so that no marked peripheral unloading effect appeared to be evident (27).

Recently, Gerstenblith et al. (19) have published a prospective, randomized, placebo-controlled study, in which nifedipine and conventional treatment were

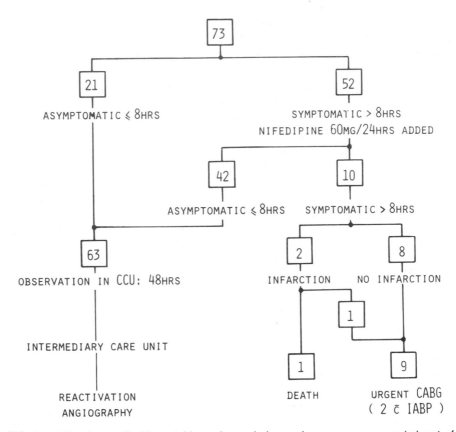

FIG. 3. In 73 patients, all with unstable angina and observed over a one-year period, out of 1,263 admissions to the coronary care unit in the University Hospital in Rotterdam, 21 became asymptomatic within 8 hr with conventional therapy consisting of bedrest, nitrates (p.o. or i.v.), and β-blockade. Of the 52, who remained symptomatic during the first 8 hr of such treatment, nifedipine was added in doses of 60 mg/24 hr. In 42 of 52, usually when the second dose had been administered orally, symptoms were completely relieved. In 10 other patients, who did not experience such relief, the subsequent arteriograms showed far advanced coronary artery disease. It is argued that the relief of increased vasomotor tone in patients with unstable angina is the deciding factor in explaining the clinical efficacy of nifedipine. CABG, coronary artery bypass grafting; IABP, intraaortic balloonpumping. (From ref. 26.)

compared in the treatment of unstable angina pectories. Thirty-eight of 68 patients given nifedipine showed success after treatment, against 27 of 70 in the control group. Success of medical treatment was defined as absence of sudden death, myocardial infarction, or need for bypass surgery within 4 months. These data provide a welcome substantiation of our observations. Similar data for a comparison of diltiazem with propanolol were shown by André-Fouët et al. (1a) favoring this Ca²⁺ antagonist over propanolol in the majority of their patients with unstable angina. In stable exertional angina pectoris, Broustet and co-workers (10) have shown that when nifedipine is used in conjunction with atenolol, the suppression of symptoms induced during exercise testing may be maximal. Schmutzler (59) has shown similar data for the combination of metroprolol and nifedipine. The explanation for the increased efficacy of the combination is readily at hand: Reduction in heart rate together with decreased afterload seem to be the main factors responsible for increased exercise tolerance, decreased incidence of angina pectoris attacks, and of diminished nitroglycerin usage.

In *unstable angina pectoris,* however, there is relatively little definite information in the literature regarding the exact mechanism of action. This is readily explicable because of the uncertainties surrounding the causes of unstable angina pectoris. Despite emphasis on the role of coronary artery spasm, a good example of which can be found in the pathological studies of Leary nearly half a century ago (39), and recently reemphasized by Maseri and co-workers (44), it has still not been generally accepted that this occurs more than in a relatively few cases. The general assumption is still that fixed organic stenosis through atherosclerotic involvement of the arterial wall is the usual cause of angina pectoris. Although it is now known that obstruction is not always concentric and, indeed, frequently may be eccentric, the concept of fixed stenosis has remained. In the majority of patients with unstable angina, however, the anatomical situation probably lies in between (Fig. 4). Particularly when eccentric lesions are present which leave part of the circumference of the vascular wall intact, vasoconstrictive stimuli may cause marked changes in the tone of that part of the vessel wall

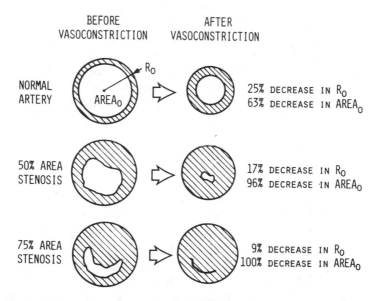

FIG. 4. Effect of changes in vasomotor tone. Note that in the second example an eccentric endothelial lesion with a 50% area stenosis can turn to a critical 96% stenosis with only minor changes in the external diameter. In other words, moderate changes in vasomotor tone can render an insignificant obstruction into a critical one.

and thus influence the coronary blood flow. Several authors have now demonstrated spontaneous changes in coronary vascular resistance independent of identifiable changes in myocardial metabolic demand. Others have seen these changes, up to complete spastic obstruction after total plexectomy, or even cardiac transplantation (7).

The *myogenic control of coronary resistance* was originally proposed by Bayliss (4) in 1902, who described the intrinsic ability of blood vessels to respond to changes in transmural pressure. This mechanism is not generally considered to have a dominant role, but it must be pointed out that is has been difficult up to now to formulate studies capable of defining the importance of this mechanism in atherosclerotic blood vessels. Berne and co-workers (5) have tested different vasoactive agents such as adenosine, nitroglycerin, and Ca^{2+} antagonists for their ability to affect the induced action potential of isolated large and small coronary arteries. Adenosine blocked the Ca^{2+}-dependent action potential in small coronary arteries, but had no effect on the action potential in large arteries. In contrast, nitroglycerin blocked the action potential in large coronary arteries, but not in small ones. Ca^{2+} antagonists blocked the action potential irrespective of the size of the vessel. Indeed, nifedipine is capable of completely blocking the autoregulation of the renal vascular bed, whereas glyceryl trinitrate fails to affect this regional autoregulation. Since autoregulation of blood flow is defined as the intrinsic regulatory mechanism of a vascular bed to maintain its blood flow at a constant rate regardless of the changes in perfusion pressure, these experimental data emphasize the *advantages of nifedipine over nitrates in affecting the coronary vascular system.* In the syndrome of unstable angina with the combination of an eccentric fixed endothelial lesion and a (hyper)sensitive, but otherwise healthy, vascular wall opposite, the influence of nifedipine is such that it promptly relaxes the excessive vascular tone. In keeping with this concept are the observations of the rapid and persistent relief of pain in the majority of patients with unstable angina pectoris reported in this study (26), and the striking results in Prinzmetal's angina (2). The specific action of nifedipine on the arteriolar tone of the major epicardial and the smaller coronary arteries, over the 48-hr observation period, stabilized what had been a very brittle condition. The fact that, in 42 of the 52 patients, such relief persisted for the entire period of observation is a further strong argument in favor of this mechanism.

The hypothesis has also been put forward that there is a subset of patients with angina at rest, and with inappropriate vasoconstriction or suspected coronary artery spasm, who may worsen with β-adrenergic blockade. In fact, Yasue et al. (71) have specifically argued against β-blockers in these individuals, as they showed that β-blockade may induce vasoconstrictive action. Since in our series of patients who had remained unresponsive during 8 hr of β-blockade, the response to nifedipine was so consistent [and just as effective as had been pain relief by intraaortic balloon pumping in our previous experience (46) with the same kind of patients], there is little doubt that nifedipine was the critical agent. Recently Braunwald (8) reviewed current clinical evidence and stated that there now might very well be a preference for the use of Ca^{2+} antagonists over β-blockade in patients suspected of having abnormally increased coronary vasomotor tone.

Such an opinion is supported by several reports in the literature (17,28,54, 55,70) which indicate that angina pectoris occurring in the Prinzmetal's syndrome may also be worsened by the treatment with β-blockers, in particular propranolol. The first observation by Yasue and co-workers (71) appeared in 1976 after having postulated earlier that in Prinzmetal's syndrome β-blockade could potentially lead to further vasoconstriction and, thus, worsen symptoms. In a recent report (70), they observed 4 cases in whom periodic attacks during rest were relieved by nitroglycerin, but made more severe by propranolol. In fact, the combination of propranolol and isoproterenol infusion induced "Prinzmetal" attacks very similar to spontaneous attacks, whereas infusion of isoproterenol alone did not do so. Coronary arteriography at the time showed severe spasm of the coronary arteries. These observations are similar to those described by Fleckenstein on an isolated vascular system (17). In these experiments, Fleckenstein had proved conclusively that the addition of β-blockade caused severe vasoconstriction of the coronary arteriolar wall which could be relieved, however, by Ca^{2+} antagonists.

Fuller et al. (18) recently studied, with thallium-201 scintigraphy, the responses to nitrates, β-adrenergic blockade, Ca^{2+} flux blockade, and prostaglandin inhibition. The painful episodes could be prevented by oral nitrates, but not totally eliminated by the other drugs. In addition, β-adrenergic blockade appeared to be detrimental. A 69-year-old man treated by Carile and Civerra (11) with pindolol, had his attacks of angina worsen with further ECG signs of anterior ischemia. Replacement by nifedipine led to total relief. This was also the conclusion of Marx (43), who overviewed the subject in 1980. He concluded: "in spasm-induced angina, propranolol may exacerbate symptoms while calcium antagonists of various kinds would appear to be the drug of choice." This *concept of dynamic coronary obstruction* in the presence of "normal" or diseased coronary arteries implies a direct role for coronary vasodilators in patients with any form of angina pectoris, even when frank coronary spasm is absent.

Also implicit in the hypothesis is the concept that dynamic and fixed components (Fig. 5) to obstruction may contribute variably to the degree of obstruction in different patients, and it should not be surprising that in patients with largely fixed obstructions, benefit will mainly come from attempts to lower myocardial O_2 uptake with nitrates and β-blocking agents. In extreme cases only, the balloon catheter dilation of the coronary artery or bypass surgery can provide adequate relief.

SIDE-EFFECTS AND DOSAGES

Clinical experience with pharmacological agents, in general, has taught us that no drug is "perfect" or without unwanted actions. Although major side-effects have rarely been reported, thus far, with nifedipine (1,9,47,51,56), this and other agents in the group of Ca^{2+} antagonists, such as verapamil, may

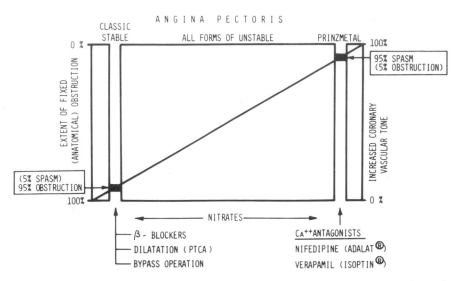

FIG. 5. The therapeutic approach to the various forms of angina pectoris depends on the clinician's awareness of the underlying pathophysiology. If "fixed" stenosis (*left*) is suspected, the first choice of therapy will be different than if spasm (*right*) is the most likely cause of symptoms. Most cases will lie in between, and therefore require, as always in clinical circumstances, individual assessment of the situation in order to achieve optimal choice of therapy. PTCA, percutaneous transluminal coronary angioplasty.

result in severe hypotension. In the latter, this is presumably because of its strong influence on atrioventricular conduction, and in the former, because of its primary negative inotropic action on cardiac contractile behavior. One can readily visualize situations, for example, in acute myocardial infarction, with an attendant hypotensive state, in which the negative inotropic characteristics of these drugs override their other actions. By and large, the side-effects (see references for details) are few, readily reversible upon interrupting the drug, and also predictable as they seem to occur exclusively at end-stages of cardiac disease.

The daily dosage of nifedipine (Adalat®, Bayer) ranges from 30 to 120 mg in divided doses, 60 mg/day our average. An intravenous solution is available, but as the drug is rapidly and fully absorbed, oral dosing is usually sufficient. Verapamil is given in the same manner in dosages between 240 and 360 mg/day, while diltiazem is effective at dosages between 180 and 360 mg. As the biological half-life ranges between 3 and 7 hr, divided doses 4 to 6 times a day usually suffice. Unavoidable side-effects relate to their mode of action: Headache, flushing, and gastrointestinal symptoms are dose-related, usually minor, and rarely a contraindication. Particular caution should be given to the use of verapamil in hypotensive states or in situations where the negative inotropic action is unwanted, i.e., in congestive heart failure when also β-blockade is given. With nifedipine, hypotensive episodes have also been described, but they are rare, given the hundreds of patient years of treatment.

PRACTICAL AND PERSONAL RECOMMENDATIONS

Treatment depends on the cause, and three main causes have been implicated in the development of angina pectoris.

The first is *fixed stenosis,* a permanent narrowing of the coronary arteries, with pain occurring only on exertion. This condition is called chronic stable angina, which is usually predictable and reverses when exertion is stopped.

The second cause, the focus of much recent interest, is *spasm,* in which dynamic changes in vessel diameter cause transient arterial obstruction. Here the manifestations may be nonexertional pain, or even silent ischemic episodes evidenced by ST-T-segment changes and arrhythmias. In its extreme form, the manifestations correspond to Prinzmetal's (variant) angina, which can occur even when there is no fixed coronary artery obstruction.

Third, excessive *platelet aggregation* can lead to partial, and occasionally total, coronary vessel blockage and myocardial infarction, often coincident with excessive thromboxane A_2 release and spasm. All of these causes may interact to produce unstable angina—the main focus of this chapter.

The first decision the physician has to make is to ascertain which of the three conditions exists: stable angina pectoris, unstable angina pectoris, or Prinzmetal's syndrome. Efforts at diagnosis should first include a detailed history, which, if inconclusive, should lead to an exercise test in ambulatory males. Various aspects of the hemodynamic and electrocardiographic response to exercise should be evaluated. Only if a suspicion of angina pectoris persists in the face of a negative exercise electrocardiogram should a thallium-201 exercise test be carried out. If positive and there is *stable angina pectoris,* we would recommend a therapeutic trial either with nitroglycerine, nifedipine, or β-blockade. The choice of the initial agent depends on the frequency and variety of the attacks, the preliminary diagnosis of the cause of angina pectoris, and ancillary signs and symptoms. For example, in a hypertensive patient with tachycardia, we would prefer to begin with a combination of β-blockade and nifedipine, rather than with nitroglycerin tablets. Contrariwise, in an elderly patient with infrequent attacks, nitroglycerin tablets sublingually might be sufficient. At any rate, an individual assessment of that patient's cause for angina pectoris and his response to that therapy should be the basis for initial management. If a response is not adequate, rather than persist, we would change the drug, since it could well be that the pathophysiology is different than suspected. Consider the schemes illustrated in Figs. 5 and 6.

When *unstable angina pectoris,* including Prinzmetal's angina, is suspected, it is our current view that nifedipine (or diltiazem) should be given at the outset with the usual supportive therapy. Certainly when attacks of myocardial ischemia are repeatedly evident, this would be the first line of attack. When the clinician is not sure of the exact pathophysiological mechanism at work, then the initial pharmacological therapy should be with nitroglycerin tablets and isosorbide dinitrate. When further therapy is required, adequate β-blockade with an effective agent such as propranolol, acebutolol, or metoprolol, with

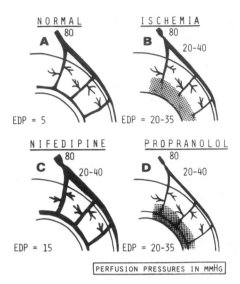

FIG. 6. Schematic drawing of hemodynamic conditions in the normal coronary vascular tree **(A)**. During ischemia **(B)**, perfusion pressure distal to the obstruction drops to 20 mm Hg. When intraventricular diastolic pressure rises, it can readily be understood why the subendocardial layers are not perfused adequately. During nifedipine treatment **(C)**, coronary vascular tone is relaxed and perfusion via the penetrating arteries and the capillary bed is enhanced. As afterload is reduced, end-diastolic pressures will be lowered which results in still better perfusion of the subendocardial layers. When propranolol is given **(D)**, there is no direct effect on coronary vascular tree and diastolic pressures remain high, so that there is no major reduction in subendocardial ischemia (*stippled area*). EDP, end-diastolic pressure.

which we have the most experience, should be introduced. Then if further therapy is required, nitrates and β-blockade should be combined with nifedipine. Only when such combination therapy is not successful (obviously assuming that appropriate doses have been given), coronary artery bypass grafting must be considered. In a small subset of patients, percutaneous transluminal coronary artery dilation will be the appropriate therapy.

From the long-term point of view, in the *post-hospital phase,* particular emphasis should be given to combination therapy: Our current experience indicates that a combination of relatively small doses of nifedipine (20–30 mg/day) with an effective β-blocker leads to marked symptom relief in most of the patients and a considerable reduction in the incidental use of nitroglycerin sublingually. This would seem the more advisable as some patients with angina pectoris have coexistent hypertension. The ultimate decision of the relative roles of β-blockade and Ca^{2+} antagonists will have to await the results of further large randomized, double-blind, and placebo-controlled studies, one of which is currently in progress in The Netherlands (30), while other trials are certain to come in various acute ischemic conditions, such as those during open-heart surgery (13).

SUMMARY

Although the effect of the three major Ca^{2+} antagonists (nifedipine, verapamil, and diltiazem) on vascular and cardiac muscle is similar, they are not identical; there exist major differences, for example, in the antiarrhythmic properties. Experimental data on the isolated rat heart and the intact working heart of the pig show that the detrimental metabolic effects of ischemia can be aborted or mitigated by these agents.

All three Ca^{2+} antagonists are effective in treating patients with coronary spasm, variant angina, and unstable angina. In our experience with 73 patients with unstable angina, 21 became asymptomatic within 8 hr of therapy with nitrates and β-blockers. Of the remaining 52, who were refractory to such therapy, the addition of 10 mg nifedipine orally every 2 hr to a maximum of 60 mg rendered 42 of 52 asymptomatic within a further 8 hr. It is argued that the timely administration of nifedipine to these and similar patients, will reduce or delay the incidence of arrhythmias and myocardial infarction.

REFERENCES

1. Anastassiades, C. J. (1980): *Br. Med. J.*, 281:1251–1252.
1a. André-Fouët, X., Usdin, J. P., Gayet, C., Wilner, C., Thizy, J. F., Viallet, M., Apoil, E., Fernant, P., and Pont, M. (1983): *Eur. Heart J.*, 4 (*in press*).
2. Antman, E., Muller, J., Goldberg, S., MacAlpin, R., Rubenfire, M., Tababsnik, B., Liang, C., Heupler, F., Achuff, S., Reichek, N., Geltman, E., Kerin, N. Z., Neff, R. K., and Braunwald, E. (1980): *N. Engl. J. Med.*, 302:1269–1273.
3. Atkinson, D. E. (1977): *Cellular Energy Metabolism and Its Regulation.* Academic Press, New York.
4. Bayliss, W. M. (1902): *J. Physiol.*, 28:220–232.
5. Berne, R. M., Belardinelli, L., Harder, D. R., Sperelakis, N., and Rubio, R. (1980): In: *Calcium Antagonismus,* edited by A. Fleckenstein and H. Roskamm, pp. 208–220. Springer Verlag, Berlin.
6. Bertrand, M. E., Lablanche, J. M., and Tilmant, P. Y. (1980): *Eur. Heart J.*, (Suppl. B) 1:65–69.
7. Bertrand, M. E., Lablanche, J. M., and Tilmant, P. Y. (1981): *Am. J. Cardiol.*, 47:174–178.
8. Braunwald, E. (1980): *Am. J. Cardiol.*, 46:1045–1046.
9. Brooks, N., Carrell, M., Pidgeon, J., and Balcon, R. (1980): *Br. Med. J.*, 281:1324.
10. Broustet, J. P., Rumeau, P., Guern, P., Cherrier, A., Pic, A., and Bonnet, J. (1980): *Eur. Heart J.*, (Suppl. B) 1:59–64.
11. Carile, L., and Civerra, C. (1980): *Clin. Ter.*, 94:351–361.
12. Carr, C. J., Talbot, J. M., and Fisher, K. D. (1975): *Life Sci. Res. Office, Fed. Am. Soc. Exp. Biol.* Bethesda.
13. Clark, R. E., Christlieb, J. Y., Henry, P. D., Fisher, A. E., Mora, J. D., Williamson, J. R., and Sobel, B. E. (1979): *Am. J. Cardiol.*, 44:825–831.
14. Engel, H. J., Wolf, R., Hudeshagen, H., and Lichtlen, P. R. (1980): *Eur. Heart J.*, (Suppl. B) 1:53–58.
15. Fagbemi, O., and Parratt, J. R. (1981): *Eur. J. Pharmacol.*, 75:179–185.
16. Fleckenstein, A., and Fleckenstein-Grun, G. (1980): *Eur. Heart J.*, (Suppl. B) 1:15–21.
17. Fleckenstein, A., Fleckenstein-Grun, G., Byon, Y. K., Haastert, H. P., and Spah, F. (1979): *Arzneim. Forschung.*, 29:230–246.
18. Fuller, C. M., Raizner, A. E., Chahine, R. A., Nahormek, P., Isihimori, T., Verani, M., Nitishin, A., Nokotoff, C., and Luchi, R. J. (1980): *Am. J. Cardiol.*, 46:500–506.
19. Gerstenblith, G., Ouyang, P., Achuff, S. C., Bulkley, B. H., Becker, L. C., Mellits, E. D., Baughman, K. L., Weiss, J. L., Flaherty, J. T., Kallman, C. H., Llewellyn, M., and Weisfeldt, M. L. (1982): *N. Engl. J. Med.*, 306:885–889.
20. Goldberg, S., Reichek, N., Wilson, J., Hirshfeld, J. W., Jr., Muller, J., and Kastor, J. A. (1979): *Am. J. Cardiol.*, 44:804.
21. Hearse, D. J., Humphrey, S. M., and Bullock, G. R. (1978): *J. Mol. Cell. Cardiol.*, 10:641–668.
22. Heeger, H., Kahn, P., and Aldor, E. (1975): In: *Proceedings of the 2nd International Adalat Symposium,* pp. 204–210. Springer Verlag, Berlin.
23. Henry, P. O. (1980): *Am. J. Cardiol.*, 46:1047–1058.
24. Heupler, F. A., and Proudfit, W. L. (1979): *Am. J. Cardiol.*, 44:798–803.
25. Higgins, T. J. C., Allsopp, D., and Bailey, P. J. (1980): *J. Mol. Cell. Cardiol.*, 12:909–927.

26. Hugenholtz, P. G., Michels, H. R., Serruys, P. W., and Brower, R. W. (1981): *Am. J. Cardiol.,* 47:163–173.
27. Hugenholtz, P. G., Serruys, P. W., and Balakumaran, K. (1982): *J. Cardiovasc. Med.,* 7:373–378.
28. Hugenholtz, P. G., Serruys, P. W., and Simoons, M. L. (1982): *Hartbulletin,* 13:171–177.
29. Ichihara, K., Ichihara, M., and Abiko, Y. (1979): *Arzneim. Forsch./Drug Res.,* 29:1539–1544.
30. *Interuniversitary Cardiological Institute, The Netherlands.* (Study design available upon request.)
31. Jong, J. W. de (1979): In: *The Pathophysiology of Myocardial Perfusion,* edited by W. Schaper, pp. 719–750. Elsevier/North-Holland, Amsterdam.
32. Jong, J. W. de, Harmsen, E., Tombe, P. P. de, and Keijzer, E. (1982): *Eur. J. Pharmacol.,* 81:89–96.
33. Jong, J. W. de, Harmsen, E., Tombe, P. P. de, and Keijzer, E. (1982): *Eur. Heart J.,* (Suppl. C) 4:520–531.
34. Jong J. W., de, Harmsen, E., Tombe, P. P. de, and Keijzer, E. (1982): *Adv. Myocardiol.,* 4:339–345.
35. Joshi, P. I., Dalal, J. J., Ruttley, M. S. J., Sheridan, D. J., and Henderson, A. H. (1981): *Br. Heart J.,* 45:457–459.
36. Kaltenbach, M., Schulz, W., and Kober, G. (1979): *Am. J. Cardiol.,* 44:832–838.
37. Koch, G. (1980): In: *Proceedings of the 4th International Adalat Symposium,* edited by P. Puech and R. Krebs, pp. 131–142. Excerpta Medica, Amsterdam.
38. Kohler, J. A. (1975): In: *Proceedings of the 2nd International Adalat Symposium,* pp. 234–235. Springer Verlag, Berlin.
39. Leary, T. (1935): *Am. Heart J.,* 10:338–348.
40. Lydtin, H., Lohmoller, G., Lohmoller, R., Schmitz, H., and Walter, I. (1975): In: *Proceedings of the 2nd International Adalat Symposium,* edited by W. Lochner, W. Braasch, and G., Kronenberg, pp. 112–123. Springer Verlag, Berlin.
41. Maguire, M. H., Lukas, M. C., and Rettie, J. F. (1972): *Biochim. Biophys. Acta,* 262:108–115.
42. Malacoff, R. F., Lorell, B. H., Mudge, G. H., Holman, B. L., Idoine, J., Bifolck, L., and Cohn, P. F. (1982): *Circulation,* 65:I-32 (Abstract).
43. Marx, L. J. (1980): *Science,* 208:1127–1130.
44. Maseri, A., L'Abbate, A., Baroldi, G., Chiercha, S., Marzilli, M., Ballestra, A. M., Severi, S., Parodi, P., Biagini, A., Distante, A., and Pesola, A. (1978): *N. Engl. J. Med.,* 299:1271–1277.
45. Merillon, J. P., Morgant, C., Zygelman, M., Beaufils, P., Patart, O., Chapuy, J. Y., and Gourgon, R. (1978): *Arch. Mal. Coeur,* 8:913–921.
46. Michels, R., Haalebos, M., Kint, P. P., Hagemeijer, F., Balakumaran, K., Brand, M. vd, Serruys, P. W., and Hugenholtz, P. G. (1980): *Eur. Heart Jr.,* 1:31–43.
47. Motte, G., Chanu, B., Sebag, C., and Benaim, P. (1980): *Nouv. Presse Med.,* 9:379–380.
48. Nayler, W. G., Ferrari, R., and Williams, A. (1980): *Am. J. Cardiol.,* 46:242–248.
49. Nayler, W. G., and Poole-Wilson, P. (1981): *Basic Res. Cardiol.,* 76:1–15.
50. Opie, L. H. (1980): *Lancet,* 1:806–810.
51. Opie, L. H., and White, D. A. (1980): *Br. Med. J.,* 281:1462.
52. Perez, J. E., Sobel, B. E., and Henry, P. D. (1980): *Am. J. Physiol.,* 239:H658–H663.
53. Previtali, M., Salerno, J. A., Tavazzi, L., Ray, M., Medici, A., Chimienti, M., Specchia, G., and Bobba, P. (1980): *Am. J. Cardiol.,* 45:825–830.
54. Robertson, D., Robertson, R. M., Nies, A. S., Oates, J. A., and Friesinger, G. C. (1979): *Am. J. Cardiol.,* 43:1080–1085.
55. Robertson, R. M., Wood, A. J. J., Vaughn, W. K., and Robertson, D. (1982): *Circulation,* 65:281–285.
56. Robson, R. H., and Vishwanath, M. C. (1982): *Br. Med. J.,* 284:104.
57. Rousseau, M. F., Pouleur, H., Detry, J. M. R., and Brasseur, L. A. (1980): *Eur. Heart J.,* (Suppl. B) 1:37–41.
58. Schaefer, J., Schwarzkopf, H. J., Schoettler, M., and Wilms, R. (1975): In: *Proceedings of the 2nd International Adalat Symposium,* edited by W. Lochner, W. Braasch, and G. Kronenberg, pp. 140–144. Springer Verlag, Berlin.
59. Schmutzler, H. (1981): In: *Coronary Heart Disease—Calcium Antagonist Adalat, A Worldwide Success,* pp. 87–93. Bayer, Leverkusen.
60. Serruys, P. W., Brower, R. W., Katen, H. J. ten, Bom, A. H., and Hugenholtz, P. G. (1981): *Circulation,* 63:584–591.

61. Serruys, P. W., Hooghoudt, T. E. H., Brand, M. vd, and Hugenholtz, P. G. (1981): *Eur. Heart J.,* (Suppl. A) 2:51.
62. Serruys, P. W., Jong, J. W. de, Harmsen, E., and Hugenholtz, P. G. (1982): In: *Abstracts of the 5th International Adalat Symposium,* Berlin, p. 32.
63. Servi, S. de, Mussini, A., Specchia, G., Bramucci, E., Gavazzi, A., Falcone, C., Ardissino, D., Guagliumi, G., and Bobba, P. (1980): *Eur. Heart J.,* (Suppl. B) 1:43–47.
64. Serruys, P. W., Vanhaleweijck, G., and Hugenholtz, P. G. (1983): *Ann. Int. Med.* (*in press*).
65. Simonsen, S., and Nitter-Hauge, S. (1978): *Acta Med. Scand.,* 204:179–184.
66. Stone, P. H., Antman, E. M., Muller, J. E., and Braunwald, E. (1980): *Ann. Int. Med.,* 93:886–904.
67. Verdouw, P. D., Cate, F. J. ten, Hartog, J. M., Scheffer, M. G., and Stam, H. (1982): *Basic Res. Cardiol.,* 77:26–33.
68. Verdouw, P. D., Cate, F. J. ten, and Hugenholtz, P. G. (1980): *Eur. J. Pharmacol.,* 63:209–212.
69. Verdouw, P. D., Hartog, J. M., Cate, F. J. ten, Schamhardt, H. D., Bastiaans, O. L., Bremen, R. H. van, Serruys, P. W., and Hugenholtz, P. G. (1981): In: *Drug Treatment of Myocardial Infarction,* edited by P. A. van Zwieten, P. G. Hugenholtz, and E. Schonbaum. *Prog. Pharmacol.,* 4:91–100.
70. Yasue, H., Omote, S., Takizawa, A., Nagao, M., Miva, K., and Tanaka, S. (1979): *Circulation,* 59:938–948.
71. Yasue, H., Touyama, M., Kato, H., Tanaka, S., and Akiyama, F. (1976): *Am. Heart J.,* 91:149–155.
72. Zimmerman, A. N. E., Daems, W., Hulsmann, W. C., Snijder, J., Wisse, E., and Durrer, D. (1967): *Cardiovasc. Res.,* 1:201–209.

LITERATURE ON INTERACTION BETWEEN NIFEDIPINE AND β-BLOCKER

Dargie, H. J., Lynch, P. G., Krikler, D. M., Harris, L., and Krikler, S. (1981): *Am. J. Med.,* 71:676–682.
Dean, S., and Kendall, M. J. (1981): *Br. Med. J.,* 282:1322.
Ekelund, L. G., and Orö, L. (1976): In: *Proceedings of the 3rd International Adalat Symposium,* pp. 218–225. Excerpta Medica, Amsterdam.
Ekelund, L. G., and Orö, L. (1979): *Clin. Cardiol.,* 2:203–211.
Fox, K. M., Jonathan, A., and Selwyn, A. P. (1981): *Clin. Cardiol.,* 4:125–129.
Lynch, P., Dargie, H., Krikler, S., and Krikler, D. (1980): *Br. Med. J.,* 281:184–187.
Moses, J. W., and Wertheimer, J. H. (1981): *Ann. Intern. Med.,* 94:425–429.
Oakley, D., Fox, K. M., Dargie, H. J., and Selwyn, A. P. (1979): *Br. Med. J.,* 1:1540.
Staffurth, J. S., and Emery, P. (1981): *Br. Med. J.,* 282:225.
Tweddel, A. C., Beattie, J. M., Murray, R. G., and Hutton, L. (1981): *Br. J. Clin. Pharmacol.,* 12:229–233.

OTHER RECOMMENDED LITERATURE

Books

Adelman, A. G., and Goldman, B. S. (editors) (1981): *Unstable Angina, Recognition and Management.* Martinus Nijhoff, The Hague.
Bertrand, M. E. (editor) (1979): *Coronary Artery Spasm.* Laboratoire Dausse. Proceedings of an European Symposium in Lille. Bayer Pharma, France.
Rafflenbeul, W., Lichtlen, P. R., and Balcon, R. (editors) (1981): *Unstable Angina Pectoris.* International Symposium Hannover. Georg Thieme Verlag, Stuttgart.

Articles

Brugmann, U., Dirschinger, J., Blasini, R., and Rudolph, W. (1982): *Herz,* 7:235–242.
Hopf Becker, H. J., Kober, G., Dowinsky, S., and Kaltenbach, M. (1982): *Herz,* 7:221–234.
Morad, M., and Tung, L. (1982): *Am. J. Cardiol.,* 49:584–594.

*Calcium Antagonists and Cardiovascular
Disease,* edited by L. H. Opie.
Raven Press, New York © 1984.

Chapter 24

Calcium and Acute Myocardial Infarction

James T. Willerson, Amal Mukherjee, Kenneth Chien,
Carlos Izquierdo, and *L. Maximilian Buja

*Department of Internal Medicine (Cardiovascular Division) and *Department of Pathology,
University of Texas Health Science Center and Parkland Memorial Hospital,
Dallas, Texas 75235*

Fixed coronary arterial occlusion of 1 hr or longer and temporary coronary arterial occlusion lasting at least 40 min followed by reflow are associated with the development of alterations in cell membrane integrity (15,23–26,45,49). Alterations in sarcolemmal and subcellular membrane integrity are associated with significant derangements in cellular ultrastructure. With relatively short periods of coronary arterial occlusion, only a minority of myocardial cells are altered, but as the period of myocardial ischemia is prolonged, more muscle cells demonstrate changes. Severe injury following temporary ischemia and reperfusion is characterized by cell and mitochondrial swelling, marked myofibrillar hypercontraction, and the distortion of cellular architecture including segmentation of edematous cytoplasm into subsarcolemmal blebs and vacuoles (15,23–26,45,49). Cell swelling and interstitial edema are most prominent with temporary coronary occlusion followed by reperfusion, but cell swelling without interstitial edema also occurs with longer periods of fixed coronary arterial occlusion. In most experimental models of ischemia and in patients, the initial cellular alterations occur in subendocardial tissue with subsequent spread into epicardial regions (35,38). The development of abnormal myocardial fluid retention and the loss of cell volume regulation appear to precede the development of extensive myocardial necrosis (49). Direct evidence of altered cell membrane integrity following temporary and fixed coronary arterial occlusion for periods lasting up to one hour comes from the demonstration of structural breaks in cell membrane integrity, the electron microscopic identification of the development of mitochondrial edema, and the accumulation of various tracers ordinarily excluded from the intracellular space including lanthanum, various molecular weight proteins, and technetium-99m stannous pyrophosphate (Tc-99m-PPi) (10,26,27,42,44,45,49).

With relatively short periods of temporary coronary arterial occlusion followed by reperfusion and with longer periods of fixed coronary arterial occlusion, Ca^{2+} accumulates intracellularly in damaged myocardial cells, especially in the mitochondrial of such cells (5,16,20,39). Some of the alterations that occur in sarcolemmal membrane structure and function during the period of Ca^{2+}-loading of injured myocardial cells are now documented (9,10,13). The consequences of accumulation of Ca^{2+} as regards alterations in mitochondrial function are also known (11,28,30). In addition, it is possible to detect irreversibly injured myocardial tissue with myocardial scintigraphy by virtue of excessive Ca^{2+} deposition (1,8,31,46).

This chapter reviews the sarcolemmal alterations that occur in association with increased Ca^{2+} permeability during experimental myocardial ischemia, potential consequences of cell loading with Ca^{2+} in this setting, and the ability to detect increased Ca^{2+} accumulation in injured tissue using noninvasive, scintigraphic imaging methods. Finally, some insight will be provided into the efficacy of administering selected Ca^{2+} antagonists to protect ischemically injured myocardial tissue from accumulating excessive Ca^{2+}.

SARCOLEMMAL ALTERATIONS THAT OCCUR IN ASSOCIATION WITH INCREASED CALCIUM PERMEABILITY DURING EXPERIMENTAL MYOCARDIAL ISCHEMIA

Phospholipid Metabolism

A variety of experimental findings suggest that a disturbance in phospholipid metabolism may be one of the critical alterations that occurs in association with the development of irreversible cellular injury during myocardial ischemia and infarction (12,13). In studies performed by Chien et al. at our institution, experimental myocardial ischemia was produced in dogs by proximal left anterior descending coronary arterial (LAD) ligation. After 3 hr of fixed LAD occlusion, there was a 10% decrease in total phospholipid content (13); silica gel chromatography revealed this decrease to be the result of decreases in phosphatidylcholine and phosphatidylethanolamine. If Tc-99m-PPi, a marker of irreversible cellular injury, was injected intravenously after various intervals of LAD occlusion and 10 min prior to 1.5 hr of reflow, there was a close temporal and topographical correlation between the extent of phosphatidylethanolamine depletion and Tc-99m-PPi uptake (13). Furthermore, Chien et al. have demonstrated that treatment of purified cardiac sarcolemmal membranes with an exogenous phospholipase (either phospholipase A or C, 0.01 mg/ml) causes a similar decrease in total phospholipid content which is associated with more than a 50% increase in net Ca^{2+} efflux from sarcolemmal vesicles preloaded by $Na^{+}:Ca^{2+}$ exchange (13). In addition, sarcolemmal vesicles isolated from ischemic myocardium after 3 hr of proximal LAD occlusion have an increased Ca^{2+} permeability and phosphatidylcholine depletion compared to vesicles obtained from the corresponding nonischemic myocardium. These studies suggest that an alteration in phospholipid metabolism is related closely to the development of irreversible damage in ischemic canine myocardium and to alterations in Ca^{2+} permeability (13). We believe that the biochemical mechanism responsible for this relationship may be the degradation of sarcolemmal membrane phospholipids and an associated increase in sarcolemmal Ca^{2+} permeability.

Alterations in Lanthanum Permeability

Studies have also been performed by Burton et al. (10) at our institution to evaluate alterations in sarcolemmal membrane function occurring with or prior to the development of irreversible cellular injury during one of the component parts of myocardial ischemia, i.e., hypoxia. Sixty-seven isolated feline right ventricular papillary muscles were used to evaluate alterations in ultrastructure and contractile parameters. Hypoxia was provided by gasing these muscles with 100% nitrogen for varying intervals. An ionic La^{3+} probe technique was employed as a cytochemical marker to monitor the progression of cellular injury (10). Marked depression of developed tension and the rate of tension development occurred after 30 min of hypoxia (10). Contractile function showed significant recovery with reoxygenation after 1 hr and 15 min of hypoxia, but remained depressed when reoxygenation was provided after 2 or 3 hr of hypoxia. Examination by transmission and analytical electron microscopy (energy dispersive X-ray microanalysis) revealed La^{3+} deposition only in extracellular regions in control muscles and muscles subjected to 30 min of hypoxia. After hypoxic intervals of more than 1 hr, abnormal intracytoplasmic and intramitochondrial localization of La^{3+} were detected. After 1 hr and 15 min of hypoxia, abnormal intracellular La^{3+} accumulation was associated with only minimal ultrastructural evidence of injury. Muscles, provided reoxygenation after 1 hr and 15 min of hypoxia, showed improved ultrastructure and did not exhibit intracellular La^{3+} deposits with exposure to La^{3+} during the reoxygenation period (10) (Fig. 1). After 2 to 3 hr of hypoxia, abnormal intracellular La^{3+} accumulation was associated with ultrastructural evidence of severe muscle injury which persisted after reoxygenation. More recently, abnormal La^{3+} accumulation was found to occur with progressive ischemic injury in isolated perfused myocardium (9). In this model, pretreatment with chlorpromazine exerted a protective effect on the progression of membrane and cellular injury (9), possibly by retarding the degradation of membrane phospholipids (12). Thus, the data from these studies support the conclusion that cellular and subcellular membrane alterations responsible for abnormal intracellular La^{3+} deposition precede the development of irreversible injury, but evolve at a transitional stage in the progression from reversible to irreversible injury induced by hypoxia and ischemia in isolated muscle preparations (9,10).

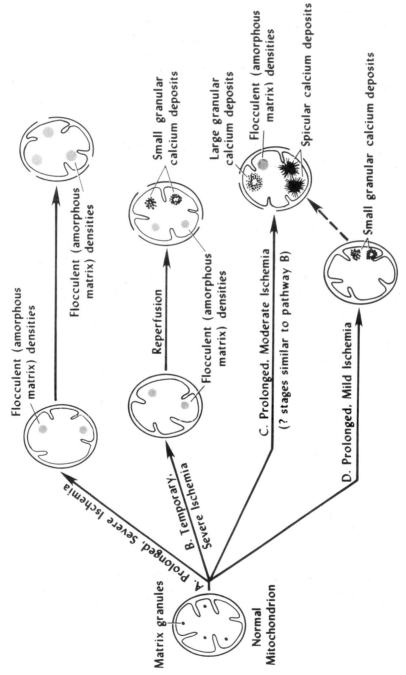

FIG. 1. The different types and conditions under which mitochondrial matrix granules occur are shown. (From ref. 18.)

Matrix granules

Normal
Mitochondrion

A. Prolonged, Severe Ischemia

B. Temporary,
Severe Ischemia

C. Prolonged, Moderate Ischemia
(? stages similar to pathway B)

D. Prolonged, Mild Ischemia

Flocculent (amorphous
matrix) densities

Flocculent (amorphous
matrix) densities

Flocculent (amorphous
matrix) densities

Reperfusion

Flocculent (amorphous
matrix) densities

Small granular
calcium deposits

Large granular
calcium deposits

Flocculent (amorphous
matrix) densities

Spicular calcium deposits

Small granular calcium deposits

CALCIUM DEPOSITION IN ISCHEMICALLY INJURED
MYOCARDIAL TISSUE

Irreversible cellular injury developing during myocardial ischemia may be associated with Ca^{2+} accumulation in damaged mitochondria (5,8,16,20,23, 26,39,43,49). There are several mitochondrial inclusions that occur normally and following irreversible cellular damage with myocardial ischemia (Fig. 1) (5,20). Small matrix granules occur in normal mitochondria and appear to represent organic material without detectable Ca^{2+} (Fig. 1) (5,20). In established myocardial infarcts necrotic myocardial cells contain at least two types of mitochondrial inclusions (Fig. 1) (5,20). Inclusions of the first type are characterized by the presence of variable amounts of electron-dense material and often exhibit a structure consisting of aggregates of granules and thin spicules. The spicular inclusions range from 500 to 4,000 Å in diameter (5). Inclusions of the second type are composed of moderately electron-dense amorphous material. These are devoid of very electron-dense spicular material (Fig. 1). The amorphous inclusions range from 750 to 2,000 Å in diameter (5). Analytical electron microscopic studies performed at our institution have demonstrated the presence of Ca^{2+} in the spicular inclusions, but not in the amorphous matrix (flocculent) densities (5,20). We believe that the amorphous matrix densities represent precipitates of phospholipids and denatured protein, and that the mitochondrial inclusions containing very electron-dense spicular material represent advanced stages of mitochondrial calcification. Such calcification appears to be localized to the peripheries of the infarcts and can be explained by the dual requirements of cellular injury and persistent tissue perfusion allowing delivery of serum Ca^{2+} to damaged myocardial cells (5,20,23,25,26,39,42,43,45). Mitochondrial calcification appears to develop selectively in a subpopulation of Ca^{2+}-loaded myocardial cells with impaired plasma membrane integrity and sufficient mitochondrial function to initiate the accumulation and precipitation of calcium phosphate (5,8,20,23,25,26,45). The spicular quality of the mitochondrial inclusions suggests that they represent apatite-like crystalline material (2,3,5,17,20,43,47).

Inclusions composed of finely granular material have been found in mitochondria obtained from necrotic cells in a variety of conditions (2) and have also been described in cardiac muscle cells irreversibly injured by prolonged intervals of temporary coronary artery occlusion followed by reperfusion (17,23,26,39). This type of inclusion also has been observed in mildly altered muscle cells with abnormal lipid accumulation located in the outermost regions of established myocardial infarcts ("border zone" regions) (8). These annular granular inclusions are usually smaller (less than 1,000 Å) than the spicular inclusions. It has been suggested previously that the granular inclusions represent a readily soluble subcrystalline precursor of a Ca^{2+}-deficient hydroxyapatite (2,3,5,20, 39,43). Mitochondrial inclusions composed of apatite-like, needle-shaped crystals have been found in structurally intact muscle cells subjected to Ca^{2+} overloading (2,3), as well as in cardiac muscle cells from patients following cardiovascular surgery (17). Studies from our laboratory have demonstrated the presence of large granular and finely spicular types of Ca^{2+}-containing precipitates in mitochondria of necrotic muscle cells injured during experimental canine myocardial infarction (5,8,20).

More recent studies from our institution utilizing analytical electron microscopy with quantitative analyses of Ca^{2+} in mitochondria of irreversibly damaged cells have indicated the concentration of Ca^{2+} in such mitochondria is 300 to 500 mmoles/kg dry wt (i.e., 300–500 nmoles/mg) and that these mitochondria contain equimolar concentrations of phosphate (4,18,19).

CONSEQUENCES OF EXCESSIVE CALCIUM ACCUMULATION IN ISCHEMICALLY INJURED MYOCARDIAL TISSUE

We and others have evaluated the influence of Ca^{2+} accumulation on oxidative phosphorylation in isolated mitochondria (11,28,30,33). Exogenous calcium chloride (50–270 nmoles/mg protein) severely depresses oxidative phosphorylation in mitochondria in ethyldiaminetetraacetate (EDTA)-free medium (30). The addition of calcium chloride (150–170 nmoles/mg protein) completely abolishes mitochondrial oxidative phosphorylative ability (30). Electron microscopy demonstrates significant alterations, morphologically, in mitochondria incubated with calcium chloride at 200 nmoles/mg protein (30). These amounts of Ca^{2+} are within the range of those documented to exist in irreversibly damaged cells during severe hypoxia and ischemia (4,18,19). The addition of exogenous phosphate also depresses the function of isolated canine cardiac mitochondria severely, such that the accumulation of 5 to 50 mmoles phosphate severely impairs oxidative phosphorylation (30).

Therefore, the accumulation of either Ca^{2+} or phosphate in mitochondria may seriously impair mitochondrial oxidative phosphorylation; Ca^{2+} accumulation may also cause structural damage to mitochondrial membranes. We have shown that the amounts of Ca^{2+} and phosphorous required to produce both functional and morphological alterations do accumulate during irreversible cellular injury caused by one of the component parts of the ischemic process, i.e., severe hypoxia. Thus, accumulation of Ca^{2+} (and phosphate) may be important factors in causing irreversible cellular injury as a result of their seriously impairing the ability of mitochondria to generate high-energy phosphates for metabolic purposes and for the maintenance of normal membrane integrity and function. These considerations indicate the potential importance of abnormal Ca^{2+} accumulation in cellular injury. However, further work is needed to provide direct confirmation that excess intracellular Ca^{2+} accumulation occurs during initial stages of acute myocardial infarction in the intact animal, and that such accumulation plays a major role in the genesis of the wavefront of necrosis in the evolving infarct.

MYOCARDIAL SCINTIGRAPHIC DETECTION OF CALCIUM DEPOSITION IN INJURED MYOCARDIAL TISSUE

Tc-99m-PPi myocardial scintigrams provide a means to detect and localize acute myocardial infarction. These scintigrams are expected to be abnormal with acute myocardial infarcts of at least 3 g in weight, if serial imaging is utilized and proper attention to technique is provided (1,31,46,47). We have found a close temporal and topographical relationship between Ca^{2+} accumulation and Tc-99m-PPi uptake responsible for scintigraphic detection of acute myocardial infarction in experimental animals subjected to fixed or temporary proximal left anterior descending coronary artery occlusion (6,8,13,32,47).

Recent studies performed at our institution have provided insight into the sites and mechanisms of localization of Tc-99m-PPi in acute myocardial infarcts (8). Autoradiographic studies with ³H-diphosphonate have revealed extensive labeling in the infarct periphery in regions containing necrotic muscle cells with features of severe Ca^{2+} overloading, including widespread hypercontraction as well as more selective formation of mitochondrial calcific deposits (8). These same studies also have demonstrated ³H-diphosphonate labeling of a small population of damaged border zone muscle cells which exhibit prominent accumulation of lipid droplets and focal early mitochondrial calcification. These findings have been confirmed recently by Tomoike et al. who reported autoradiographic localization of Tc-99m-PPi in myocardial infarcts (41). We have also shown that the most marked Tc-99m-PPi uptake occurs in irreversibly damaged myocardial cells receiving 10 to 40% of control blood flow values (7). Therefore, we have proposed the pathophysiological schemes shown in Figs. 2 and 3 to explain Tc-99m-PPi incorporation into irreversibly damaged myocardial cells caused by acute myocardial infarction.

Tc-99m-PPi myocardial imaging does provide a sensitive way to detect acute myocardial infarction amounting to 3 g or more of irreversibly damaged tissue with acute myocardial infarction. Tomographic imaging with single-photon emitters (such as Tc-99m) indicate that one may detect even smaller amounts of myocardial necrosis, i.e., 1 g. We and others have utilized imaging techniques

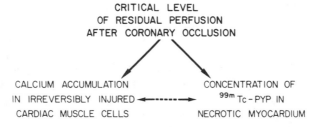

FIG. 2. The relationship between collateral coronary blood flow, pathological calcification, and the concentration of Tc-99m-PPi in necrotic myocardium is shown.

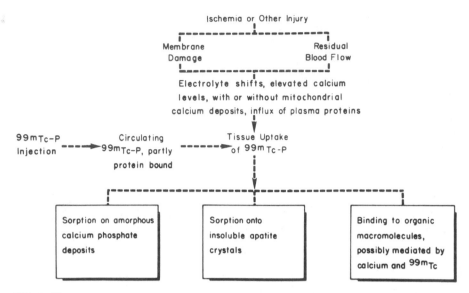

FIG. 3. The proposed pathophysiological factors involved in the concentration of increased Tc-99m-PPi in damaged myocardium following coronary arterial occlusion are described. (From ref. 8.)

extensively to detect and localize acute myocardial infarction, and to estimate the relative size of acute transmural anterior or anterolateral myocardial infarcts (1,6–8,29,31,32,34,40,41,46–48).

INFLUENCE OF CALCIUM ANTAGONISTS ON REGIONAL MYOCARDIAL BLOOD FLOW, MYOCARDIAL NECROSIS, AND SEGMENTAL VENTRICULAR FUNCTION

We and others have evaluated the influence of Ca^{2+} antagonists in terms of their ability to reduce myocardial necrosis, improve blood flow, and protect ventricular function during experimental canine myocardial infarction (14,21,37). We have used nifedipine or verapamil, Ca^{2+} antagonists, in mongrel dogs instrumented with ultrasonic crystals, left ventricular catheter-tipped manometers (Konigsberg P22), left atrial catheters, and an occlusive device positioned around the proximal left anterior descending coronary artery to produce myocardial infarction when desired. The animals were instrumented with at least five sets of ultrasonic crystals positioned within and around the left ventricular (LV) ischemic region so as to monitor segmental function expressed as net systolic thickening; we use segmental net systolic thickening as a measure of regional ventricular contractility (36–38).

In these studies, we administered nifedipine or verapamil beginning 5 min after permanent proximal occlusion of the left anterior descending coronary artery in awake, unsedated dogs and continued the infusion for 6 hr (22). Nifedi-

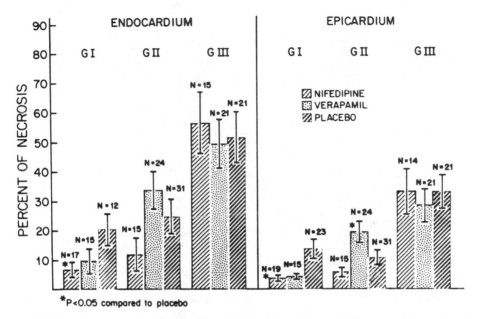

FIG. 4. The influence of two "slow-channel" Ca^{2+} antagonists, nifedipine and verapamil, on the extent of myocardial necrosis after experimental myocardial infarction is shown. Both nifedipine and verapamil tended to decrease the extent of necrosis at mildly dysfunctional left ventricular sites (GI), but neither reduced the extent of necrosis at moderately dysfunctional (GII), or at severely dysfunctional sites (GIII).

pine was given in an intravenous dose that slightly decreased systolic blood pressure and slightly increased heart rate, but these parameters were not changed by more than 15 mm Hg or 10 beats/min, respectively. Nifedipine was protected from light during its preparation and administration. Verapamil was given intravenously at a dose that decreased systolic blood pressure 10 to 15 mm Hg, and decreased heart rate by approximately 10 beats/min.

In these studies, we found that nifedipine administration reduces the extent of histological necrosis at mildly and moderately dysfunctional LV sites, but not at severely dysfunctional ones (Fig. 4) (37). Verapamil reduced necrosis only at mildly dysfunction LV sites (Fig. 4) (22,37). In addition, nifedipine administration was associated with an increase in regional myocardial blood flow to ventricular segments with mild and moderate ischemic dysfunction, but not to sites of severe segmental dysfunction. Nifedipine also improved segmental function at mildly dysfunctional segments, but it did not significantly change segmental function at either moderately or severely damaged segments (22,37) (Fig. 5). Verapamil did not increase blood flow or improve segmental function at any LV site (Fig. 5) (22,37).

Therefore, nifedipine given soon after coronary arterial occlusion and continued for the subsequent 6 hr does increase regional coronary blood flow and reduce myocardial necrosis at mildly and moderately dysfunctional segments,

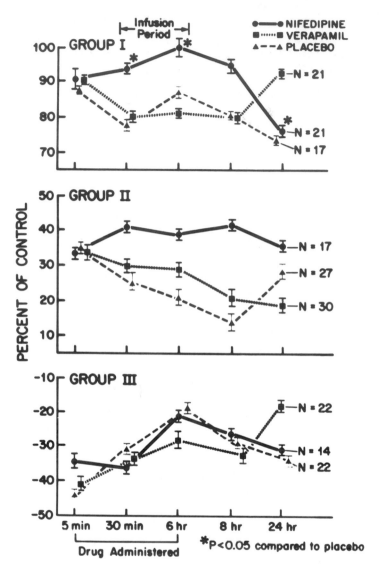

FIG. 5. The influence of two "slow-channel" Ca^{2+} antagonists, nifedipine and verapamil, in protecting segmental left ventricular function following experimental coronary arterial occlusion is shown. Nifedipine improved segmental contractility at mildly dysfunctional sites (Group I) during its infusion from 5 min to 6 hr following coronary arterial occlusion. However, nifedipine did not alter segmental function at moderately dysfunctional (Group II) or at severely dysfunctional sites (Group III). Verapamil did not alter segmental function at any of these sites.

and preserve ventricular function at mildly dysfunctional sites. However, this Ca^{2+} antagonist (and also verapamil) does not reduce the extent of myocardial necrosis at the most severely dysfunctional LV sites, nor does it preserve ventricular function at moderately or severely dysfunctional sites (22,37). Studies are in progress to evaluate the effects of these agents with shorter intervals of coronary occlusion and reflow.

SUMMARY

Ca^{2+} is deposited in the mitochondria of irreversibly damaged myocardial cells with short periods of temporary coronary artery occlusion followed by reperfusion, and with extended periods of fixed coronary artery occlusion and acute myocardial infarction. The amount of Ca^{2+} (and phosphate) that accumulates in these mitochondria is sufficient to impair mitochondrial oxidative phosphorylation. Alterations in sarcolemmal membranes occur in association with a loss of normal permeability barriers to Ca^{2+} in injured myocardial cells and are likely a factor in allowing cellular Ca^{2+} loading during myocardial infarction. Certain Ca^{2+} antagonists, such as nifedipine, possess the ability to increase coronary blood flow, reduce the extent of myocardial necrosis, and preserve ventricular function; presumably, this occurs as a consequence of their ability to improve blood flow and function and/or reduce myocardial O$_2$ demand; it may also be related to their ability to reduce the amount of Ca^{2+} entering injured cells.

ACKNOWLEDGMENTS

This study was supported in part by National Institutes of Health Ischemic Specialized Center of Research (SCOR) Grant HL 17669 and the Harry S. Moss Heart Fund.

REFERENCES

1. Bonte, F. J., Parkey, R. W., Graham, K. D., Moore, J., and Stokely, E. (1974): *Radiology,* 110:473–474.
2. Bonucci, E., Derenzini, M., and Marinozzi, V. (1973): *J. Cell. Biol.,* 59:185–211.
3. Bonucci, E., and Sadun, R. (1973): *Am. J. Pathol.,* 71:167–184.
4. Buja, L. M., Burton, K. P., Hagler, H. J., and Willerson, J. T. (1983): *Circulation (in press).*
5. Buja, L. M., Dees, J. H., Harling, D. F., and Willerson, J. T. (1976): *J. Histochem. Cytochem.,* 24:508–516.
6. Buja, L. M., Parkey, R. W., Dees, J. H., Stokely, E. M., Harris, R. A., Jr., Bonte, F. J., and Willerson, J. T. (1975): *Circulation,* 52:596–607.
7. Buja, L. M., Parkey, R. W., Stokely, E. M., Bonte, F., and Willerson, J. T. (1976): *J. Clin. Invest.,* 57:1508–1522.
8. Buja, L. M., Tofe, A. J., Kulkarni, P. V., Mukherjee, A., Parkey, R. W., Francis, M. D., Bonte, F. J., and Willerson, J. T. (1977): *J. Clin. Invest.,* 60:724–740.
9. Burton, K. P., Hagler, H. K., Willerson, J. T., and Buja, L. M. (1981): *Am. J. Physiol.,* 24:H714–723.
10. Burton, K. P., Hagler, H. K., Templeton, G. H., Willerson, J. T., and Buja, L. M. (1977): *J. Clin. Invest.,* 60:1289–1302.
11. Carafoli, E., and Crompton, M. (1976): In: *Calcium in Biological Systems,* edited by C. J. Duncan, pp. 89–115. *Symp. Soc. Exp. Biol.,* No. 30, New York.
12. Chien, K. R., Abrams, J., Serroni, A., Martin, J. T., and Farber, J. L. (1978): *J. Biol. Chem.,* 253:4809–4817.
13. Chien, K. R., Reeves, J. P., Buja, L. M., Bonte, F., Parkey, R. W., and Willerson, J. T. (1981): *Circ. Res.,* 48:711–719.

14. Clark, R. E., Christlieb, I. Y., Henry, P. D., Fischer, A. E., Nora, J. D., Williamson, J. R., and Sobel, B. E. (1979): *Am. J. Cardiol.,* 44:825–831.
15. Csapo, Z., Dusek, J., and Rona, G. (1974): *J. Mol. Cell. Cardiol.,* 6:79–83.
16. D'Agostino, A. N. (1964): *Am. J. Pathol.,* 45:633–638.
17. D'Agostino, A. N., and Chiga, M. (1970): *Am. J. Clin. Pathol.,* 53:820–824.
18. Hagler, H., Burton, K., and Buja, L. (1981): In: *Microprobe Analysis of Biological Systems,* edited by T. E. Hutchinson and A. P. Somlyo, pp. 245–281. Academic Press, New York.
19. Hagler, H. K., Lopez, L. E., Murphy, M. E., Greico, C., and Buja, L. M. (1981): *Lab. Invest.,* 45:241–247.
20. Hagler, H. K., Sherwin, L., and Buja, L. M. (1979): *Lab. Invest.,* 40:529–544.
21. Henry, P. D., Shuchleib, R., Borda, J. J., Roberts, R., Williamson, J. R., and Sobel, B. E. (1978): *Circ. Res.,* 43:372–380.
22. Izquierdo, C., Roan, P., Buja, L. M., and Willerson, J. T. (1982): *Am. J. Cardiol.,* 49:1005 (Abstract).
23. Jennings, R. B., and Ganote, C. E. (1974): *Circ. Res.,* 34,35 (Suppl. III):111–156.
24. Jennings, R. B., Hawkins, H. K., Lowe, J. E., Hill, M. L., Klotman, S., and Reimer, K. A. (1978): *Am. J. Pathol.,* 92:187–208.
25. Kloner, R. A., Ganote, C. E., and Jennings, R. B. (1974): *J. Clin. Invest.,* 54:1496.
26. Kloner, R. A., Ganote, C. E., Whalen, D. A., Jr., and Jennings, R. B. (1974): *Am. J. Pathol.,* 74:399.
27. Leaf, A. (1970): *Am. J. Med.,* 49:29.
28. Lehninger, A. L. (1970): *Biochem. J.,* 119:129–138.
29. Lewis, M., Buja, L. M., Saffer, S., Mishelevich, D., Stokely, E. M., Lewis, S., Parkey, R., Bonte, F., and Willerson, J. T. (1977): *Science,* 197:167–169.
30. Mukherjee, A., Wong, T. M., Templeton, G., Buja, L. M., and Willerson, J. T. (1979): *Am. J. Physiol.,* 237:224–238.
31. Parkey, R. W., Bonte, F. J., Meyer, S. L., Atkins, J., Curry, G., and Willerson, J. T. (1974): *Circulation,* 50:540–546.
32. Parkey, R. W., Kulkarni, P. V., Lewis, S. E., Datz, F., Gutekunst, D., Dehmer, G., Buja, L., Bonte, F., and Willerson, J. T. (1981): *J. Nucl. Med.,* 22:133–137.
33. Peng, C. F., Kane, J. J., Murphy, M. L., and Straub, K. D. (1977): *J. Mol. Cell. Cardiol.,* 9:897–908.
34. Poliner, L. R., Buja, L. M., Parkey, R. W., Stokely, E., Stone, M., Harris, R., Satten, S., Templeton, G., Bonte, F., and Willerson, J. T. (1977): *J. Nucl. Med.,* 18:517–523.
35. Reimer, K. A., and Jennings, R. B. (1979): *Lab. Invest.,* 40:633–644.
36. Roan, P. G., Buja, L. M., Izquierdo, C., Hashimi, H., Saffer, S. I., and Willerson, J. T. (1981): *Circ. Res.,* 49:31–40.
37. Roan, P. G., Izquierdo, C., Buja, L. M., Hashimi, H., and Willerson, J. T. (1981): In: *New Perspectives on Calcium Antagonists,* Clinical Physiology Series, *Am. Physiol. Soc.,* 16:211–216.
38. Roan, P., Scales, F., Buja, L. M., and Willerson, J. T. (1979): *J. Clin. Invest.,* 64:1074–1088.
39. Shen, A. C., and Jennings, R. B. (1972): *Am. J. Pathol.,* 67:417–434.
40. Stokely, E. M., Buja, L. M., Lewis, S. E., Parkey, R. W., Bonte, F., Harris, R., and Willerson, J. T. (1976): *J. Nucl. Med.,* 17:1–5.
41. Tomoike, H., Nakamura, M., Watanabe, K., et al. (1982): *J. Nucl. Med.,* 23:84–85.
42. Trump, B. F., Croker, B. P., Jr., and Mergner, W. J. (1971): In: *Cell Membranes: Biological and Pathological Aspects,* edited by G. W. Richter and D. G. Scarpelli, pp. 84–128. Williams & Wilkins, Baltimore.
43. Trump, B. F., Strum, J. M., and Bulger, R. E. (1974): *Virchows Arch. Cell Pathol.,* 16:1–34.
44. West, P. N., Connors, J. P., Clark, R. E., et al. (1978): *Lab. Invest.,* 38:677–684.
45. Whalen, D. A., Jr., Hamilton, D. G., Ganote, C. E., and Jennings, R. B. (1974): *Am. J. Pathol.,* 74:381.
46. Willerson, J. T., Parkey, R. W., Bonte, F. J., Meyer, S. L., Atkins, J., and Stokely, E. (1975): *Circulation,* 51:1046–1052.
47. Willerson, J. T., Parkey, R. W., Bonte, F. J., Lewis, S. E., Corbett, J., and Buja, L. M. (1980): *Sem. Nucl. Med.,* 10:54–69.
48. Willerson, J. T., Parkey, R. W., Stokely, E. M., Bonte, F., Lewis, S., Harris, R., Blomqvist, G., Poliker, L., and Buja, L. (1977): *Cardiovasc. Res.,* 11:291–299.
49. Willerson, J. T., Scales, F., Mukherjee, A., Platt, M., Templeton, G., Fink, G., and Buja, L. (1977): *Am. J. Pathol.,* 87:159–188.

Calcium Antagonists and Cardiovascular Disease, edited by L. H. Opie.
Raven Press, New York © 1984.

Chapter 25

Comparison of Nifedipine and Nitrates: Clinical and Angiographic Studies

C. Richard Conti, James A. Hill, Robert L. Feldman,
Jamie B. Conti, and Carl J. Pepine

*Division of Cardiology, University of Florida, JHM Health Center,
Gainesville, Florida 32610*

This chapter will deal with two studies comparing two important classes of compounds, nifedipine and nitrates. However, it should be emphasized at the outset that conclusions reached from these studies may not necessarily apply to different groups of patients, patients receiving different drug doses, or patients studied at different times after administration of the drug.

The first study will deal with the effects of nifedipine and isosorbide dinitrate on the frequency of angina and consumption of nitroglycerin in patients with proven coronary arterial spasm. The second study was performed in the cardiac catheterization laboratory to evaluate the effect of sublingual nifedipine and intracoronary nitroglycerin on coronary artery size in patients without coronary artery spasm.

COMPARISON OF NIFEDIPINE AND ISOSORBIDE DINITRATE IN PATIENTS WITH CORONARY ARTERY SPASM

The subjects for this study were 22 men and 4 women who had angina which occurred mostly at rest and was relieved by nitroglycerin. There was a 2-week lead-in phase during which Ca^{2+} antagonists and/or topical nitrates were excluded from the treatment regimen. Patients who had more than three episodes of pain per week were entered into the double-blind randomized phase (treatment with either nifedipine or isosorbide dinitrate). After dose titration (40–120 mg/day) and evaluation, they were given the alternate therapy. During the course of the trial, the effects of nifedipine and isosorbide dinitrate on the frequency of angina and consumption of nitroglycerin were evaluated by patient diary. Twenty-one patients completed all study phases. Two patients died, 1 in each group. Two patients could not tolerate isosorbide dinitrate because of headache and hypotension, and an additional patient stopped the study medication because of a poor response.

Results

In the 21 patients who completed all 3 study phases, the mean frequency of angina during the lead-in phase was 1.86 episodes/day. Compared to lead-in phase, the mean frequency of angina was significantly decreased for both nifedipine (0.71 episodes/day) and isosorbide dinitrate (0.66 episodes/day) (both $p <$ 0.05). Likewise, nitroglycerin consumption was significantly decreased in the lead-in phase (2.09 tablets/day) when compared to both nifedipine (0.90 tablets/day) and isosorbide dinitrate (0.56 tablets/day) phases (both $p <$ 0.05).

Individual responses for 19 patients are described in Hill et al. (5). Compared to the lead-in phase, angina frequency during the nifedipine phase was reduced by 50% or more in 18 of 24 patients. Six of these were asymptomatic. During isosorbide dinitrate phase, 15 of the 21 patients had a greater than 50% decrease in their angina frequency, and 4 of these were asymptomatic. Eleven patients showed this decrease in angina frequency during both nifedipine and isosorbide dinitrate phases. In addition, 6 patients on nifedipine and 6 patients on isosorbide had a less than 50% decrease in angina frequency.

When the entire group of 21 patients who completed all study phases were evaluated, 11 had a greater than 50% decrease in angina frequency on nifedipine compared to isosorbide dinitrate, and 7 had a greater than 50% decrease in angina frequency on isosorbide dinitrate compared to nifedipine. The remaining 3 patients had a similar angina frequency on both drugs.

COMPARISON OF THE EFFECT OF SUBLINGUAL NIFEDIPINE AND INTRACORONARY NITROGLYCERIN ON CORONARY ARTERY SIZE IN PATIENTS WITHOUT CORONARY SPASM

The precise mode by which nifedipine provides clinical benefit to patients with ischemic heart disease is unclear. Some have hypothesized that nifedipine works by preventing the vasoconstrictor response of coronary arteries. Several investigators have suggested nifedipine acts by dilating coronary arteries and increasing coronary blood flow. The implications are that the beneficial action is secondary, at least in part, to increase of diameter in large coronary arteries, particularly in areas of stenosis. The purpose of this investigation is to quantify the response of the left coronary artery to buccal nifedipine, compared to the response of the conventional, known, direct-acting vasodilator intracoronary nitroglycerin.

Protocol of Study

Patients with documented ischemic heart disease (effort angina plus significant coronary artery stenosis in the left coronary artery system) were selected for study. No patient had rest angina nor any evidence for coronary artery spasm. Heart rate, mean aortic pressure, and selected areas of the left coronary artery were measured in 8 patients in the control state, 15 min after 10 mg buccal nifedipine and 2 min after 200 μg of intracoronary nitroglycerin. The sequence of measurements was the same in all patients, i.e., no patient received nitroglycerin prior to buccal nifedipine.

Selective coronary angiograms were obtained using a 105 mm photo spot camera. A special eye-piece calibrated measuring device was used to assess coronary artery diameter by placing the eye-piece over a back-lighted 105 mm photo spot frame. Drugs were not administered until the effects of contrast injections on the ECG and aortic pressure returned to control values. Measurements of the coronary artery were taken at specific sites in all 8 patients in order to ensure a reasonable comparison between patients.

The left main coronary diameter was measured just proximal to the bifurcation of the left anterior descending and circumflex arteries. Diameter of the proximal circumflex was measured just prior to the first obtuse marginal branch. The middle circumflex and middle left anterior descending were measured just distal to the first obtuse marginal and second diagonal branch, respectively. The distal vessels were measured prior to the last bifurcation of the coronary artery tree.

Results

Hemodynamics: Mean aortic pressure decreased from 102 ± 18 to 96 ± 14 mm Hg ($p < 0.05$) after nifedipine, and continued to decrease to a low of 87 ± 15 mm Hg ($p < 0.05$) following nitroglycerin administration. Heart rate rose slightly from 66 ± 9 to 70 ± 6 ($p < 0.05$) after buccal nifedipine, but there was no further increase after intracoronary nitroglycerin.

Angiography: Ninety-three nonstenotic areas of the left coronary artery were

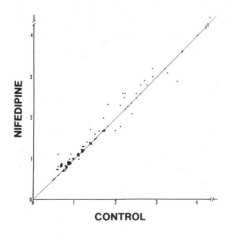

FIG. 1. Coronary artery diameter (in millimeters) before and after nifedipine. (From Feldman et al., ref. 4, with permission.)

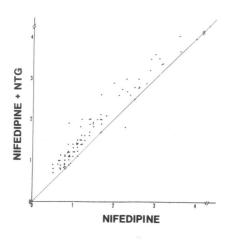

FIG. 2. Coronary artery diameters (in millimeters) after nifedipine, and after nifedipine plus intracoronary nitroglycerine (NTG). (From Feldman et al., ref. 4, with permission.)

measured. Six decreased in size, 60 were unchanged, and 27 increased in size after nifedipine. Figure 1 plots the individual data points before and after 10 mg of buccal nifedipine administration.

After intracoronary nitroglycerin was administered to the patients, measurements of coronary artery size was obtained. These measurements now represent the coronary artery diameter after the combination of 10 mg buccal nifedipine and 200 µg intracoronary nitroglycerin. Eighty-two of the coronary arteries showed increased diameters compared to diameters after nifedipine alone. One patient had a decrease in diameter of the coronary artery. These changes in diameter of the coronary artery are illustrated in Fig. 2.

In the 8 patients studied, eight coronary artery stenoses were measured prior to and after drug administration. Fifteen minutes after buccal nifedipine was administered, the diameter of three coronary stenoses increased slightly, and five were unchanged compared to control (Fig. 3). Following the administration of intracoronary nitroglycerin, four stenotic areas were noted to dilate after the combination of nifedipine and intracoronary nitroglycerin, and four did not change. These changes are summarized in Fig. 4.

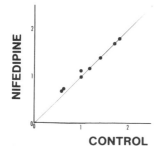

FIG. 3. Coronary stenosis diameters (in millimeters) before and after nifedipine.

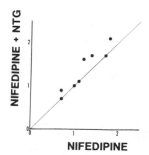

FIG. 4. Coronary stenosis diameters (in millimeters) after nifedipine, and after nifedipine plus intracoronary nitroglycerine (NTG).

DISCUSSION

Clinical experience with Ca^{2+} antagonists in the United States is still relatively modest, but widespread use of these drugs in current clinical trials in progress will eventually provide guidelines for the optimal use of Ca^{2+} antagonists alone, or in combination with other drugs for the treatment of coronary artery spasm.

An open-label study of nifedipine in patients with coronary spasm published by Antman et al. (1) stated that 87% of patients with coronary spasm had a beneficial response to nifedipine. Our data suggest a similar beneficial response to nifedipine, but the magnitude of symptom relief was somewhat less (5). Perhaps this magnitude difference can be explained by the fact that many patients in the open-label trials received long-acting nitrates in addition to nifedipine. Presumably, in many cases, nifedipine was added because of failure of nitrate therapy.

The studies described in this chapter are not an indictment against the effectiveness of nifedipine, but rather support the contention that nifedipine is an efficacious agent for the management of symptoms related to coronary artery spasm. Of course, it is also important to emphasize that isosorbide dinitrate, when given in doses comparable to nifedipine, is also effective for the management of these study patients. The message that one can take away from these data is that proper dosing of potent pharmacologic agents is the key to effective therapy.

Our data indicate that sublingual nifedipine usually does not produce significant changes in diameter of the coronary artery visualized angiographically (3). However, the dose of nifedipine used in this study of coronary artery size was modest, and the effects were measured relatively soon after drug administration. Large-dose nifedipine administered either by the sublingual or oral route might have produced changes in epicardial coronary artery diameter. If the repeat coronary angiograms were obtained during the 30 to 60 min after nifedipine administration, an important effect on coronary artery diameter might have been found. However, when these measurements were made, 15 min after nifedipine administration, important changes in aortic pressure and heart rate occurred. In addition, others have shown that important blood levels are achieved approximately 3 min after sublingual administration of nifedipine. Another consideration is the patient population being studied. None of these patients had evidence of active ischemia at the time of the angiogram. In patients who have "increased basal coronary artery tone," nifedipine might have a more important effect on the diameter of these vessels compared to the coronary arteries that do not have any "increased vasomotor tone." Brown et al. (2) have postulated that verapamil either prevented or decreased the vasoconstrictive effect on coronary artery size after isometric hand grip and ergonovine stimulation.

The beneficial actions of nifedipine in patients with ischemic heart disease is not necessarily secondary to an increase in diameter of epicardial coronary arteries, small intramural coronary arteries, or most coronary stenoses. However, since nifedipine is a potent peripheral vasodilator, its major clinical effects may be related to afterload reduction combined with the maintenance of coronary artery size, i.e., prevention of vasoconstriction in this patient population. In contrast, nitrates, which clearly dilate epicardial coronary arteries significantly, may be effective because of this action plus a marked effect on decreasing ventricular volume and ventricular end diastolic pressure. Table 1 summarizes the physiologic effects of three classes of antianginal agents on determinants of myocardial O$_2$ demands and coronary blood flow.

Thus, based on data presented in this chapter, the best way to manage patients with coronary artery spasm may be to combine nifedipine with long-acting nitrates. The combined use of nifedipine and nitrates will (a) dilate the coronary arteries to maintain coronary blood flow; (b) decrease systemic arterial pressure, and thus decrease peripheral vascular resistance; and (c) dilate peripheral veins, and thus decrease ventricular volume and pressure. When proper doses are used, the combination may be more effective than either drug alone. Of course

TABLE 1. *Physiologic effects of nitrates, β-blockers, and calcium blockers on determinants of myocardial oxygen uptake and coronary blood flow*

			Calcium antagonists		
	Nitrates	β-blockers	Diltiazem	Verapamil	Nifedipine
Myocardial oxygen uptake					
Contractility	↑	⬇	↓	↓	n.c.
Heart rate	↑	⬇	↓	↓↑	↑
LV wall tension					
Volume	⬇	↑	?	↑	↓
Systolic pressure	↓	↓	↓	↓	↓
Diastolic pressure	⬇	↑	n.c.	↑	n.c.
Coronary blood flow					
Aortic pressure	↓	↓	↓	↓	↓
Coronary resistance	⬇	↑	⬇	⬇	⬇
Epicardial artery size	⬆	↓	↑↑	↑↑	↑↑

Small arrow, minor effect; *two small arrows*, moderate effect; *large arrow*, major effect. n.c., No change.

a proper dose must be determined for the individual patient by the physician, but initial treatment with isosorbide dinitrate should begin with 10 mg every 6 hr. A similar dosing schedule can be used for nifedipine. Both drugs can be increased to higher levels, i.e., 120 mg/day, if the clinical situation warrants it.

REFERENCES

1. Antman, E., Muller, J., Goldberg, S., et al. (1980): *N. Engl. J. Med.*, 302:1269–73.
2. Brown, B. G., Pierce, C. D., Sing, B. N., Bolsen, E. L., and Dodge, H. T. (1981): *Circulation*, 64:4–50 (Abstract).
3. Conti, J. B., Feldman, R. L., Hill, J. A., Pepine, C. J., and Conti, C. R. (1982): *Am. J. Cardiol.*, 49:966 (Abstract).
4. Feldman et al. (1983): *Am. Heart J.*, 105:651–659.
5. Hill, J. A., Feldman, R. L., Pepine, C. J., and Conti, C. R. (1982): *Am. J. Cardiol.*, 49:431–438.

Calcium Antagonists and Cardiovascular Disease, edited by L. H. Opie.
Raven Press, New York © 1984.

Chapter 26

Properties of Calcium-Dependent Slow Action Potentials: Their Possible Role in Arrhythmias

Nick Sperelakis

Physiology Department, University of Cincinnati College of Medicine, Cincinnati, Ohio 45267

SOME PROPERTIES OF THE SLOW CHANNELS

Action of Positive Inotropic Agents

A number of positive inotropic agents exert an effect to increase the number of available slow channels in the myocardial cell membrane, and this action may be the predominant explanation for their increase in cardiac contractility. It is through the slow channels that Ca^{2+} influx occurs during the cardiac action potential, and the amount of Ca^{2+} ion entering the cell controls the force of contraction. The Ca^{2+} entering directly elevates $[Ca]_i$ involved in activating the myofilaments, and indirectly does so by further releasing Ca^{2+} from the intracellular sarcoplasmic reticulum stores (6). Blockade of the slow channels, and hence Ca^{2+} influx, by Ca^{2+}-antagonistic agents (such as verapamil, nifedipine, Mn^{2+}, Co^{2+}, and La^{3+}) depresses or abolishes the contractions without greatly affecting the normal fast action potential, i.e., contraction is uncoupled from excitation.

The positive inotropic agents that affect the number of available slow channels include: β-adrenergic receptor agonists (such as isoproterenol and norepinephrine), histamine (H_2 receptor), methylxanthines (such as caffeine, theophylline, and methylisobutyl-xanthine), angiotensin II, fluoride ion, and exogenous dibutyryl-cyclic AMP. The action of most of these agents is very rapid, and the peak effect often occurring within 1 to 3 min. The action of the exogenous cyclic AMP compound is relatively slow, the peak effect occurring in 15 to 30 min (26). The effect of the catecholamines is blocked by β-adrenergic blocking agents. The action of histamine in inducing the slow action potentials is blocked by H_2-receptor blocking agents (but not by H_1-receptor antagonists) (10). The action of angiotensin II in inducing slow response is blocked by specific angiotensin receptor blocking agents (8).

One method of detecting the effect of agents on the slow channels is to first block the fast Na^+ channels and excitability by tetrodotoxin, or to voltage-inactivate them by partially depolarizing the cells (e.g., to -40 mV) in elevated $[K]_o$ (e.g., 25 mM). Then, addition of agents, such as catecholamines, which rapidly increase the number of slow channels available for activation upon stimulation, causes the appearance of slowly-rising overshooting action potentials (the "slow responses") which resemble the plateau component of the normal fast action potential (Fig. 1). Both Ca^{2+} and Na^+ inward currents participate in the slow action potentials, and they are accompanied by contractions (27). The slow action potentials are blocked by agents which block inward slow current, including Mn^{2+}, La^{3+}, verapamil, and D-600 (24,27).

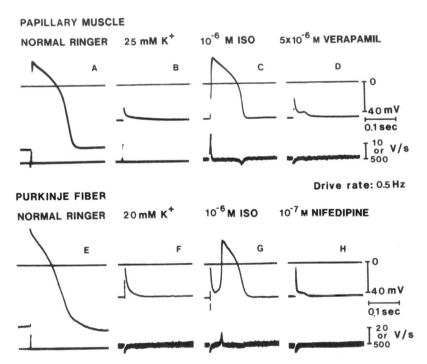

FIG. 1. Set-up for the slow action potential (AP), and block of the slow APs by Ca^{2+}-antagonistic drugs in the guinea pig. **A–D:** Papillary muscle. **E–H:** Purkinje fiber. **A, E:** Normal fast APs. **B, F:** Elevation of $[K]_o$ to 25 mM **(B)** or 20 mM **(F)** depolarized to about -45 mV and blocked excitability (shock artifacts only visible). **C, G:** Addition of isoproterenol (10^{-6} M) rapidly induced slowly-rising APs, and slow APs. **D, H:** Addition of verapamil (5×10^{-6} M) **(D)** or nifedipine (10^{-7} M) **(H)** rapidly depressed and blocked the slow APs. The driving rate for the slow APs was 0.5 Hz. The *upper straight line* in each panel is the zero potential level, and the *lower trace* is dV/dt, the peak excursion of which gives $\dot{V}_{max}$. The voltage and time calibrations are the same throughout; the *dV/dt calibration bars* represent 500 V/sec for **A** and **E**, and 10 V/sec for **B, C, D,** or 20 V/sec for **F, G, H.** (From ref. 21.)

Cyclic AMP Dependence

Cyclic AMP is somehow involved with the slow channels (26–28). Histamine and β-adrenergic agonists, subsequent to binding to their specific receptors, lead to rapid stimulation of adenylate cyclase with resultant elevation of cyclic AMP levels. The methylxanthines enter into the myocardial cells and inhibit phosphodiesterase, the enzyme that destroys cyclic AMP, thus causing an elevation of cyclic AMP. These positive inotropic agents also rapidly induce the slow action potentials, presumably by making more slow channels available in the membrane. Dibutyryl cyclic AMP also induces the slow action potentials, but only after a much longer lag period, as expected from slow penetration through the membrane.

A test of the cyclic AMP hypothesis was done by using a guanosine 5′-triphosphate (GTP) analog (5′-guanylimidodiphosphate [GPP(NH)P], an agent known to directly activate adenylate cyclase. The addition of GPP(NH)P (10^{-5}–10^{-3} M) induced the slow action potentials in cultured reaggregates of chick heart cells within 5 to 30 min (12). Another test of the cyclic AMP hypothesis was done by iontophoretically microinjecting cyclic AMP intracellularly into dog Purkinje fibers and guinea pig ventricular muscle (34). Cyclic AMP injections induced the slow action potentials in the injected cell for a transient period of 1 to 2 min. The amplitude and duration of the induced slow response was a function of the amount of cyclic AMP injected. Cyclic AMP injections potentiated (increased their rate of rise and amplitude) slow action potentials induced by theophylline. In recent experiments, using pressure injection into single ventricular myocardial cells (guinea pig papillary muscles), cyclic AMP, GPP(NH)P, and cholera toxin all rapidly induced and potentiated slow action potentials (17). These results support the hypothesis that the intracellular level of cyclic AMP controls the availability of the slow channels in the myocardial sarcolemma.

Metabolic Dependence

The induced slow action potentials are blocked by hypoxia, ischemia, and metabolic poisons (including cyanide, dinitrophenol, and valinomycin), accompanied by a lowering of the cellular ATP level (28). This suggests that interference with metabolism somehow leads to blockade of the slow channels. This effect is relatively rapid; the blockade occurs within 5 to 15 min, depending on the metabolic intervention used or the dose of metabolic poison. Under conditions in which the slow action potentials are blocked, the fast action potentials are unaffected, indicating that the fast Na^+ channels are essentially unaffected. However, the contractions accompanying the normal fast action potentials are depressed or abolished, indicating that contraction is uncoupled from excitation, as expected if the slow channels were blocked. The slow action potentials blocked by valinomycin or by hypoxia are restored by elevation of the glucose concentration, indicating that the effect of metabolic poisons or hypoxia is indeed mediated by metabolic interference. Thus, there is a differential dependence of the slow channels on metabolic energy.

With prolonged metabolic interference, e.g., 60 to 120 min of hypoxia, there is a gradual shortening of the duration of the normal fast action potential, until a relatively brief spike-like component only remains, but which is still rapidly rising. Thus, in addition to the rapid effect of metabolism on the slow channels, metabolic interference exerts a second, but much slower, effect on the membrane, namely to increase the kinetics of g_K turn-on, thereby shortening the action potential. The mechanism of this effect could be mediated by a gradual rise in $[Ca]_i$, which can cause an increase in K^+ conductance, the Ca^{2+}-activated g_K.

Phosphorylation Hypothesis

Because of the relationship between cyclic AMP and the number of available slow channels, and because of the demonstrated dependence of the functioning of the slow channels on metabolic energy, it has been postulated that a membrane protein must be phosphorylated in order for the slow channel to become available for voltage activation (28) (Fig. 2). The only well-documented effect of cyclic AMP is the activation of a cyclic AMP-dependent protein kinase (dimer split into two monomers), which phosphorylates a variety of proteins in the presence of ATP. Several myocardial membrane proteins become phosphorylated under appropriate conditions.

The protein that is phosphorylated might be a protein constituent of the slow channel itself. Phosphorylation could make the slow channel available for activation by a conformational change that either allowed the activation

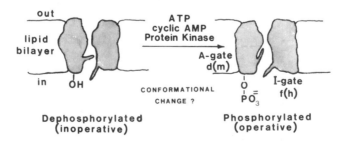

FIG. 2. Cartoon model for a slow channel in myocardial cell membrane in two hypothetical forms: dephosphorylated (or electrically silent) for (*left*) and phosphorylated form (*right*). The two gates associated with the channel, an activation (A) gate, and an inactivation (I) gate, are kinetically much slower than those of the fast Na^+ channel. The hypothesis states that a protein constituent of the slow channel must be phosphorylated in order for the channel to be in a functional state available for voltage activation. Phosphorylation occurs by a cyclic AMP-dependent protein kinase in the presence of ATP. Phosphorylation of the slow-channel protein may produce a conformation change that allows the gates to operate or increases the diameter of the water-filled pore so that Ca^{2+} and Na^+ can pass through. (From ref. 28.)

gate to be opened upon depolarization, or effectively increased the diameter of the water-filled pore (the "selectivity filter" portion) so that Ca^{2+} and Na^+ could pass through (Fig. 2). The phosphorylated form of the slow channel would be the active (operational) form, and the dephosphorylated form would be the inactive (inoperative) form. That is, only the phosphorylated form would be available to become activated upon depolarization to threshold. The dephosphorylated channels would be electrically silent. An equilibrium would probably exist between the phosphorylated and dephosphorylated forms of the slow channels for a given set of conditions, including the level of cyclic AMP. Thus, agents that act to elevate the cyclic AMP level would increase the fraction of the slow channels that are in the phosphorylated form, and hence available for voltage activation. Such agents would increase the force of contraction of the myocardium.

The role, if any, of *cyclic GMP* in the functioning of the slow channels is not fully known. Acetylcholine (ACh) depresses contractility and blocks slow action potentials in atrial cells. ACh is known to increase g_K, and this would tend to suppress the slow action potentials. It is not clear whether the effect of ACh on g_K is mediated through changes in cyclic GMP level or by some more direct mechanism. In ventricular cells, activation of the muscarinic receptor by ACh reverses the stimulation of the adenylate cyclase produced by β-adrenergic agonists (13).

There are some positive inotropic agents that do not elevate cyclic AMP, but do induce the slow channels. Angiotensin II is one example (8). Angiotensin may directly activate protein kinase. Fluoride ion (< 1 mM) is a second example. It induces the slow response and acts as a positive inotropic agent, but does not elevate cyclic AMP (32). Fluoride ion may act by inhibiting the phosphoprotein phosphatase which dephosphorylates the slow-channel protein, thereby resulting in a larger fraction of phosphorylated channels. Thus, the results with angiotensin and fluoride can be fitted within the framework of the phosphorylation hypothesis.

Selective Blockade by Acidosis

The myocardial slow channels induced by positive inotropic agents are selectively blocked by acidosis. That is, the slow action potentials induced by isoproterenol, for example, are depressed in rate of rise, amplitude, and duration as the pH of the perfusing solution is lowered below 7.0 (31). The slow action potential is completely abolished at about pH 6.1, and 50% inhibition occurs at pH 6.6. (The slow action potentials would be abolished before all the slow channels were blocked because of the requirement of a minimum density of slow channels for regenerative and propagating responses.) The contractions are depressed in parallel with the slow action potentials. Similar results of acidosis were shown in voltage-clamp experiments on cardiac muscle, namely that acid pH depressed the inward slow current (I_{si}) (1).

Acidosis has little or no effect on the normal fast action potential, i.e., the rate of rise remains fast, and the overshoot and duration are only slightly affected. However, the contractions become depressed and abolished as a function of the degree of acidosis. That is, excitation-contraction uncoupling occurs, as would be expected from a selective blockade of the slow channels.

Two different buffer systems, HCO_3^--CO_2 buffer and PIPES buffer, gave similar results. Since the PIPES buffer system should only slowly change the intracellular pH, it appears that the blockade of the slow channels occurs with acidification of the outer surface of the cell membrane. This could change the surface charge of the membrane and/or the conformation of the slow-channel proteins.

Since the myocardium becomes acidotic during hypoxia and ischemia (glycolysis is increased, and lactic acid diffuses into the interstitial fluid space), it is likely that some of the effects of these metabolic interventions on the slow channels are mediated by the accompanying acidosis, and not solely by a decrease in ATP level. Consistent with this, the effects of hypoxia on the slow action potential were almost immediately reversed, but only partially and transiently, by changing the pH of the perfusing solution to 8.0 (the responses gradually diminished further during the hypoxia even at the alkaline pH).

Protection Hypothesis

The Ca^{2+} influx of the myocardial cell can be controlled by extrinsic factors. For example, stimulation of the sympathetic nerves to the heart, or circulating catecholamines, or other hormones can have a positive inotropic action, whereas stimulation of the parasympathetic neurons has a negative inotropic effect. The mechanism for some of these effects is mediated by changes in the levels of the cyclic nucleotides. This extrinsic control of the Ca^{2+} influx is enabled by the peculiar properties of the slow channels, as, for example, the postulated requirement for phosphorylation.

However, in addition, the myocardial cell itself can exercise control over its Ca^{2+} influx, i.e., there is intrinsic control. For example, under conditions of transient regional ischemia, many of the slow channels become unavailable (or silent). This effect may be mediated by lowering the ATP level of the affected cells and by the accompanying acidosis (since slow-channel blockade during hypoxia occurs faster at acid pH than at alkaline pH). Acidosis blocks the slow channels directly (presumably), and metabolic interference causes indirect inactivation of the slow channels. Both effects are relatively selective for the slow channels.

Thus, *the myocardial cell can partially or completely suppress its Ca^{2+} influx under adverse conditions.* This causes the affected cells to contract weakly or not at all, and since most of the work done by the cell is mechanical, this conserves ATP. Such a mechanism may serve to protect the myocardial cells under adverse conditions, such as transient regional ischemia. If the myocardial cell could not control its Ca^{2+} influx, then the ATP level might drop so low under such conditions that irreversible damage would be done, i.e., the cells would die. Because of the peculiar properties of the slow channels, they become inactivated, thus uncoupling contraction from excitation and conserving ATP. The cells could then recover fully when the blood flow returns to normal. The almost normal resting potentials and fast action potentials would allow propagation through the ischemic area to be normal thus minimizing the chances for the induction of arrhythmias.

The action potential region of prolonged ischemia may not be a slow-channel action potential but rather a depressed fast-channel action potential. The depression of the rate of rise is caused by the partial depolarization of the cells due to K^+ accumulation in the interstitial space and perhaps to depression of electrogenic Na^+ pumping. (Depolarization voltage inactivates a fraction of the fast Na^+ channels due to closing of their inactivation (I) gates.) The slow channels would be expected to be nearly completely blocked because of the acidosis and lowered ATP level; if so, the action potential could not be dependent on an inward slow current (I_{si}). The effect of metabolic interference on shortening the action potential (due to enhanced kinetics for g_K turn-on that terminates the action potential) would also help to shut off I_{si} more quickly, thereby reducing the total Ca^{2+} influx per impulse, and so helping to conserve ATP.

BLOCKADE OF SLOW CHANNELS BY CALCIUM ANTAGONISTS: POSSIBLE MECHANISMS

The Ca^{2+} antagonistic drugs, such as verapamil, D-600, nifedipine, diltiazem, and bepridil, block the voltage-dependent slow channels (Ca^{2+}, Ca^{2+}-Na^+, and Na^+ types) found in myocardial cells, Purkinje fibers, nodal cells, and vascular smooth muscle cells (and even in skeletal fibers). Some Ca^{2+} antagonists, such as verapamil and D-600, are not specific for Ca^{2+} or Ca^{2+}-Na^+ types of slow channels, but also block slow Na^+ channels (24).

To be a member of this class of compounds, a drug must block the slow channel by a direct action on the cell membrane channel itself (and not indirectly via metabolic depression or acidosis, for example), and this action must be relatively specific for the slow channel in contrast to the other types of voltage-dependent ion channels (e.g., fast Na^+ channel or delayed rectifier K^+ channel).[1] Thus, this definition would distinguish Ca^{2+} antagonists from local anesthetics or metabolic poisons, for example.

In addition, some Ca^{2+} antagonists, such as bepridil, may exert a second action, e.g., intracellularly to depress Ca^{2+} uptake into or release from the sarcoplasmic reticulum (33). The evidence for a second effect of bepridil was the fact that it depressed cardiac contractile force more than could be accounted for by the depression of the inward slow Ca^{2+} current. In addition, bepridil

---

[1] Some use a looser definition of Ca^{2+} antagonists to include compounds that do not have a prominent blocking effect on the slow channels.

and verapamil enter the myocardial cells, the order of uptake being: bepridil > verapamil >> nifedipine > diltiazem (23). This order of uptakes is consistent with the order of lipid solubilities. Since bepridil and verapamil enter into the myocardial cells, they have the possibility of having a second site of action. In addition, Ca^{2+} antagonists that readily enter the cells have the possibility of exerting their effect on the slow channels from the inner surface of the cell membrane.

Ca^{2+} binding to isolated sarcolemmal membranes (vesicles) was inhibited by verapamil and bepridil in a dose-dependent manner, verapamil being the more potent of the two, as it is in inhibition of I_{si} (22). Since Ca^{2+} binding to the outer mouth of the slow channel (as depicted in Fig. 3) is probably the first step in ion permeation through the channel, Ca^{2+} displacement could be one possible mechanism for blockade of Ca^{2+} entry, although this may not easily account for the frequency-dependency of the effect of these two drugs. On the other hand, the frequency-independent block of Ca^{2+} entry by Mn^{2+}, Co^{2+}, or La^{3+} ions could be by such a mechanism. Nifedipine and diltiazem did not inhibit Ca^{2+} binding. Thus, there are great differences in properties of the Ca^{2+}-antagonistic drugs, and they may block the slow channels by different molecular

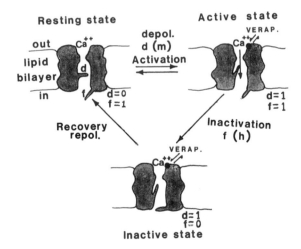

FIG. 3. Cartoon model for the three hypothetical states of a slow channel, patterned after the Hodgkin-Huxley states for the fast Na^+ channel. In the resting state (*upper left*), the d(m) gate is closed and the f(h) gate is open (d = 0; f = 1). Depolarization to the threshold activates the slow channel to the active state (*upper right*), the d gate opening rapidly and the f gate still being open (d = 1; f = 1). The activated channel spontaneously inactivates to the inactive state (*bottom*) due to closure of the f gate (d = 1; f = 0). The recovery process upon repolarization returns the channel from the inactive state back to the resting state, which is again available for reactivation. The Ca^{2+} ion is depicted as being bound to the outer mouth of the channel and poised for entry down its electrochemical gradient when both gates are in the open position (active state of channel). Also depicted is the possible binding of verapamil to the outer mouth of the slow channel (*solid circle*) in the active state or inactive state, and thereby either blocking the activated channel or slowing the recovery process for converting from the inactive state back to the resting state. (From ref. 30.)

mechanisms, as might be predicted from their widely different chemical structures.

Apparent reversal of the block of the slow action potentials and contractions by the Ca^{2+} antagonists by *elevation of* $[Ca]_o$ may result from either of two mechanisms: (a) competition between Ca^{2+} and drug for binding to the outer mouth of the channel, and (b) the increased electrochemical driving force for Ca^{2+} influx through the fraction of slow channels not blocked by the drug. The latter mechanism probably operates in all cases, whereas the former mechanism may be involved with some of the drugs, such as verapamil and bepridil.

The effects of some Ca^{2+}-antagonistic drugs (e.g., nifedipine, diltiazem) are more readily reversed upon *washout of the drug,* whereas the effects of other drugs (e.g., bepridil and verapamil) are more difficult to reverse (e.g., 30–60 min washout required). It might be expected that those drugs that exert their primary or secondary effects intracellularly (e.g., on the inner surface of the cell membrane) may be more difficult to wash out. Since the $t_{1/2}$ for uptakes of bepridil (31 min) and verapamil (27 min) is much longer than those for nifedipine (6 min) and diltiazem (2 min), the washouts would be expected to be in the reverse order.

The effect of most of the Ca^{2+}-antagonistic drugs on depression of the inward slow Ca^{2+} current (I_{si}) is *frequency-dependent.* That is, the higher the frequency of stimulation, the greater the blocking effect on the slow channels. For example, a dose of drug that completely blocks the slow action potentials at a drive rate of 1 Hz may exhibit no effect at 0.1 Hz. This effect is prominent in the action of all this class of drugs, although nifedipine seems to have a lesser frequency-dependence than the other drugs. In contrast, Ca^{2+} entry blockers, such as Mn^{2+}, Co^{2+}, and La^{3+}, do not exhibit a frequency-dependency. That is, the effect of Mn^{2+} is present even to the first stimulation after equilibration of the Mn^{2+} under resting conditions.

This frequency-dependency of effect suggests that *the Ca^{2+}-antagonistic drugs do not act as simple plugs for the Ca^{2+} slow channels,* as perhaps Mn^{2+} or La^{3+} might act. Rather, this property suggests that the drug might act to slow the recovery process of the slow channel from the inactive state back to the resting state (Fig. 3). If so, then a slow drive rate or a long quiescent period (e.g., 20–60 sec) would allow complete recovery of the drugged slow channel before the next excitation occurred. To exert such an effect on the gate recovery kinetics, the drugs could bind anywhere on the channel protein or in the central pore of the channel, if such binding were only to occur in the inactive state. An alternative possibility is that the drug binds to the channel only in the active state (membrane also depolarized) to block it (e.g., by plugging) and then dissociates before conversion of the channel to the sequential states. There is some evidence that binding of the drug is voltage-dependent, hyperpolarization favoring unbinding. Any drug that affected the phosphorylation of the slow channels by some direct means would also effectively block the slow channels selectively.

The degree of frequency dependency of the drugs in blocking the Ca^{2+}-dependent action potentials (slow) and contractions in vascular smooth muscle cells is not clear. However, the inhibition of the Ca^{2+} entry can account for the vasodilating, antianginal, and antihypertensive properties of these drugs.

A number of other chemicals and drugs also block the myocardial slow channels, including local anesthetics (11) and volatile general anesthetics (18). The local anesthetics, lidocaine and procainamide, however, blocked the slow channels nonspecifically; that is, the dose-response curve for the slow action potentials was identical to that for the fast action potentials. In contrast, depressed fast action potentials, produced in 10 mM $[K]_o$, were about 10-fold more sensitive to lidocaine (29). Halothane and enflurane are more selective for the slow channels of the heart than for the fast Na^+ channels (18).

EXCITATION AND CONDUCTION OF THE SLOW ACTION POTENTIALS

The slow action potentials have a stimulation threshold nearly 10 times higher than that for the fast action potentials, i.e., the slow action potentials have a lower excitability. The threshold potential (V_{th}) for the slow action potentials is at an E_m of about -35 mV, whereas that for the fast action potentials is about -55 mV, i.e., the critical depolarization required to excite is larger for the slow action potentials (assuming an unchanged resting potential of -80 mV). Since the slow action potentials are dependent on an inward current carried through the slow channels, tetrodotoxin has no effect on them, whereas Ca^{2+}-antagonistic drugs or agents, such as verapamil or Mn^{2+}, block them. The slow action potentials propagate at a velocity of about 4 to 10 cm/sec, a value similar to that for visceral smooth muscle. It is not known to what degree decremental conduction may occur, i.e., decreasing propagation velocity and response amplitude as a function of the distance along the muscle.

In a simple cable (25), *conduction velocity* (Θ) should vary directly with the square root of the $\dot{V}_{max}$. That is, the faster the rate of rise of the action potential, the faster should the action potential propagate. (There are exceptions to this in cardiac muscle when comparing transverse propagation versus longitudinal propagation.) Thus, if the fast action potential in cardiac muscle propagates at 0.40 m/sec for a $\dot{V}_{max}$ of 150 V/sec, then if $\dot{V}_{max}$ is reduced to 15 V/sec for the slow action potential, Θ should be reduced by $\sqrt{10}$ times or to 0.127 m/sec. However, propagation velocity is decreased more than the predicted amount in both myocardium (12.7 cm/sec predicted versus 4–10 cm/sec actual) and Purkinje fibers (0.2 m/sec predicted versus <0.1 cm/sec actual) (5). The latter authors attributed the discrepancy to the fact that a higher effective membrane capacitance (C_m), i.e., a higher capacitive reactance (X_c), should be associated with the slow action potential.

A recent study has focused on the *ability of propagating fast action potentials to trigger slow action potentials.* In rabbit, left atrial strips (composed of homogeneous parallel bundles of fibers) compartmentalized into three functional segments, the left (test) segment being exposed to 12.7 mm $[K]_o$ and 1 mM $[Ba]_o$ to depolarize sufficiently to block the fast action potentials, Masuda et al. (20) found that Θ of the slow action potentials was 0.04 to 0.08 m/sec. High-frequency (0.63–2.5 Hz) stimulation caused 2:1 block due to fatigue of the slow action potential (slowness of recovery of excitability). However, low-frequency (0.13–0.4 Hz) stimulation also produced complete block. Therefore, there was a limited frequency range in which a normal fast action potential could stimulate slow action potentials at a sustained 1:1 ratio. The low-frequency block was attributed to the observed reduced amplitude and duration of the atrial fast action potential, since acetyl-choline, which shortens the plateau of the atrial action potential, also blocked the development of the slow action potential in the test compartment when it was added to the middle compartment. Hence, the amplitude and duration and frequency of the fast action potentials determined whether they served as effective stimuli for the slow action potentials in the depolarized region.

Cukierman and Paes de Carvalho (4) studied the properties of "membrane" (nonpropagated) slow action potentials induced (stimulated with a suction electrode) in short (2–3 mm) atrial trabeculae from rabbit left atrium by 1 mM $[Ba]_o$ and 10 mM $[K]_o$. The resting potential in the high K^+-Ba^{2+} solution was -55 mV, the amplitude of the slow action potentials was 60 mV, and the APD_{50} was 84 msec. Chronaxie of the slow action potential (0.9 msec) was about 10 times higher than that for the fast action potential. The slow action potential upstroke was always initiated from a small subthreshold depolarizing step; accommodation to this "subliminal response" did not occur. The slow action potential was all-or-none, and had a V_{th} of about -35 mV. The slow action potential fatigued at high pacing rates (>1 Hz), and a fully developed slow action potential could only be obtained within a certain frequency range, as found in the long strip preparation of Masuda et al. (20).

POSSIBLE ROLE OF SLOW ACTION POTENTIALS IN ARRHYTHMIAS

Slow action potentials have been implicated in the genesis of arrhythmias (2,3,4,20). Slow conduction in a pathway allows circus movement of excitation around that pathway, and may lead to reentrant type of arrhythmias. There is a requirement of one-way conduction through the depressed area, and the length of the reentry loop is critical, depending on velocity. In an ischemic or infarcted zone, and the surrounding border zone, there is a depressed area with slowed conduction. Partial depolarization of the cells in this area occurs because of a high $[K]_o$ due to the hypoxia/ischemia and consequent impaired metabolism. In addition, there is norepinephrine release from the sympathetic nerve terminals. Because norepinephrine elevates cyclic AMP and increases the number of available slow channels, this would tend to increase the slow inward current carried primarily by Ca^{2+} ions, in these cells in the ischemic zone. However, the hypoxia/

ischemia tends to depress the slow inward current because of the accompanying lowered ATP level and the metabolic dependence of the slow channel functioning.

Therefore, the ischemic action potential can be either (a) a depressed fast action potential (i.e., an action potential whose inward current is carried through fewer fast Na^+ channels) due to the partial depolarization and the h_∞ versus E_m relationship), or (b) a pure slow action potential (i.e., an action potential whose inward current is carried only through slow channels) if the K^+ depolarization is great enough such that complete voltage inactivation of all (or most) fast Na^+ channels has occurred (at about -55 mV). There is some evidence for both possibilities. The evidence for a true slow action potential has been summarized by Cranefield (2). The evidence that the ischemic action potential depressed fast action potential includes the facts that tetrodotoxin blocks the action potential, whereas verapamil does not (9,15,35). Additional points supporting the view that the ischemic action potential is a depressed fast action potential and not a slow action potential are: (a) the metabolic dependence of the functioning of the slow channels, and (b) the dyskinesis or akinesis of the ischemic area.

Although local anesthetics depress and block slow action potentials at the same concentrations that depress the normal fast action potentials, the depressed fast action potentials are nearly 10-fold more sensitive to these drugs (29). Thus, lidocaine and procainamide and related antiarrhythmic agents can relatively selectively suppress depressed fast action potentials in ischemic/infarcted regions, and thereby suppress arrhythmias.

The action potentials in the ischemic area have slow upstroke velocities ($\dot{V}_{max}$), are conducted slowly (ca. 0.05 m/sec), and about 35% of the action potentials have notched upstrokes or two peaks (3). There are delays and possibly decremental conduction. The depressed area exhibits one-way block, frequency-dependent block, and the Wenckebach phenomenon. There is a low safety factor for conduction, causing the impulse to be prone to block at impediments. Structural inhomogeneities/asymmetries and pathological changes can act as impediments to conduction. In addition, premature excitation can unmask asymmetries, and so a premature impulse may travel more easily in one direction than the other. Such unidirectional block of a premature impulse sets up one condition necessary for circus movement, namely one-way conduction. Increase in resistance of the cell-to-cell junctions (or in junctional cleft width) during hypoxia/ischemia were suggested as causes of conduction impediment (3).

DELAYED AFTER-DEPOLARIZATION

A depolarizing after-potential following a conventional hyperpolarizing after-potential was first described in cultured embryonic chick heart cells (monolayers) (16). The authors were able to turn trains of spontaneous action potentials on and off by applying hyperpolarizing current pulses of various intensities, and thereby demonstrated that each action potential in a train was triggered by the preceding action potential via the delayed depolarizing after-potential. Subsequently, this phenomenon was described in mammalian heart (7) and called a delayed after-depolarization (DAD). Cardiac glycosides potentiated the delayed after-depolarization, pointing to its possible importance in arrhythmogenesis.

There is a relationship between Ca^{2+} ion and the delayed after-depolarizations. Elevated $[Ca]_o$ enhances the delayed after-depolarization, and Ca^{2+}-antagonistic drugs depress and abolish the delayed after-depolarization. However, it has been shown (14) that the delayed after-depolarization is not directly produced by an inward Ca^{2+} current, but rather indirectly by release of Ca^{2+} from the sarcoplasmic reticulum which, in turn, produces an increase in a nonspecific leakage-type conductance for an inward depolarizing current. In voltage-clamp experiments, this inward current associated with delayed after-depolarization and concomitant after-contractions is known as the transient inward current (I_{Ti}). The transient inward current is enhanced by digitalis and catecholamine and K^+-free solution and by increased $[Ca]_o$, and is depressed by D-600 and verapamil and Mn^{2+}. Tetrodotoxin has no effect on the transient inward current, which is abolished by pretreatment with caffeine (10 mM) to release the sarcoplasmic reticulum stores of Ca^{2+}. The delayed after-depolarization or transient inward current is progressively potentiated during a train of impulses. The reversal potential (E_{rev}) for the transient inward current is about -5 mV, and is sensitive to $[Na]_o$ but not to $[Ca]_o$ and $[Cl]$.

In accordance with the view that the transient inward current is not caused by a Ca^{2+} influx, but is indirectly produced by an elevated $[Ca]_i$, ouabain potentiates the transient inward current by inhibiting the Na^+-K^+ pump, thereby increasing $[Na]_i$, which increases $[Ca]_i$ via the Ca^{2+}-Na^+ exchange system. The elevated $[Ca]_i$, in turn, triggers an oscillatory release of Ca^{2+} from the sarcoplasmic reticulum by the Ca^{2+}-trigger-Ca^{2+} mechanism (7). The oscillatory release can account for the damped oscillations in the transient inward current (and in delayed after-depolarizations and after-contractions) sometimes observed. The increase in $[Ca]_i$ opens a nonspecific voltage-independent postsynaptic type of ion channel (that presumably allows both Na^+ and K^+ to pass through). This type of channel would be somewhat analogous to the Ca^{2+}-activated K^+ channel ($g_{K(Ca)}$).

Thus, $[Ca]_i$ has profound effects on membrane electrical properties. For example, elevation in $[Ca]_i$ activates at least two different types of ion channels: (a) the nonspecific channel conductance (g_i) that underlies the transient inward current as discussed above, and which may be important in genesis of delayed after-depolarizations and dysrhythmias and even in cardiac plateau formation; (b) the Ca^{2+}-activated (Sr^{2+} and Ba^{2+} can substitute for Ca^{2+}) K^+ channel conductance ($g_{K(Ca)}$), which has been shown to be present in nerve and cardiac muscle, and which may be important in shortening of the cardiac action potential. In addition, there is some evidence that elevation of $[Ca]_i$ but not Sr^{2+} increases the voltage-dependent slow inward current in Purkinje fibers, and that this might mediate some of the effects of cardiac glycosides (19). The mechanism of this effect of $[Ca]_i$ is not known, but could involve the Ca^{2+}-calmodulin-activated protein kinase and phosphorylation of the slow channels. This positive feedback of $[Ca]_i$ may be limited in extent because higher $[Ca]_i$ could inhibit Ca^{2+} entry (negative feedback), either by somehow blocking the channels and/or decreasing the electrochemical gradient for Ca^{2+} entry.

SUMMARY

Slow action potentials have been implicated in the genesis of reentrant types of arrhythmias in ischemic zones, but there is opposing evidence that some ischemic action potentials are depressed fast action potentials rather than true slow action potential (namely, tetrodotoxin blocks the ischemic action potentials whereas Ca^{2+}-antagonist drugs do not). Regardless whether the ischemic action potential is a depressed fast action potential or a slow action potential, propagation velocity will be slow and there will be conduction disturbances that can predispose to dysrhythmias. Although local anesthetics depress and block slow action potentials and fast action potentials at the same concentrations, depressed fast action potentials are nearly 10-fold more sensitive to these drugs.

Delayed depolarizing after-potentials have also been implicated in genesis of arrhythmias of the triggered automaticity type. Any condition, such as hypoxia/ischemia or digitalis or catecholamines, that elevates $[Ca]_i$ potentiates the depolarizing after-potential, and hence the possible triggering of action potential trains from these ectopic foci and producing arrhythmias. Ca^{2+}-antagonistic drugs suppress these after-potentials and prevent such arrhythmogenesis.

ACKNOWLEDGMENTS

The work of the author and his colleagues reviewed and summarized in this article was supported by grants from the National Institutes of Health (HL-18711 and HL-19242), Muscular Dystrophy Association, Wallace Laboratories, and Smith, Kline and French Laboratories.

REFERENCES

1. Chesnais, J. M., Coraboeuf, E., Sauviat, M. P., and Vassas, J. M. (1975): *J. Mol. Cell. Cardiol.*, 7:627–642.
2. Cranefield, P. F. (1975): *The Conduction of the Cardiac Impulse.* Futura, Mt. Kisco, New York.
3. Cranefield, P. F., and Dodge, F. A. (1980): In: *The Slow Inward Current and Cardiac Arrhythmias,* edited by D. P. Zipes, J. C. Bailey, and V. Elharrar, pp. 149–171. Martinus Nijhoff, The Hague.
4. Cukierman, S., and Paes de Carvelho, A. (1982): In: *Normal and Abnormal Conduction in the Heart,* edited by A. Paes de Carvalho, B. F. Hoffman, and M. Lieberman, pp. 413–428. Futura, Mt. Kisco, New York.

5. Dodge, F. A., and Cranefield, P. F. (1982): In: *Normal and Abnormal Conduction in the Heart,* edited by A. Paes de Carvelho, B. F. Hoffman, and M. Lieberman, pp. 379–396. Futura, Mt. Kisco, New York.
6. Fabiato, A., and Fabiato, F. (1979): *Annu. Rev. Physiol.,* 41:473–484.
7. Ferrier, G. R., and Moe, G. K. (1973): *Circ. Res.,* 33:508–515.
8. Freer, R. J., Pappano, A. J., Peach, M. J., Bing, K. T., McLean, M. J., Vogel, S. M., and Sperelakis, N. (1976): *Circ. Res.,* 39:178–183.
9. Gilmour, R. F., Jr., and Zipes, D. P. (1982): *Circ. Res.,* 50:599–609.
10. Josephson, I., Renaud, J. F., Vogel, S., McLean, M., and Sperelakis, N. (1976): *Eur. J. Pharmacol.,* 35:393–398.
11. Josephson, I., and Sperelakis, N. (1976): *Eur. J. Pharmacol.,* 40:201–208.
12. Josephson, I., and Sperelakis, N. (1978): *J. Mol. Cell. Cardiol.,* 10:1157–1166.
13. Josephson, I., and Sperelakis, N. (1982): *J. Gen. Physiol.,* 79:69–86.
14. Kass, R. S., Tsien, R. S., and Weingart, R. (1978): *J. Physiol. (Lond.),* 281:209–226.
15. Lazzara, R., and Scherlag, B. (1980): In: *The Slow Inward Current and Cardiac Arrhythmias,* edited by D. P. Zipes, J. C. Bailey, and V. Elharrar, pp. 399–416. Martinus Nijhoff, The Hague.
16. Lehmkuhl, D., and Sperelakis, N. (1967): In: *Factors Influencing Myocardial Contractility,* edited by R. D. Tanz, F. Kavaler, and J. Roberts, pp. 245–278. Academic Press, New York.
17. Li T., and Sperelakis, N. (1983): *Circ. Res.,* 52:111–117.
18. Lynch, C., Vogel, S., and Sperelakis, N. (1981): *Anesthesiology,* 55:360–368.
19. Marban, E., and Tsien, R. W. (1982): *J. Physiol.,* 329:589–614.
20. Masuda, M. O., Paula-Carvalho, M., and Paes de Carvalho, A. (1982): In: *Normal and Abnormal Conduction in the Heart,* edited by A. Paes de Carvalho, B. F. Hoffman, and M. Lieberman, pp. 397–412. Futura, Mt. Kisco, New York.
21. Molyvdas, P. A., and Sperelakis, N. (1983): *J. Cardiovasc. Pharmacol.,* 5:162–169.
22. Pang, D. C., and Sperelakis, N. (1982): *Eur. J. Pharmacol.,* 81:403–409.
23. Pang, D. C., and Sperelakis, N. (1983): *Eur. J. Pharmacol.,* 87:199–207.
24. Shigenobu, K., Schneider, J. A., and Sperelakis, N. (1974): *J. Pharmacol. Exp. Therap.,* 190:280–288.
25. Sperelakis, N., Mayer, G., and Macdonald, R. (1970): *Am. J. Physiol.,* 219:952–963.
26. Shigenobu, K., and Sperelakis, N. (1972): *Circ. Res.,* 31:932–952.
27. Schneider, J. A., and Sperelakis, N. (1975): *J. Mol. Cell. Cardiol.,* 7:249–273.
28. Sperelakis, N., and Schneider, J. A. (1976): *Am. J. Cardiol.,* 37:1079–1085.
29. Sperelakis, N., Belardinelli, L., and Vogel, S. M. (1979): *Proceedings of 8th World Congress of Cardiology,* Tokyo, edited by S. Hayase and S. Murao, pp. 229–236. Excerpta Medica, Amsterdam.
30. Sperelakis, N. (1982): In: *The Coronary Artery,* edited by S. Kalsner, pp. 118–167. Croom Helm, London.
31. Vogel, S., and Sperelakis, N. (1977): *Am. J. Physiol.,* 233:C99–C103.
32. Vogel, S., Sperelakis, N., Josephson, I., and Brooker, G. (1977): *J. Mol. Cell. Cardiol.,* 9:461–475.
33. Vogel, S., Crampton, R., and Sperelakis, N. (1979): *J. Pharmacol. Exp. Ther.,* 210:378–385.
34. Vogel, S., and Sperelakis, N. (1981): *J. Mol. Cell. Cardiol.,* 13:51–64.
35. Zipes, D. P., Rinkenberger, R. L., Heger, J. J., and Prystowsky, E. N. (1980): In: *The Slow Inward Current and Cardiac Arrhythmias,* edited by D. P. Zipes, J. C. Bailey, and V. Elharrar, pp. 481–506. Martinus Nijhoff, The Hague.

Calcium Antagonists and Cardiovascular Disease, edited by L. H. Opie. Raven Press, New York © 1984.

Chapter 27

Evidence for a Role of Calcium in the Genesis of Early Ischemic Cardiac Arrhythmias

William T. Clusin, Maurice Buchbinder, Michael R. Bristow, and Donald C. Harrison

Division of Cardiology, Stanford University School of Medicine, Stanford, California 94305

There is increasing evidence that the electrophysiological effects of cardiac ischemia are mediated by Ca^{2+}. Myocardial ischemia is accompanied by impaired sequestration of intracellular Ca^{2+} during diastole, often described as "intracellular Ca^{2+} overload" (26). Drugs such as Ca^{2+} channel blockers, which alleviate this condition, have been reported to "preserve" ischemic myocardium, especially when administered beforehand. This myocardial preservation can occur independently of changes in coronary blood flow (16,21), and is accompanied by beneficial electrophysiological effects, including reduction of ischemic ECG changes, and suppression of early ischemic arrhythmias in experimental animals. It is likely that the same mechanisms operate in patients with coronary artery disease.

Quite apart from these developments, there has been increasing awareness of the diverse role which Ca^{2+} ions play in the membrane permeability processes that lead to electrical excitability in cardiac and other tissues (10). Cardiac cell membranes have been shown to contain specific inward current channels that are activated by the presence of Ca^{2+} at the inner surface of the cell membrane (11). In addition, extrusion of Ca^{2+} across the surface membrane in exchange for Na^+ appears to involve net inward movement of positive charge (34). These mechanisms presumably mediate the depolarizing afterpotentials that occur in digitalis (24,25) and appear to operate during other conditions where intracellular Ca^{2+} is increased (6).

The purpose of this chapter is to suggest a mechanism whereby increased intracellular Ca^{2+} might directly mediate the development of early ischemic cardiac arrhythmias. We present preliminary evidence that the antifibrillatory effect of Ca^{2+} channel blockers is related to amelioration of the effects of ischemia on the cardiac action potential, with resultant diminution of "injury" current across the ischemic border. These observations are supported by voltage-clamp experiments in which the effects of metabolic inhibition on cardiac membrane potential appear to be mediated by intracellular Ca^{2+}.

ANTIFIBRILLATORY EFFECTS OF CALCIUM CHANNEL BLOCKERS AND RELATED AGENTS

The ability of a Ca^{2+} channel blocker to suppress early ischemic ventricular arrhythmias was first appreciated by Kaumann and Aramendia nearly 15 years ago (28). In their study, 10 of 11 control animals developed ventricular fibrillation after occlusion of the left anterior descending artery, while 9 of 10 verapamil-treated animals survived. The antifibrillatory effect of verapamil has been confirmed in several subsequent studies (4,14,37). Verapamil not only reduces the incidence of spontaneous ventricular fibrillation, but diminishes the fall in ventricular fibrillation threshold during ischemia (4,14,37). Similar protective effects have been demonstrated for other Ca^{2+} channel blockers, including D-600 (36), diltiazem (8,37), nifedipine (13), and several other dihydropyridines (13).

A particularly sensitive method of quantifying the antifibrillatory effect is to measure the time between coronary occlusion and the onset of ventricular fibrillation. We have found that when the proximal left anterior descending and circumflex arteries of dogs are occluded during rapid right ventricular pacing, ventricular fibrillation occurs predictably, with a latency that is nearly constant during consecutive trials at 15 min intervals (8). Mean ventricular fibrillation latency remains constant during 6 control occlusions, increases approximately 100% during diltiazem infusion, and returns toward the control values when the infusion ceases. Occlusions performed during diltiazem infusion sometimes fail to elicit ventricular fibrillation within an arbitrary period of 360 sec. The coronary occluders are then released to permit further trials. The changes in ventricular fibrillation latency are highly significant, ($p < 10^{-6}$, Friedman's test), and have now been demonstrated in 15 dogs. Ventricular fibrillation latency is closely correlated with simultaneous measurements of atrioventricular conduction delay and serum diltiazem concentration.

The antifibrillatory effect of Ca^{2+} channel blockers was initially interpreted as a lessening of the ischemic insult, rather than a primary electrophysiological phenomenon. Although Ca^{2+} channel blockers may reduce ischemia through improvement of coronary perfusion, or reduction of myocardial energy consumption, neither of these mechanisms adequately explains the antifibrillatory effect. In the ventricular fibrillation latency model, significant residual coronary perfusion is unlikely to occur because both arteries that supply the left ventricle are occluded proximally. This impression has been confirmed in 5 dogs in which coronary blood flow was measured by a thermodilution catheter placed in the coronary sinus (8). Although diltiazem significantly increased base line coronary sinus flow, flow during occlusion was nearly absent, and was not increased by diltiazem in any animal. The possible role of changes in energy consumption has also been investigated in the ventricular fibrillation latency model by calculation of left ventricular work (8). In 5 animals, diltiazem *increased* preischemic left ventricular work by $56 \pm 24\%$ ($p < 0.001$), presumably because of afterload reduction. Coronary occlusion produced complete electromechanical dissociation both in the presence and absence of diltiazem. However, work performed in the presence of diltiazem never fell below that measured in the absence of the drug. Thus, the prolongation of ventricular fibrillation latency by diltiazem cannot be ascribed to a reduction in mechanical work.

Two additional observations suggest that the antifibrillatory effects of Ca^{2+} channel blockers are a direct result of reduced Ca^{2+} influx. First, Thandroyen (37) has measured the effects of Ca^{2+} channel blockers on high-energy phosphate stores in rat myocardium, and found that the antifibrillatory effect is not contingent upon improvement of myocardial energetics. Second, an antifibrillatory effect similar to that of diltiazem is observed when serum ionized Ca^{2+} is reduced by infusion of sodium citrate (8). Ventricular fibrillation latency remains constant during 6 control occlusions, increases progressively during increasing infusions of sodium citrate, and returns toward the control level when the citrate infusion is discontinued. The changes in ventricular fibrillation latency and serum ionized Ca^{2+} are both statistically significant ($p < 0.01$, Friedman's test). Moreover, changes in ventricular fibrillation latency are closely correlated with the accompanying reduction of ionized Ca^{2+} ($R = 0.84$, $p < 10^{-6}$).

REDUCTION OF ISCHEMIC "INJURY" CURRENTS BY A CALCIUM CHANNEL BLOCKER

Early ischemic arrhythmias must ultimately arise from the effects of ischemia on the cellular transmembrane potential. In myocardial cells, ischemia produces a reduction of the resting potential, which leads to a diastolic "injury" current across the ischemic border. This diastolic current produces "T-Q depression" on the DC epicardial electrogram. At the same time, reduction of action potential duration in ischemic cells produces a systolic current in the opposite direction. This systolic current is manifested as "true" ST elevation in the DC electrogram.

There is increasing evidence that the flow of "injury" current during ischemia is directly responsible for initiation of early ischemic arrhythmias. Katzung et al. (27) found that the "injury" current resulting from localized application of high K^+ to mammalian papillary muscles can induce premature beats in the untreated region. They postulate that a similar mechanism operates during ischemia. Their hypothesis has been supported by studies in which the ventricular activation sequence is determined by epicardial mapping during ischemia. In two such studies (18,20), the initiating beat of ventricular fibrillation was found to invariably originate from the normal edge of the ischemic boundary.

Since Ca^{2+} channel blockers retard ischemic arrhythmias through a direct action on the myocardium, they might also diminish the effects of ischemia upon the ventricular action potential. This deduction can be tested by recording DC epicardial electrograms during ischemia, as illustrated in Fig. 1. In this

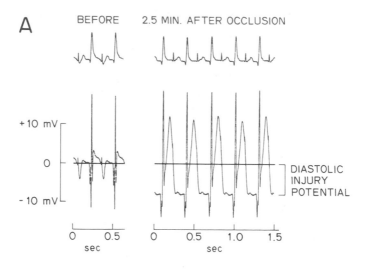

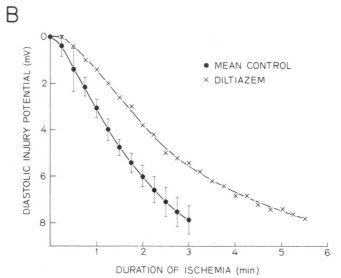

FIG. 1. Reduction of the epicardial injury potential by diltiazem. **A** is an epicardial potential (*lower trace*) recorded before (*left*) and 150 sec after (*right*) occlusion of the proximal left anterior descending (LAD) and circumflex coronary arteries. The recording is obtained using a DC differential amplifier with Ag/AgCl electrodes sutured to the left ventricular epicardium. The positive electrode is positioned within the ischemic zone, while the reference lead covers a small nonischemic region supplied by a diagonal branch arising from the LAD proximal to the site of occlusion. The diastolic injury potential (*indicated by bracket*) is measured as depression of the pre-QRS segment below the original isoelectric line. Elevation of the T wave above this line represents the systolic injury potential. The left atrium is paced at 200 beats/min throughout the occlusion. The *top trace* is the standard electrocardiographic lead II. In **B,** the diastolic injury potential is plotted against duration of ischemia for occlusions performed before and after diltiazem administration. *Filled circles* show the mean and standard deviation of the injury potential during 6 consecutive control occlusions performed 15 min apart. Data points beyond 3 min have not been obtained owing to the development of ventricular fibrillation. *Crosses* show the diastolic injury potential after a 25 min infusion of diltiazem (0.02 mg/kg/min). Ventricular fibrillation is prevented by diltiazem, and the injury potential develops more slowly. (W. Clusin and M. Buchbinder, *unpublished data*).

experiment, Ag/AgCl electrodes have been sutured to the epicardium of a dog prior to occlusion of the left anterior descending and circumflex coronary arteries. During coronary occlusion, the "injury" current is proportional to the voltage difference between the ischemic and nonischemic epicardial regions, as shown in Fig. 2A. In Fig. 2B, the diastolic "injury" potential (T-Q depression) is plotted as a function of the duration of ischemia. The time course with which this potential develops is nearly constant during six consecutive control occlusions (*filled circles*). However, infusion of diltiazem (0.02 mg/kg/min for 25 min) markedly reduces the diastolic potential during the next occlusion (*crosses*).

A similar reduction of "injury" current by diltiazem has been demonstrated in several other dogs. This diminution of "injury" current is not confined to the diastolic component (T-Q depression), but affects the systolic component (ST elevation) to approximately the same extent (not illustrated). The reduction of "injury" current is correlated with the increase in ventricular fibrillation latency. This observation is consistent with the hypothesis of Katzung et al. (27) and suggests that the antifibrillatory effect of diltiazem could be causally related to reduction of the diastolic current. As noted above, the reduction of "injury" currents in this model cannot be ascribed to improvement of coronary perfusion or reduction of cardiac work. Failure of diltiazem to alter perfusion near the ischemic electrode can be directly tested in this model by infusion of radioactively labeled microspheres. Our results indicate that diltiazem directly alleviates the effects of ischemia on the resting and action potential of ventricular muscle.

DOES CALCIUM OVERLOAD CAUSE ISCHEMIC DEPOLARIZATION?

An attractive explanation for the ability of diltiazem to diminish the electrophysiological effects of ischemia is that these effects are a direct consequence of intracellular Ca^{2+} overload (9). This explanation has become especially plausible in view of the role that Ca^{2+}-mediated permeability changes appear to play in cardiac excitation.

In order to determine how ischemia modifies cardiac transmembrane potentials, it would be desirable to study the effects of ischemia on individual membrane currents under voltage clamp. This is, of course, not possible because the voltage-clamp technique can only be utilized in small, isopotential preparations. However, the electrophysiological effects of ischemia can be faithfully reproduced *in vitro* by metabolic inhibitors. Fig. 2A shows the effects of 0.1 mM dinitrophenol (DNP) plus 0.1 mM iodoacetate (IAA) on the transmembrane potential of an isopotential chick embryonic myocardial cell aggregate. Addition of metabolic inhibitors causes reduction of the diastolic potential and action potential duration within 1 min. Because the preparation beats spontaneously, the depolarizing effect is initially manifested by an increase in beat frequency, which is perceptible within seconds, and persists until the preparation arrests.

The mechanism of depolarization during metabolic inhibition can be studied in this preparation using the voltage-clamp technique (7). In Fig. 2B, an aggregate

A

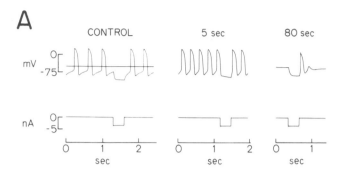

B

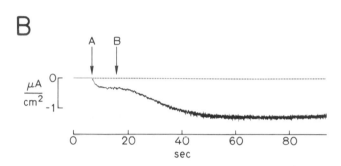

FIG. 2. Effects of metabolic inhibitors on action potentials and membrane current in tissue cultured chick myocardial cell aggregates. In **A**, a spontaneously beating aggregate is abruptly superfused with 0.1 mM dinitrophenol (DNP) plus 0.1 mM iodoacetate (IAA) following the control recording. Beat-frequency increases markedly within 5 sec, and the aggregate arrests within 60 sec in a partly depolarized state. Hyperpolarizing current pulses (*bottom trace*) then elicit action potentials of reduced duration. The resting potential at 80 sec is indicated on the control record by a *horizontal line*. In **B**, a cell aggregate is voltage-clamped at −65 mV beginning at *arrow A*, and then exposed to DNP + IAA, beginning at *arrow B*. DNP + IAA evoke a sustained depolarizing (inward) current. The experiment has been performed in 10 mM Ca²⁺, which accentuates the metabolic inhibitor-induced inward current. This and several other properties of the inward current suggest that it results from a permeability change that is activated by increased intracellular free Ca²⁺. (From ref. 7.)

is clamped at a potential in the pacemaker range (−65 mV) beginning at *arrow A*, and then superfused with dinitrophenol + iodoacetate at *arrow B*. Addition of metabolic inhibitors induces a depolarizing (inward) current that is perceptible within several seconds, and reaches its maximum value within about 30 sec. Several properties of this inward current suggest that it results from an effect of increased intracellular free Ca²⁺ on membrane permeability:

1. Like known Ca²⁺-activated inward currents in cardiac cells, the metabolic inhibitor current is abolished by removal of extracellular Na⁺.

2. The metabolic inhibitor current is also abolished by prior reduction of extracellular Ca^{2+} to 0.1 mM, which reduces intracellular Ca^{2+} to the extent that contraction no longer occurs during action potentials.

3. Conversely, the metabolic inhibitor current is augmented by maneuvers that increase intracellular Ca^{2+}. These include elevation of extracellular Ca^{2+} to 10 mM, intermittent rapid pacing by current pulses, and intoxication with acetylstrophanthidin.

The Ca^{2+}-activated inward current that occurs in digitalis toxicity is initiated by abnormal release of sequestered intracellular Ca^{2+}, which may then open Ca^{2+}-activated channels, or be extruded electrogenically. Several considerations suggest that these mechanisms also operate during metabolic inhibition. Jundt et al. (22) showed that exposure of mammalian cardiac fibers to cyanide caused a prompt increase in Na^+-dependent $^{45}Ca^{2+}$ efflux. More recently, Dahl and Isenberg (12) recorded intracellular Ca^{2+} activity with Ca^{2+}-sensitive intracellular electrodes and found that exposure of myocardial fibers to dinitrophenol produces a 100-fold increase in intracellular Ca^{2+} activity within 3 min, which parallels the decline in resting potential. The Ca^{2+} that appears in the myoplasm during metabolic inhibition could be released either from mitochondria or from the sarcoplasmic reticulum. Cyanide is known to release Ca^{2+} from isolated cardiac mitochondria within a few seconds (22). Moreover, exposure of cultured myocardial cell aggregates to caffeine, which releases Ca^{2+} from the sarcoplasmic reticulum, induces an inward current similar in magnitude to that produced by metabolic inhibition (6).

While there are a number of differences between ischemia and metabolic inhibition, the mechanisms described above may be sufficient to explain the rapid depolarization of myocardium during ischemia. Since treatment of myocardium with Ca^{2+} channel blockers reduces intracellular Ca^{2+} stores, amelioration of ischemic depolarization by these drugs would also be explained.

DOES CALCIUM OVERLOAD SHORTEN THE ACTION POTENTIAL DURING ISCHEMIA?

The depression of the systolic "injury" current by diltiazem suggests that abbreviation of the action potential duration during ischemia is also related to intracellular Ca^{2+} overload. There is considerable evidence that action potential duration can be regulated by intracellular Ca^{2+}. Conditions that increase intracellular Ca^{2+} while shortening the action potential, include metabolic inhibition, digitalis toxicity, increased extracellular Ca^{2+}, increased beat frequency, and direct intracellular injection of Ca^{2+} with microelectrodes (19,29). Conversely, the action potential is lengthened by injection of the Ca^{2+} chelating agent, ethylene bis (oxyethylenenitrilo) tetraacetic acid (EGTA) (19). EGTA injection also normalizes plateau duration during digitalis toxicity (29).

While the control of plateau duration by intracellular Ca^{2+} is well established experimentally, this phenomenon has been difficult to interpret at the subcellular level. The effects of Ca²⁺ injection on the plateau were initially taken as evidence that the repolarizing K⁺ current flows through a Ca²⁺-activated K⁺ channel (2,5,19), as frequently occurs in the nervous system (10). However, direct characterization of cardiac K⁺ channels by membrane patch recording has failed to support this inference so far. Furthermore, Kass (23) has shown that Ca²⁺ influx in Purkinje fibers can be suppressed without apparent effect on the repolarizing K⁺ current.

An alternative explanation for the effects of intracellular Ca²⁺ on plateau duration has to do with the contribution of Ca²⁺-activated *inward* current during the action potential. While descriptions of Ca²⁺-activated inward current in heart were initially limited to conditions of abnormal Ca²⁺ loading, Clusin subsequently noted several situations in which intracellular Ca²⁺ appeared to induce inward current in otherwise normal cardiac cells (5). Based on such observations, it has been proposed that the increase in intracellular Ca²⁺ during each action potential induces a depolarizing current that contributes to the maintenance of the plateau (1,5,6,31,32). This contribution would be particularly important during the later portion of the plateau, when depolarization-induced inward currents had inactivated.

There are two ways in which Ca²⁺ overload could shorten the plateau in the above scheme. First, although the diastolic level of free Ca²⁺ is necessarily increased during "Ca²⁺ overload," phasic Ca²⁺ release may be impaired, as evidenced by a decline in developed tension. This reduction in systolic free Ca²⁺ could diminish the inward current contributing to the plateau. Secondly, the Ca²⁺-activated inward current channels that have been isolated from embryonic cardiac cells "desensitize" during prolonged exposure of their cytoplasmic aspect to elevated Ca²⁺ concentrations (11). Thus, "intracellular Ca²⁺ overload" could reduce the proportion of these channels available to contribute to the plateau.[1]

While much remains to be learned about the role of intracellular Ca²⁺ during the normal cardiac action potential, it is foreseeable that these phenomena will largely account for the early electrophysiological effects of ischemia, as well as their amelioration by drugs that prevent intracellular Ca²⁺ overload.

THERAPEUTIC IMPLICATIONS

A principal objective of therapy for coronary artery disease is to reduce the incidence of sudden cardiac death. β-Adrenergic blockers are reported to have antifibrillatory effects during experimental ischemia (28,33), and to reduce the incidence of early postinfarction arrhythmias (17), and sudden cardiac death (3,38), when administered prophylactically after myocardial infarction. While some of the arrhythmias of coronary artery disease are not produced by acute ischemia, β-adrenergic blockers appear to be more effective in preventing sudden

---

[1] We are indebted to Prof. Harald Reuter for suggesting this mechanism.

death than in suppressing chronic extrasystoles or recurrent ventricular tachycardia.

In light of the above evidence, the antifibrillatory effect of β-blockers may be due to improvement of Ca^{2+} overload in the ischemic myocardium. β-blockers produce this effect by reducing Ca^{2+} influx during each action potential, and by reducing heart rate. However, there are variety of other ways in which the same result could be achieved. α-Adrenergic blockers, for example, reportedly improve Ca^{2+} sequestration by the sarcoplasmic reticulum (30), and also suppress early ischemic arrhythmias in experimental animals (35).

Perhaps the most important implication of our formulation is that treatment of the electrophysiological effects of ischemia may not always require improvement of myocardial energetics or reduction of myocardium at risk. Many years ago, Fozzard and Das Gupta noted that "currents generating the ST-segment changes may be the basis for producing arrhythmias that could compromise cardiac function or kill the patient, and interruption of these currents could help the patient, regardless of infarct size (15)." It now seems possible that an appreciable reduction of cardiovascular mortality could be achieved in this manner.

SUMMARY

Early ischemic arrhythmias are suppressed by drugs that retard the development of intracellular Ca^{2+} overload. To explain this, we propose that the rapid depolarization of ischemic myocardium, and resulting diastolic injury current are caused by effects of intracellular Ca^{2+} on the ionic permeability of the cell membrane. Our hypothesis is supported by voltage-clamp experiments in cultured heart cells, and by recordings of injury current and arrhythmia onset after coronary occlusion in dogs.

REFERENCES

1. Allen, D. G., and Eisner, D. A. (1982): *J. Physiol.,* 330:95P.
2. Bassingthwaighte, J. B., Fry, C. H., and McGuigan, J. A. S. (1976): *J. Physiol.,* 262:15–38.
3. Beta Blocker Heart Attack Trial Research Group (1982): *JAMA,* 247:1707–1712.
4. Brooks, W. W., Verrier, R. L., and Lown, B. (1980): *Cardiovasc. Res.,* 14:295–302.
5. Clusin, W. T. (1980): In: *Drug-Induced Heart Disease,* edited by M. R. Bristow, pp. 103–126. Elsevier, Amsterdam.
6. Clusin, W. T. (1982): *Nature,* 301:248–250.
7. Clusin, W. T. (1983): *Proc. Natl. Acad. Sci. (USA),* 80:3865–3869.
8. Clusin, W. T., Bristow, M. R., Baim, D. S., et al. (1982): *Circ. Res.,* 50:518–526.
9. Clusin, W. T., Buchbinder, M., and Harrison, D. C. (1983): *Lancet,* I:272–274.
10. Clusin, W. T., Spray, D. C., and Bennett, M. V. L. (1975): *Nature,* 256:425–427.
11. Colquhoun, D., Neher, E., Reuter, H., and Stevens, C. F. (1981): *Nature,* 294:752–754.
12. Dahl, G., and Isenberg, G. (1980): *J. Membr. Biol.,* 53:63–75.
13. Fagbemi, O., and Parratt, J. R. (1981): *Eur. J. Pharmacol.,* 75:179–185.
14. Fondacaro, J. D., Han, J., and Yoon, M. S. (1978): *Am. Heart J.,* 96:81–86.
15. Fozzard, H. A., and DasGupta, D. S. (1976): *Circulation,* 54:533–537.
16. Higgins, T. J. C., Alsopp, D., and Bailey, P. (1980): *J. Mol. Cell. Cardiol.,* 12:909–927.

17. Hjalmarson, A., Elmfeldt, D., Herlitz, J., *et al. Lancet,* ii:823–827.
18. Ideker, R. E., Klein, G. J., Harrison, L. *et al.* (1981): *Circulation,* 63:1371–1379.
19. Isenberg, G. (1977): *Pfluegers Arch.,* 371:51–59.
20. Janse, M. J., van Capelle, F. J. L., Morsink, H., *et al.* (1980): *Circ. Res.,* 47:151–165.
21. Jolly, S. R., Menahan, L. A., and Gross, G. J. (1981): *J. Mol. Cell. Cardiol.,* 13:359–372.
22. Jundt, H., Porzig, H., Reuter, H., and Stucki, J. W. (1975): *J. Physiol.,* 246:229–253.
23. Kass, R. S. (1982): *J. Pharmacol. Exp. Ther.,* 223:446–456.
24. Kass, R. S., Lederer, W. J., Tsien, R. W., and Weingart, R. (1978): *J. Physiol.,* 281:187–208.
25. Kass, R. S., Tsien, R. W., and Weingart, R. (1978): *J. Physiol.,* 281:209–226.
26. Katz, A. M., and Reuter, H. (1979): *Am. J. Cardiol.,* 44:188–190.
27. Katzung, B. G., Hondeghem, L. M., and Grant, A. O. (1975): *Pflueger's Arch.,* 360:193–197.
28. Kaumann, A. J., and Aramendia, P. (1968): *J. Pharmacol. Exp. Ther.,* 164:326–332.
29. Matsuda, H., Noma, A., Kurachi, Y., and Irisawa, H. (1982): *Circ. Res.,* 51:142–151.
30. Niedergerke, R., and Page, S. (1981): *Proc. R. Soc. Lond. (Biol.),* 213:325–344.
31. Niedergerke, R., and Page, S. (1982): *J. Physiol.,* 228:17P.
32. Noble, S., and Shimoni, Y. (1981): *J. Physiol.,* 310:57–75.
33. Patterson, E., and Lucchesi, B. R. (1982): *J. Pharmacol. Exp. Ther.,* 223:144–152.
34. Reeves, J. P., and Sutko, J. L. (1980): *Science,* 208:1461–1464.
35. Sheridan, D. J., Penkoske, P. A., Sobel, B. E., and Corr, P. B. (1980): *J. Clin. Invest.,* 65:161–171.
36. Schoenberger, A. S., Verrier, R. L., and Lown, B. (1979): *Proc. Soc. Exp. Biol. Med.,* 161:56–59.
37. Thandroyen, F. T. (1982): *J. Mol. Cell. Cardiol.,* 14:21–32.
38. The Norwegian Multicenter Study Group (1981): *N. Engl. J. Med.,* 304:801–807.

Calcium Antagonists and Cardiovascular
Disease, edited by L. H. Opie.
Raven Press, New York © 1984.

Chapter 28

Calcium Channel Antagonists as Antiarrhythmic Agents: Contrasting Properties of Verapamil and Diltiazem versus Nifedipine

Lionel H. Opie, Francis T. Thandroyen, Cecilia A. Muller, and
Christian W. Hamm

*MRC-UCT Ischaemic Heart Disease Research Unit, Department of Medicine, Groote
Schuur Hospital and University of Cape Town, South Africa*

The slow inward current, carried predominantly by Ca^{2+} ions (8,22), is considered to be responsible for the development of slow-response action potentials with reduced resting membrane potentials and a slow rate of propagation. Under physiological conditions, these slow-response action potentials appear to play an important role in the propagation of impulses within nodal tissue, especially the atrioventricular muscle (27,45,48). The inhibition of atrioventricular conduction by Ca^{2+} channel antagonists (45,48) (Fig. 1) is indirect evidence that the slow inward Ca^{2+} current is of major importance in the generation of atrioventricular nodal action potentials.

Paroxysmal supraventricular tachycardias are usually associated with reentrant circuits involving the atrioventricular node and/or bypass tracts (7,12, 13,47). Verapamil, the prototype Ca^{2+} antagonist, is the treatment of choice in such supraventricular tachycardias (17,23,31,34,35); its antiarrhythmic action is by inhibition of conduction through the atrioventricular node. Verapamil is also of value in the control of a rapid ventricular response in atrial flutter or fibrillation (17,35,37,38).

During acute myocardial ischemia or infarction, slow-response action potentials, arising in ischemic ventricular cells, are currently considered to be one electrophysiological mechanism underlying the development of ventricular fibrillation (8,28; Chapter 26; *this volume*). An important reservation is that such slow responses have not yet been found in experimental preparations with regional ischemia (developing infarction); and in one model of ischemia in explanted hamster tissue, slow responses sensitive to verapamil could not be elicited

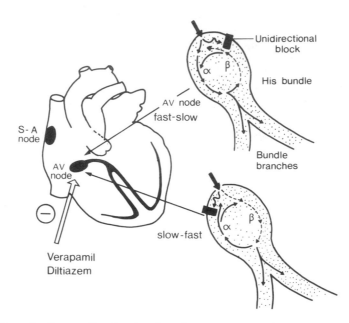

FIG. 1. The major therapeutic site of action of verapamil and diltiazem in supraventricular tachycardias is an inhibition of conduction through the atrioventricular (AV) node. This effect is not reversed by external Ca^{2+} but by β-agonists.

(14). Experimentally, Ca^{2+} channel antagonists inhibit some slow-response potentials and may improve conduction delay in ischemic myocardium (16). In certain experimental animal models (dog and rat, but not the pig), Ca^{2+} channel antagonists exhibit ventricular antiarrhythmic activity. Protection against ventricular fibrillation during acute myocardial infarction in man by Ca^{2+} antagonists has not been documented. Details of the above electrophysiological effects of the three major Ca^{2+} antagonists, nifedipine, verapamil and diltiazem, will now be reviewed. Some reference will also be made to lidoflazine and other Ca^{2+}-antagonist compounds.

ELECTROPHYSIOLOGICAL EFFECTS OF CALCIUM ANTAGONISTS

A primary and major site of the electrophysiological action of verapamil (9) and diltiazem is the atrioventricular node (Fig. 1).

Atrioventricular Node

Verapamil prolongs conduction time and refractoriness in the atrioventricular node in the atrioventricular (anterograde = antegrade) direction (31,40). In general, verapamil infrequently prolongs retrograde conduction time or refractoriness in the atrioventricular node (21). Thus, verapamil exhibits its antiarrhythmic action in the control of supraventricular tachycardia by way of antero-grade (= antegrade) atrioventricular conduction block (40), for example, by inhibition of one arc of the reentrant circuit.

Diltiazem and tiapamil also inhibit conduction in the atrioventricular node and, in preliminary reports, appear to control supraventricular tachycardias (15,20).

Nifedipine, in clinically relevant concentrations, has not been shown to prolong atrioventricular conduction time nor to terminate supraventricular tachycardia (32); a slight direct negative effect on atrioventricular conduction is offset by enhanced sympathetic tone (20).

Sinoatrial Node

Theoretically, verapamil and related compounds should inhibit conduction through the sinus node (sinoatrial conduction). The rate of spontaneous depolarization depends on three currents, I_k, I_{si}, and I_f. If the latter current, recently described by Noble's group from Oxford, is found even in the presence of the verapamil analog D600 and responds to β-adrenoceptor agonists (3), the potential of verapamil for a direct negative chronotropic effect is therefore limited, unless other nonspecific (i.e., not Ca^{2+} antagonist) properties of verapamil are involved. In addition, reflex sympathetic stimulation and some reflex withdrawal of parasympathetic tone as a result of the peripheral vasodilator effect of Ca^{2+} antagonists limit any direct negative chronotropic effects. The end result may, in fact, be that the sinus rate increases.

In patient studies, where the above reflexes can occur, verapamil is without effect on sinus node recovery time or sinoatrial conduction time (21,38), although an increased corrected sinus node recovery time has been found (19).

Diltiazem has a more marked and consistent bradycardiac effect, presumably by altering the pacemaker current, which, in turn, may imply an effect beyond that of Ca^{2+} antagonism. Similar arguments hold for lidoflazine.

In the presence of preexisting sinus node disease (sick sinus syndrome) or significant sinus node depression (by β-adrenergic blockade or excess of digitalis glycosides), intravenous verapamil and diltiazem are contraindicated, while oral administration should be only with care. Nifedipine is apparently less active against nodal tissue; it does not cause sinus node depression and may be combined with β-adrenergic blockade more safely than verapamil (43). Despite its powerful peripheral vasodilator action, nifedipine only causes a very modest tachycardia (L. Jee and L. Opie, *unpublished data*).

Atrial, His-Purkinje, and Intravenous Conduction

Verapamil does not slow interatrial, His-Purkinje, or intravenous conduction (19,33,39).

Bypass Tract

Verapamil is usually without effect on retrograde or anterograde conduction through the bypass tract. Rarely, anterograde conduction may be accelerated with undesirable consequences as a result of a reduced refractory period (39). Electrophysiological studies may be needed to exclude this possibility.

VENTRICULAR ARRHYTHMIAS

Reperfusion Ventricular Arrhythmias

During severe attacks of coronary artery vasospasm, transmural ischemia may give rise to ventricular arrhythmias typical of hyperacute myocardial infarction. In that case, any of the three standard Ca^{2+} antagonists, verapamil, diltiazem, or nifedipine, should relieve the arrhythmias by relief of spasm. In reality, very few clinical studies on this rather rare condition have been reported. Following relief of spasm, reperfusion of the acutely ischemic myocardium occurs with the theoretical danger of *reperfusion arrhythmias*. Reports on the experimental effects of Ca^{2+} antagonists on reperfusion ventricular arrhythmias vary: In rat hearts, nifedipine is effective (11,24). In the dog models, data conflict: Nifedipine and diltiazem are without effect according to Sheehan and Epstein (36), whereas verapamil protects (2), as does nifedipine according to Coker and Parratt (5). Therefore, the situation regarding reperfusion arrhythmias is open to further investigation.

Ischemic Ventricular Arrhythmias

In 1976, Podzuweit et al. postulated that the increase of intracellular cyclic AMP in the ischemic myocardium could promote the development of ventricular fibrillation (29). Electrophysiological evidence supporting this hypothesis was that cyclic AMP could promote the formation of slow-response action potentials (28,30) which are considered to underlie the development of reentrant ventricular arrhythmias (44,45). Furthermore, dibutyryl cyclic AMP (an analog of cyclic AMP which penetrates the cell membrane more easily) can cause after-depolarizations (10), considered to be another mechanism in the genesis of ventricular arrhythmias and also held to be Ca^{2+}-mediated. In addition, cyclic AMP mediates electrical uncoupling of cells in hypoxic muscle, and thereby may predispose to ventricular fibrillation (46). If all these arguments are correct, then abnormalities of Ca^{2+} ion movements are the ultimate mediator of ventricular fibrillation and Ca^{2+} antagonists (like β-blockers) should prevent ventricular fibrillation.

However, there are two problems with this line of reasoning. First, from the clinical point of view, Ca^{2+} channel antagonists have, thus far, been used against supraventricular arrhythmias (verapamil), or their effects on ventricular arrhythmias have not yet been well recognized (nifedipine, diltiazem). Second, the genesis of ventricular arrhythmias is probably multifactorial and exceedingly complex (41).

A Role for Calcium Ions in Ventricular Fibrillation?

In the isolated Langendorff-perfused rat heart, our *unpublished data* suggest that Ca^{2+} ions appear to mediate catecholamine-induced ventricular fibrillation, and also appear to play a role in the genesis of ventricular fibrillation during acute myocardial ischemia and adrenergic stimulation. Our data do not provide direct proof for this hypothesis because Ca^{2+} channel-antagonist agents not only inhibit transmembrane Ca^{2+} ion flux but some may, in addition, possess nonspecific effects. Thus, racemic verapamil may possess Na^+ channel-antagonist activity (1), while verapamil and diltiazem may possess α-adrenergic-antagonist activity (26). However, nifedipine does not possess α-adrenergic-antagonist activity in the rat myocardium (26); hence, it may be considered a "pure" Ca^{2+} antagonist in contrast to verapamil and diltiazem. Furthermore, Clusin et al. (4) have shown that the inhibitory effects of diltiazem on ischemic ventricular fibrillation latency in the dog are similar to the effects of reducing ionized serum Ca^{2+} by an infusion of sodium citrate. The common factor to all these observations is the Ca^{2+}-antagonist effect of the agents tested. In the coronary-ligated rat heart, Thandroyen (42) has shown that the protective effect of Ca^{2+} antagonists is not dependent on tissue contents of high-energy phosphate, total coronary flow, or heart rate; changes in the regional distribution of the coronary flow were not sought and must still be excluded as a possible mechanism. In the setting of acute myocardial ischemia or infarction, Ca^{2+} ions do not appear to be the only factor involved in the genesis of ventricular fibrillation. This conclusion is based on the findings that the "pure Ca^{2+}-antagonist agents," $l(-)$-verapamil and nifedipine, only partially prevented the fall in the ventricular fibrillation threshold during acute myocardial ischemia, and the d-isomer of verapamil was nearly as effective as the l-isomer. Our results in the isolated rat heart, therefore, do not fully support the hypothesis that Ca^{2+} ions mediate the electrophysiological alterations underlying ventricular arrhythmias.

Reservations

The Langendorff-perfused isolated rat heart, used by Thandroyen (42) is a preparation which has a number of obvious defects: (a) There is no integrated control with an intact autonomic nervous system and there are no circulating catecholamines; (b) the coronary flow is very high because of the absence of hemoglobin in the perfusate; (c) there is a marked species difference between rats and other animals in the nature of cardiac action potential, which is very abbreviated in the rat due to the rapidity of Ca^{2+} ion influx during the slow phase of the action potential; and (d) no external mechanical work is performed.

Pig Studies

To overcome the objections to the Langendorff-perfused isolated rat heart preparations, we carried out further studies on pigs, which have a coronary anatomy much closer to man. Ligation of the anterior descending coronary artery in the anesthetized, open-chest pig model resulted in a high incidence of ventricular fibrillation. Neither *dl*-verapamil 0.2 mg/kg, nor diltiazem 2 mg/ kg, prevented ventricular fibrillation. These studies demonstrate that even large doses of verapamil and diltiazem are ineffective in preventing ventricular fibrillation during acute regional myocardial ischemia of the left ventricle. We cannot exclude that the Ca^{2+} antagonists delayed the development of ventricular fibrillation, as found in a dog model with severe ischemia (4). The differences between rat and pig models are not just a species problem because nifedipine is effective against ventricular arrhythmias in a dog model (5). Thus, despite the theoretical and experimental evidence implicating a role for Ca^{2+} ions in the genesis of ventricular fibrillation (Chapter 27, *this volume*), Ca^{2+} channel-antagonist agents, and hence by inference, transsarcolemmal Ca^{2+} ion fluxes, do not appear to play a primary role in the genesis of ventricular fibrillation during acute myocardial infarction in the anesthetized pig.

Genesis of Ventricular Fibrillation

Hence, in both isolated rat heart and the pig heart *in situ*, Ca^{2+} channel-antagonist agents were either not specifically effective (rat) or ineffective (pig) in preventing ventricular fibrillation. This conclusion does not disprove a role for Ca^{2+} in ventricular fibrillation. First, in a model of severe ischemia, such as the pig, many other factors are at work. A very high extracellular K^+ concentration (18), up to 18 mM, can of itself, cause slow responses (28) and, if higher, actually stop Ca^{2+} influx (complete absence of action potential in highly depolarized myocardium). Second, accumulating lysophospholipids could also contribute to the development of slow responses and other electrophysiological abnormalities (6). Other factors provoking arrhythmias and not directly involving transsarcolemmal Ca^{2+} influx include the effects of circulating or endogenous free fatty acids.

It is important to stress that coronary artery ligation in our pig model results in severe ischemia, as evidenced by a decrease in blood flow in the ischemic zone to less than 10% of the preligation control value, and marked epicardial ST-segment elevation (25), the latter probably reflecting very high extracellular K^+ concentrations which result from severe ischemia. In the presence of excessive extracellular K^+, the inward Ca^{2+} current may be completely inhibited. Under these circumstances, the Ca^{2+}-antagonist agents would, therefore, find no role as antiarrhythmic agents. Such complex factors (Fig. 2) may explain the apparent failure of Ca^{2+}-antagonists in the pig model.

Proposals

It may be that Ca^{2+}-dependent mechanisms (Table 1) may play a role in the genesis of ventricular fibrillation in some models of mild ischemia (rat, dog), whereas Ca^{2+}-independent mechanisms are probably of importance in some

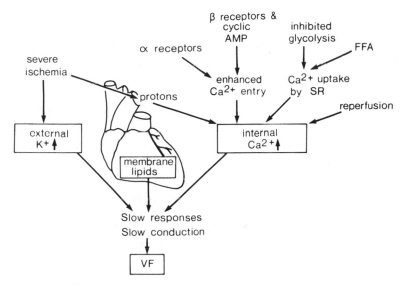

FIG. 2. This figure shows some of the numerous possible mechanisms contributing to ventricular fibrillation (VF). Although a rise in internal Ca²⁺ is regarded as important, inhibition of transmembrane Ca²⁺ influx by Ca²⁺ antagonists will only be one mechanism contributing to the postulated (but not proven) arrhythmogenic effects of the rise of internal Ca²⁺ ion concentrations.

models of severe ischemia (pig). Also, the ventricular antiarrhythmic activity of Ca²⁺ antagonists should be carefully assessed in several experimental models before any conclusion can be reached as to their efficacy in the control of ventricular fibrillation.

TABLE 1. *Ventricular fibrillation: Postulated calcium-dependent and calcium-independent mechanisms*

Ca²⁺-dependent mechanisms (? prominent in rat)
  Provocation of slow response
    Cyclic AMP rise in ischemic zone
    Severe tissue acidosis
    Severe extracellular hypokalemia
    Catecholamine effects not involving cyclic AMP (? α-receptor)
  Slow conduction
    Promoted by above factors
  Other electrophysiological mechanisms[a]
    Ischemic depolarization
    Shortening of action potential duration

Ca²⁺-independent mechanisms (? prominent in pig)
  Arrhythmogenic membrane-derived lipids (lysophospholipids)
  Excess circulating catecholamines (? fatty acids too)
  Inhibition of glycolysis
  Na⁺ channel activity
  Anatomical factors (degree of coronary flow change across border zone)

---

[a] From W. Clusin et al., Chapter 27, *this volume.*

SUMMARY

At present, it is useful to distinguish between the proven effect on supraventricular tachycardias of both verapamil and diltiazem, and those Ca^{2+} antagonists, such as nifedipine, which have a predominant effect on vascular smooth muscle and not on nodal tissue. All Ca^{2+} antagonists may inhibit ventricular arrhythmias, including ventricular fibrillation, in some models, but nonspecific (α-adrenoceptor blockade, Na^+ channel inhibition) and species-specific (rat and dog versus pig) effects are not yet fully excluded as an explanation for the effect against ventricular arrhythmias.

ACKNOWLEDGMENTS

This work was supported by the Medical Research Council of South Africa and the Chris Barnard Fund. F. T. Thandroyen was the recipient of the Guy Elliot Scholarship.

REFERENCES

1. Bayer, R., Kalusche, D., Kauffmann, R., and Mannhold, J. (1975): *Naunyn Schmiedebergs Arch. Pharmacol.,* 290:81–97.
2. Brooks, W. W., Verrier, R. L., and Lown, B. (1980): *Cardiovasc. Res.,* 14:295–302.
3. Brown, H., and Di Francesco, D. (1980): *J. Physiol.,* 308:331–351.
4. Clusin, W. T., Bristow, M. R., Bain, D. S., Schroeder, O. S., Jaillon, P., Brett, P., and Harrison, D. (1982): *Circ. Res.,* 50:518–528.
5. Coker, S. J., and Parratt, J. R. (1983): *J. Cardiovasc. Pharmacol.,* 5:406–417.
6. Corr, P. B., Gross, R. W., and Sobel, B. E. (1982): *J. Mol. Cell. Cardiol.,* 14:619–626.
7. Coumel, P. (1975): *Electrocardiology,* 8:79–90.
8. Cranefield, P. F. (1975): In: *The Conduction of the Cardiac Impulse,* p. 75. Futura, Mount Kisco, New York.
9. Cranefield, P. F., Aronson, R. S., and Wit, A. L. (1973): *Circ. Res.,* 34:204–213.
10. Daries, P. S., Saman, S., and Opie, L. H. (1981): *J. Mol. Cell. Cardiol.,* 13 (Suppl. 1): 19.
11. Fagbemi, O., and Parratt, J. R. (1981): *Eur. J. Pharmacol.,* 75: 179–185.
12. Farshidi, A., Josephson, M. E., and Horowitz, L. N. (1978): *Am. J. Cardiol.,* 41:1052–1060.
13. Gillette, P. C. (1977): *Am. J. Cardiol.,* 40:848–850.
14. Gilmour, R. F., Jr., and Zipes, D. P. (1982): *Circ. Res.,* 50:599–609.
15. Gmeiner, R., Ng, C. K., and Gstöttner, M. (1979): *Eur. J. Clin. Pharmacol.,* 16:155–164.
16. Hamamoto, H., Peter, T., Fujimoto, T., and Mandel, W. J. (1981): *Am. Heart J.,* 192:350–358.
17. Heng, M. K., Singh, B. N., Roche, A. H. G., Norris, R. M., and Mercier, C. J. (1975): *Am. Heart J.,* 90:487–498.
18. Hirche, H. J., Franz, C., Bös, L., Bissig, R., Lang, R., and Schramm, M. (1980): *J. Mol. Cell. Cardiol.,* 12:579–593.
19. Husaini, M. H., Kvasnicka, J., Ryden, L., and Holmberg, S. (1973): *Br. Heart J.,* 35:734–737.
20. Kawai, C., Konishi, T., Matsuyama, E., and Okazaki, H. (1981): *Circulation,* 63:1035–1043.
21. Klein, G. J., Gulamhusein, S., Prystowsky, E. N., Carruthers, G. S., Donner, A. P., and Ko, P. T. (1982): *Am. J. Cardiol.,* 49:117–123.
22. Kohlhardt, M., Bauer, B., Krause, H., and Fleckenstein, A. (1972): *Pfluegers Arch.,* 335:309–322.
23. Krikler, D. M., and Spurrell, R. A. J. (1974): *Postgrad. Med. J.,* 50:447–453.
24. Lubbe, W. F., McLean, J. A., and Nguyen, T. (1983): *Am. Heart J.,* 105:331–333.

25. Muller, C. A. (1981): *Ph.D. Thesis, University of Cape Town,* South Africa.
26. Nayler, W. G., Thomson, J. E., and Jarrott, B. (1982): *J. Mol. Cell. Cardiol.,* 14:182–185.
27. Noma, A., Yanagihara, K., and Irisawa, H. (1977): *Pfluegers Arch.,* 372:43–51.
28. Opie, L. H., Nathan D., and Lubbe, W. F. (1979): *Am. J. Cardiol.,* 43:131–148.
29. Podzuweit, T., Lubbe, W. F., and Opie, L. H. (1976): *J. Mol. Cell. Cardiol.,* 10:81–94.
30. Reuter, H. (1974): *J. Physiol. (Lond.),* 242:429–451.
31. Rinkenberger, R. L., Prystowsky, E. N., Heger, J. J., Troup, P. J., Jackman, W. M., and Zipes, D. P. (1980): *Circulation,* 62:996–1010.
32. Rowland, E., Evans, T., and Krikler, D. (1979): *Br. Heart J.,* 42:124–127.
33. Roy, P. R., Spurrell, R. A. J., and Sowton, G. E. (1974): *Postgrad. Med. J.,* 50:270–275.
34. Schamroth, L. (1980): *Am. Heart J.,* 100:1070–1075.
35. Schamroth, L., Krikler, D. M., and Garrett, C. (1972): *Br. Med. J.,* 1:660–662.
36. Sheehan, F. H., and Epstein, S. E. (1982): *Am. Heart J.,* 103:973–978.
37. Singh, B. N. (1975): *NZ Med. J.,* 82:339–343.
38. Singh, B. N., Ellrodt, G., and Peter, C. T. (1978): *Drugs,* 15:169–197.
39. Spurrell, R. A. J., Krikler, D. M., and Sowton, E. (1974): *Am. J. Cardiol.,* 33:590–595.
40. Sung, R. J., Elser, B., McAllister, R. G., Jr. (1980): *Ann. Int. Med.,* 93:682–689.
41. Surawicz, B. (1982): *Am. Heart J.,* 103:698–706.
42. Thandroyen, F. T. (1982): *J. Mol. Cell. Cardiol.,* 14:21–32.
43. Winniford, M. D., Markham, R. V., Firth, B. G., Nicod, P., and Hillis, L. D. (1982): *Am. J. Cardiol.,* 50:704–710.
44. Wit, A. L., and Bigger, J. T. (1977): *Postgrad. Med. J.,* 53 (Suppl. 1): 98–112.
45. Wit, E. L., and Cranefield, P. F. (1974): *Circ. Res.,* 35:413–425.
46. Wojtczak, J. (1982): *J. Mol. Cell. Cardiol.,* 14:259–265.
47. Wu, D., Denes, P., Amat-y-Leon, F., Dhingra, R., Wyndham, C. R. C., Bauernfeind, R., Latif, P., and Rosen, K. M. (1978): *Am. J. Cardiol.,* 41:1045–1050.
48. Zipes, D. P., and Fischer, J. C. (1974): *Circ. Res.,* 34:184–192.

Calcium Antagonists and Cardiovascular Disease, edited by L. H. Opie. Raven Press, New York © 1984.

Chapter 29

Calcium Influx-Dependent Vasoconstrictor Mechanisms in Essential Hypertension

Fritz R. Bühler, Peter Bolli, and U. Lennart Hulthén

Department of Research and Department of Medicine, University Hospital, Basel, Switzerland

Elevated vascular resistance is a hallmark of established essential hypertension. There is increasing evidence that besides adaptive structural changes (20) and neurogenic factors (9,31), a disturbance of the membrane control of intracellular electrolyte composition may contribute to the development and maintenance of elevated arteriolar tone. As found by some investigators in hypertensive patients, an abnormal transmembraneous Na^{2+} transport results in increased intracellular Na^+ content (8,22,26,34). Since intracellular Ca^{2+} concentration is regulated to a great extent through a Na^+-Ca^{2+} exchange mechanism (40), any reduction in the transmembraneous Na^+ gradient consequent to a rise in intracellular Na^+ hinders the outward transport of Ca^{2+}. The increased intracellular Na^+ content leads to an increase in intracellular free Ca^{2+} concentration which ultimately determines the contractile process in vascular smooth muscle cells (13,14). Accordingly, an increased intracellular Ca^{2+} concentration has been observed in spontaneously hypertensive rats (18,25) and in hypertensive patients (39). Therefore, since the influx of Ca^{2+} into the cells through voltage-dependent and possibly receptor-operated (27) slow channels primarily determines the intracellular free Ca^{2+} concentration (1), drugs which antagonize Ca^{2+} slow-channel influx (19, 24,42) induce vasodilatation (2,41).

ENHANCED CALCIUM-INFLUX-DEPENDENT VASOCONSTRICTION IN ESSENTIAL HYPERTENSION

An increased dependency of Ca^{2+} influx for contraction activation, as well as a greater relaxation in the presence of the Ca^{2+} antagonists, verapamil and nifedipine, has been demonstrated in blood vessels from spontaneously hypertensive rats as compared to normotensive rats (28,33,36,37). Similarly, administration of nifedipine decreased blood pressure in hypertensive patients, but not in normotensive subjects (5,35). Together, this points towards an enhanced Ca^{2+} slow-channel influx-dependent vasoconstriction in hypertension including the so-called "essential type."

To assess the dependency of arteriolar tone on Ca^{2+} influx in patients with essential hypertension as compared to normotensive subjects, we measured the verapamil-induced increase in forearm blood flow and related it to the nonspecific vasodilator response of sodium nitroprusside, which is not considered to inhibit Ca^{2+} influx (17,32,44). The study population consisted of 11 normotensive women without a family history of hypertension, and 11 age-matched women with uncomplicated essential hypertension with a casual diastolic pressure (Korotkoff phase V) $\geq$ 100 mm Hg on several occasions. Forearm blood flow was measured by venous occlusion plethysmography, using a mercury in silastic strain gauge (9) before and after the intraarterial infusions of step-wise increased doses of verapamil of 1 to 75 μg/min/100 ml forearm tissue for 1 min, and sodium nitroprusside at a dose of 0.6 μg/min/100 ml forearm tissue for 2 min. In preceding dose-finding studies, this dose of sodium nitroprusside was found to produce a maximal vasodilator effect in the forearm without causing systemic effects.

Starting from similar basal forearm flow values (ml/min/100 ml tissue) in normotensives (1.8 ± 0.3) and hypertensives (2.1 ± 0.2), the intraarterial infusion of verapamil 1 to 75 μg/100 ml tissue induced a stepwise increase in forearm flow in both groups reaching highest values in normotensives (19.2 ± 2.2) and hypertensives (27.3 ± 3.8) at a dose of 75 μg/100 ml tissue; the increase in forearm flow was greater in hypertensives than in normotensives at each dose of verapamil. The forearm flow following sodium nitroprusside infusion was somewhat greater in hypertensives (21.3 ± 3.5) than in normotensives (15.5 ± 2.2), but less ($p < 0.001$) than that achieved by verapamil 75 μg/100 ml tissue. When the increase in forearm flow to verapamil was adjusted to that induced by sodium nitroprusside, it was also significantly greater in hypertensives than in normotensives (Fig. 1). Accordingly, the molar ratio of verapamil and sodium nitroprusside having an equal vasodilator effect was 18:1 in normotensives and 10:1 in hypertensives. In hypertensives, but not in normotensives, mean blood pressure was significantly reduced after the infusion of the two highest doses of verapamil (40 and 75 μg/100 ml tissue), a feature that was not observed with sodium nitroprusside.

Basal plasma epinephrine correlated positively with the increase in forearm blood flow following all doses of verapamil in hypertensives ($r = 0.733$ to 0.944; $p < 0.001$ to < 0.05) but no significant correlations were found in normotensives. In hypertensives, there was also a negative correlation between basal plasma renin activity, plasma angiotensin II, and the vasodilatory response at the higher dose levels of verapamil.

The greater maximal vasodilatory response to verapamil as compared to so-

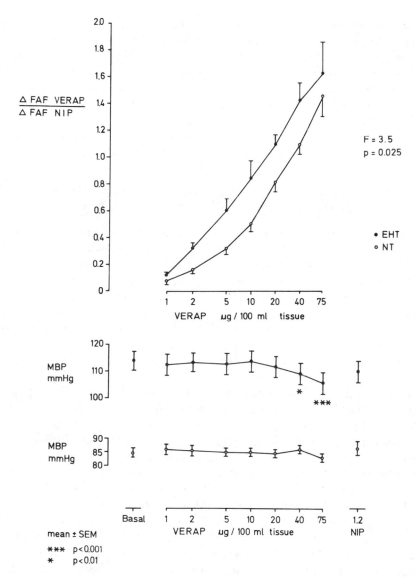

FIG. 1. *Top:* Increase in forearm flow (ΔFAF) to incremental dosages of verapamil (Verap) as adjusted for the ΔFAF to sodium nitroprusside (Nip) 1.2 μg/100 ml tissue in 11 patients with essential hypertension (EHT, *solid circles*) and 11 normotensive (NT, *open circles*) subjects. *Bottom:* Intraarterial mean blood pressure measured under basal conditions and 2 min after the infusion of incremental dosages of verapamil (Verap) and sodium nitroprusside (Nip) in the same patients and subjects.

dium nitroprusside in patients with essential hypertension, as well as in normotensive subjects, suggests that slow-channel Ca^{2+} influx is of major importance for the state of tension in the vascular smooth muscle cell. The finding that the verapamil-induced vasodilation was greater in hypertensives than in normotensives, as well as the fall in blood pressure in hypertensives with higher doses of verapamil, which was not observed in normotensives, indicate a functional abnormality in essential hypertension with enhanced dependency of arteriolar tone on Ca^{2+} influx. This abnormality seems to have a direct relationship to the activity of the sympathetic and renin-angiotensin systems.

RELATIVE CONTRIBUTION OF CALCIUM INFLUX TO VASCULAR RESISTANCE IN ESSENTIAL HYPERTENSION

Mechanisms other than, and perhaps related or unrelated to, slow-channel Ca^{2+} influx contribute to elevated vascular resistance in essential hypertension, e.g., structural vascular changes (20), an enhanced α-adrenoceptor-mediated vasoconstrictor component (9), and a blunted β-adrenoceptor-mediated dilator force (11). In order to investigate the relative contribution of these components to vascular resistance we compared, intraindividually, the vasodilator response to two different Ca^{2+} antagonists, verapamil, and the dihydropyridine derivative, nicardipine, to the nonspecific sodium nitroprusside, to the postsynaptic α_1-adrenoceptor blockade with prazosin, and to total ischemia following arterial occlusion.

Forearm blood flow as described above, measured in another set of 11 patients with essential hypertension and 10 normotensive subjects with a similar sex and age distribution, before and after a 1-min intraarterial infusion of verapamil (75 μg/min/100 ml tissue), nicardipine (40 μg/min/100 ml tissue), a 2-min infusion of sodium nitroprusside (0.6 μg/min/100 ml tissue), a 10-min infusion of prazosin (0.5 μg/min/100 ml tissue), and after a 10-min forearm ischemia by arterial occlusion; these procedures have proven earlier to result in maximal regional vasodilation without causing systemic effects.

Here again, similar basal forearm blood flow values (ml/min/100 ml forearm tissue) were found in hypertensives (2.9 $\pm$ 1.4) and in normotensives (2.5 $\pm$ 1.2). On the other hand, the increases in forearm blood flow to verapamil and nicardipine were practically of the same magnitude and similar to the vasodilatory response to 10 min arterial occlusion (Fig. 2), while the increase in flow to sodium nitroprusside was about one-third, and to prazosin about one-fourth of that produced by the Ca^{2+} antagonists. In hypertensive patients, as compared to normotensive subjects, the increase in forearm blood flow was greater after intraarterial infusion of both Ca^{2+} antagonists, verapamil and nicardipine ($p < 0.01$), as well as following postsynaptic α_1-blockade with prazosin ($p < 0.05$). In contrast, the increase in flow to nonspecific vasodilation with arterial occlusion and with sodium nitroprusside did not differ between the two groups.

The comparable increase in forearm blood flow to verapamil and nicardipine

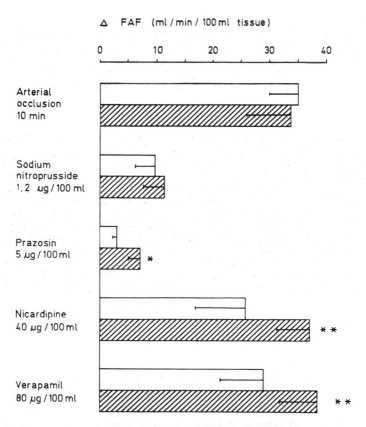

FIG. 2. Increase in forearm blood flow (ΔFAF) to nonspecific vasodilation following a 1-min arterial occlusion and with sodium nitroprusside (1.2 μg/100 ml tissue) as well as to α₁-blockade with prazosin (5 μg/100 ml tissue) and to slow Ca²⁺ channel blockade with nicardipine (40 μg/100 ml tissue) and verapamil (80 μg/100 ml tissue) in 11 patients with essential hypertension (EHT) (*hatched bars*) and 10 normotensive (NT) subjects (*open bars*). Mean ± SD. *p < 0.05; **p < 0.01.

indicates that the relaxation effect on the smooth muscle cell of these two Ca²⁺ antagonists is practically the same. The similar vasodilator effect of the Ca²⁺ antagonists to that following ischemia—which is considered to induce the greatest vasodilation that can be achieved in the human forearm (43)—emphasizes the paramount importance of Ca²⁺ influx for the regulation of arteriolar resistance, while cellular Ca²⁺ extrusion or its handling by the cytoplasmatic reticulum seem to contribute less to arteriolar tone, and thus vascular resistance does not seem to be different in the vascular bed of patients with hypertension and normotensive subjects. In relation to the maximal vasodilation induced by arterial occlusion, and as judged from the vasodilator response to prazosin, the neurogenic, α-adrenoceptor-mediated vasoconstrictor component contributes in hypertensive patients about one-quarter and in normotensive subjects about one-sixth to overall control of forearm vascular resistance. The observation that Ca^{2+} antagonists and prazosin induced a significantly greater increase in forearm flow in hypertensive patients, as compared to normotensive subjects, indicates that *both an enhanced Ca^{2+} influx-dependent and an enhanced α-adrenoceptor-mediated vasoconstrictor component contribute to increased vascular resistance in essential hypertension.* Since the vascular effect obtained with sodium nitroprusside and with arterial occlusion did not differ significantly between hypertensives and normotensives, yet at comparable flow values the vasodilatory response was significantly different in the two groups with prazosin and with Ca^{2+} antagonists, the indication is that these differences probably cannot be attributed to structural vascular changes.

CALCIUM INFLUX-DEPENDENT VASODILATION: ITS POSSIBLE RELATIONSHIP TO SYMPATHETIC TONE

Considering plasma epinephrine as a marker of sympathetic activity (4,6, 15,21), the positive correlation found in hypertensive patients between basal plasma epinephrine and the increase in forearm blood flow to verapamil suggests that the vasodilator response to verapamil in essential hypertension is augmented with increasing activity of the sympathetic nervous system. This is analogous to the findings that in essential hypertension the increase in forearm blood flow after α-adrenoceptor blockade with prazosin and phentolamine correlates positively to plasma epinephrine and plasma norepinephrine, respectively (9,30). Therefore, both enhanced Ca^{2+} influx-dependent and enhanced α-adrenoceptor-mediated vasoconstriction are related to sympathetic activity in essential hypertension. This tallies with the observation that increased Ca^{2+} influx plays a major role for α-adrenoceptor-mediated vasoconstriction (1) and α-adrenoceptor blocking activity of verapamil has been reported *in vivo* (23) and *in vitro* (12). However, the small increase in forearm blood flow to prazosin relative to the great response induced by Ca^{2+} antagonists suggests a direct rather than an α-adrenoceptor-mediated influence of catecholamines on Ca^{2+} channels. Alternatively, these quantitative differences would be in accord with the view that α-adrenoceptor-mediated effects form a part of the receptor-operated slow-channel Ca^{2+} influx-dependent vasoconstriction. On the other hand, a specific binding of the α-adrenoceptor antagonist WB-4101 to Ca^{2+} channels in rat brain membranes, and inhibition of Ca^{2+}-mediated depolarization by WB-4101 in neuroplastoma-glioma hybrid cells, was also reported (10).

PRESSURE-, AGE- AND RENIN-RELATED ANTIHYPERTENSIVE EFFICACY OF CALCIUM ANTAGONISTS

The demonstration of an increased dependency of arteriolar tone on Ca^{2+} influx in essential hypertension as compared to normotensive subjects, provides a rationale for the use of Ca^{2+} antagonists in antihypertensive therapy, and thereby may correct a primary derangement in cellular Ca^{2+} handling in patients with essential hypertension. Therefore, it follows that there is a direct relationship between the degree of antihypertensive response and the height of pretreatment blood pressure, and that Ca^{2+} antagonists lower blood pressure in hypertensives, but not in normotensives. A possible relationship between the vasodilating effect of Ca^{2+} antagonists and the renin-angiotensin system may be suggested by the finding that the increase in forearm blood flow to doses of verapamil, which caused a fall in blood pressure, correlated indirectly with basal plasma renin activity and angiotensin II values. This could indicate a compensatory increase in renin release in patients with higher basal plasma renin activity (38) leading to an attenuation of the verapamil-induced vasodilation. Therefore, the basal activity of the renin-angiotensin system might be one factor determining the vasodilatory and antihypertensive effect of verapamil. Furthermore, considering that an increased intracellular free Ca^{2+} concentration is brought about primarily by a disturbance of transmembraneous Na^+ transport (8,22,26,34), the observation that mainly elderly patients of low renin type essential hypertension show a Na^+ extrusion defect (7) may indicate that patients with a low plasma renin activity might be particularly susceptible to the antihypertensive effect of Ca^{2+} channel blockade.

In order to define the antihypertensive effect of verapamil as related to age, pretreatment blood pressure, and renin, 43 patients with essential hypertension (23 males, 20 females) aged 20 to 86 (mean 53) years with a casual diastolic blood pressure (Korotkoff V) $\geq$ 100 mm Hg in the sitting position were treated in a placebo-controlled open study with the slow release preparation of verapamil 240 to 720 (mean 427) mg/day. Verapamil lowered blood pressure from $171 \pm 16/108 \pm 6$ to $152 \pm 14/93 \pm 9$ mm Hg (both $p < 0.001$) and to the target pressure <95 mm Hg diastolic in about half of the patients. The change in mean blood pressure to verapamil correlated directly with pretreatment mean blood pressure and the age of the patients (Fig. 3). This observation tallies with the notion that Ca^{2+} antagonists correct a derangement in cellular Ca^{2+} handling by reducing Ca^{2+} influx. They are also in accordance with the known positive relations between increasing age and increasing pressure and plasma norepinephrine (11,29). However, there was a negative correlation between decreasing mean blood pressure to verapamil and pretreatment renin ($r = -0.532$; $p < 0.05$) which is in keeping with the known inverse relationship of age, blood pressure, and norepinephrine to renin (29). Hence, patients of older age with a higher blood pressure, and often lower plasma renin activity, respond best to verapamil treatment. In intraindividual comparisons, antihypertensive responses to verapamil paralleled those achieved by diuretic agents, and were inversely related to those observed with β-blocker monotherapy (3).

That this response pattern does not seem to be unique for verapamil is suggested by a most recent analysis in an older group of 63 patients with essential hypertension, including a considerable fraction of low renin patients (16). Here too, the Ca^{2+} antagonist, nifedipine, proved most effective when given alone,

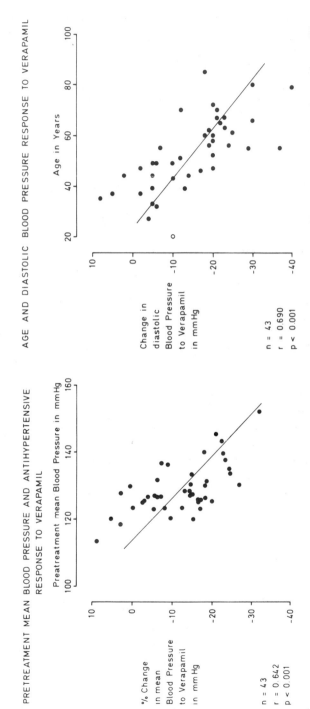

FIG. 3. The patient's pretreatment mean blood pressure and age correlates directly with the percent change in mean blood pressure and the change in diastolic pressure, respectively. A similar correlation also exists for the change in mean blood pressure and the patient's age.

but in 13 of them, side-effects such as headaches and, in some, ankle edema, were responsible for the discontinuation of the drug. In the remaining 50 patients, the antihypertensive effectiveness of nifedipine was directly related to the patient's pretreatment blood pressure, and indirectly related to pretreatment renin. In an intraindividual comparison, the antihypertensive responses to nifedipine were similar to those observed with verapamil. Thus, Ca^{2+} antagonists represent a new partner to the β-blocker in a modern treatment strategy where β-blockers are given first in the younger patients, and Ca^{2+} antagonists—to some great extent replacing diuretic agents—are the first choice for the older patients, or those not responding satisfactorily to a β-blocker.

SUMMARY

Slow-channel Ca^{2+} influx is a major determinant of the free intracellular Ca^{2+} concentration which finally triggers the contractile process of the vascular smooth muscle cell, and thereby determines arteriolar resistance. Inhibition of slow-channel Ca^{2+} influx with two different Ca^{2+} antagonists, nicardipine and verapamil, was used to demonstrate an enhanced Ca^{2+} influx-dependent vasoconstrictor mechanism in the forearm circulation of patients with essential hypertension, as compared with normotensive subjects. These effects correlated directly with plasma epinephrine concentrations, and indirectly with renin and angiotensin II. Effects were comparable to those obtained by arterial ischemia and about four times those produced by α_1-adrenoceptor blockade. The role of Ca^{2+} influx-dependent vasoconstriction was also tested pharmacotherapeutically. Ca^{2+} antagonists normalize blood pressure in at least one-third of patients with essential hypertension; the effects of verapamil and nifedipine were similar, but correlated directly with the patient's age and pretreatment blood pressure and indirectly with renin. Therefore, Ca^{2+} antagonists may form the first partner to β-blockers in a pathophysiology-oriented treatment plan.

ACKNOWLEDGMENTS

This work was supported by Swiss National Funds No. 3.807.80.

REFERENCES

1. Bolton, T. B. (1979): *Physiol. Rev.*, 59:606–718.
2. Brittinger, W. E., Schwarzbeck, A., Wittenmeier, K. W., Twittenhoff, W. D., Stegaru, B., Huber, W., Ewald, R. W., v. Henning, G. E., Fabricius, M., and Strauch, M. (1970): *Dtsch. Med. Wochenschr.*, 95:1871–1877.
3. Bühler, F. R., Hulthén, U. L., Kiowski, W., and Bolli, P. (1982): *Clin. Sci.*, 63:4395–4425.
4. Bühler, F. R., Kiowski, W., van Brummelen, P., Amann, F. W., Bertel, O., Landmann, R., Lütold, B. E., and Bolli, P. (1980): *Clin. Exp. Hypertens.*, 2:409–426.
5. Conen, D., Bertel, O., and Dubach, U. C. (1982): *J. Cardiovasc. Pharmacol.*, 4:5378–5382.
6. Cousineau, D., Lapointe, L., and De Champlain, J. (1978): *Am. Heart J.*, 96:229–234.
7. Edmondson, R. P. S., and MacGregor, G. A. (1981): *Br. Med. J.*, 282:1267–1269.

8. Edmondson, R. P. S., Thomas, R. D., Hilton, P. J., Patrick, J., and Jones, N. F. (1975): *Lancet*, 1:1003–1005.
9. Amann, F. W., Bolli, P., Kiowski, W., and Bühler, F. R. (1980): *Hypertension*, 3:I119–123.
10. Atlas, D., and Adler, M. (1981): *Proc. Natl. Acad. Sci.*, 78:1237–1241.
11. Bertel, O., Bühler, F. R., Kiowski, W., and Lütold, B. E. (1980): *Hypertension*, 2:130–138.
12. Blackmore, P. F., El-Rafai, M. F., and Exton, J. H. (1979): *Mol. Pharmacol.*, 15:598–606.
13. Blaustein, M. P. (1977): *Am. J. Physiol.*, 232(3):C165–C173.
14. Bohr, D. F. (1973): *Circ. Res.*, 32:665–672.
15. Bolli, P., Amann, F. W., Hulthén, U. L., Kiowski, W., and Bühler, F. R. (1981): *Clin. Sci.*, 61 (Suppl. 7):161s–164s.
16. Erne, P., Hulthén, U. L., Bolli, P., and Bühler, F. R. (1982): *Hypertension* (*in press*).
17. Fermum, R., Meisel, P., and Klinner, U. (1977): *Acta Biol. Med. Ger.*, 36:245–255.
18. Fitzpatrick, D. F., and Szentivanyi, A. (1980): *Clin. Exp. Hypertens.*, 2:1023–1037.
19. Fleckenstein, A. (1977): *Annu. Rev. Pharmacol. Toxicol.*, 17:149–166.
20. Folkow, B. (1971): *Clin. Sci. Mol. Med.*, 41:1–12.
21. Franco-Morselli, R., Elghozi, J. L., Joly, E., Diginilio, S., and Meyer, P. (1977): *Br. Med. J.*, ii:1251–1254.
22. Garay, R. P., and Meyer, P. (1979): *Lancet*, 1:349–352.
23. Greenberg, S., and Wilson, W. R. (1974): *Can. J. Physiol. Pharmacol.*, 52:266–271.
24. Henry, P. D. (1980): *Am. J. Cardiol.*, 46:1047–1058.
25. Holloway, E. T., and Bohr, D. F. (1973): *Circ. Res.*, 33:678–685.
26. Hulthén, U. L., Bolli, P., Kiowski, W., and Bühler, F. R. (1983): *J. Gen. Pharmacol.*, 14:193–196.
27. Hulthén, U. L., Landmann, R., Bürgisser, E., and Bühler, F. R. (1982): *J. Cardiovasc. Pharmacol.*, 4:S291–S293.
28. Jones, A. W. (1974): *Circ. Res.*, 34,35 (Suppl. 1):117–122.
29. Kiowski, W., Bertel, O., and Bühler, F. R. (1979): In: *Nervous System and Hypertension*, edited by P. Meyer and H. Schmitt, pp. 318–325. Flammarion, Paris.
30. Kiowski, W., Bühler, F. R., van Brummelen, P., and Amann, F. W. (1981): *Clin. Sci.*, 60:483–489.
31. Korner, P. I., Shaw, J., Utker, J. B., West, M. J., McRitchie, R. J., and Richards, J. G. (1973): *Circulation*, 48:107–117.
32. Kreye, V. A. W., and Gross, F. (1977): In: *Handbook of Experimental Pharmacology XXXIX*, edited by F. Gross, pp. 418–430. Springer Verlag, Berlin.
33. Lederballe Pedersen, O., Mikkelsen, E., and Andersson, K.-E. (1978): *Acta Pharmacol. Toxicol.*, 43:137–144.
34. Losse, H., Wehmeyer, H., and Wessels, F. (1960): *Klin. Wochenschr.*, 38:393–395.
35. MacGregor, G. (1982): *J. Cardiovasc. Pharmacol.*, 4:S358–S362.
36. Mochizuki, A., Aoki, K., Kondo, S., Mizuno, T., and Hotta, K. (1979): *Jpn. Heart J.*, 20:(Suppl. I):225–227.
37. Mulvany, M. J., Nyborg, N., and Nilsson, H. (1980): *Clin. Sci.*, 59:203s–205s.
38. O'Malley, K., Velaso, M., Wells, J., and McNay, J. L. (1975): *J. Clin. Invest.*, 55:230–235.
39. Postnov, Y. V., Orlov, S. N., and Pokudin, N. I. (1980): *Pfluegers Arch.*, 388:89–91.
40. Reuter, H., Blaustein, M. P., and Häusler, G. (1973): *Philos. Trans. R. Soc. Lond.* (*Biol.*), 265:87–94.
41. Robinson, B. F., Dobbs, R. J., Kelsey, C. R. (1980): *Br. J. Clin. Pharmacol.*, 10:433–438.
42. Singh, B. N., Ellrodt, G., and Peter, C. T. (1978): *Drugs*, 15:169–197.
43. Takeshita, A., and Mark, A. L. (1980): *Hypertension*, 2:610–616.
44. Thorens, S., and Häusler, G. (1979): *Eur. J. Pharmacol.*, 54:79–91.

Calcium Antagonists and Cardiovascular
Disease, edited by L. H. Opie.
Raven Press, New York © 1984.

Chapter 30

Calcium Channel Blockers and Hypertension

C. Rosendorff

*MRC/University Circulation Research Unit and Departments of Physiology and Medicine,
University of the Witwatersrand Medical School, Parktown 2193,
Johannesburg, South Africa*

This chapter is a review of the use of Ca^{2+} channel blockers in the therapy of arterial hypertension. The first section will deal with the antihypertensive mechanism of action of Ca^{2+} channel blockers at a cellular level, and then clinical studies will support the suggestion that Ca^{2+} antagonists are an important addition to our list of antihypertensive drugs.

ROLE OF CALCIUM IONS

The role of Ca^{2+} in vascular smooth muscle contraction is unclear, and much of what we know, or believe we know, is based on slender evidence or on extrapolations from other contractile tissue, particularly myocardium. There is probably a close interaction in vascular smooth muscle between the transmembrane flux of Na^+, K^+, and Ca^{2+} (Fig. 1).

What we do know is that there are *two major stimuli* to the movement of Ca^{2+} ions from the outside to the inside of vascular smooth muscle cells (40,50). One is related to depolarization of the membrane and depends on a raised extracellular K^+ concentration ("voltage-dependent channels"). The second mechanism for increasing intracellular Ca^{2+} is an activation of "receptor-operated channels," particularly by norepinephrine (20,21) and, perhaps quantitatively less important, the norepinephrine-induced release of Ca^{2+} from intracellular stores. Present evidence, such as it is, supports the idea that smooth muscle contraction elicited by membrane depolarization, as occurs when extracellular K^+ concentration is increased, depends to a greater extent on Ca^{2+} influx than that induced by norepinephrine (9).

A third mechanism for increasing vascular smooth muscle tone was proposed in 1977 by Blaustein (8). This relates to another linked transport mechanism,

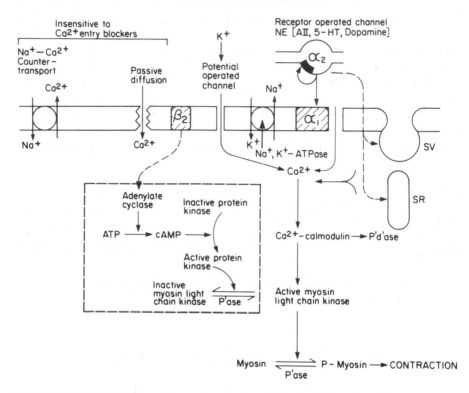

FIG. 1. Possible mechanisms of increasing cytoplasmic Ca^{2+}, and the action of Ca^{2+} on contractile proteins, in vascular smooth muscle. Two Ca^{2+} channels are insensitive to Ca^{2+} entry blockers: a Ca^{2+}-Na^+ countertransport channel, and a passive diffusion channel. Two channels are sensitive to Ca^{2+} entry blockers: a potential (voltage)-operated channel sensitive to the extracellular concentration of K^+, and a receptor-(α_1) modulated channel sensitive to norepinephrine (NE). NE also activates prejunctional α_2-receptors, causing feedback inhibition of NE release from adrenergic nerve terminals. Dopamine is also inhibitory to NE release, while angiotensin II (AII) and 5-hydroxytryptamine (5-HT) are facilitatory. The role of released Ca^{2+} from surface vehicles (SV) and sarcoplasmic reticulum (SR) is unclear. Intracellular Ca^{2+} induces the sequence: Ca^{2+}-calmodulin complex formation, activation of myosin light chain kinase, phosphorylation of myosin and contraction. Relaxation depends upon the dephosphorylation of myosin by a phosphatase and/or the inactivation of myosin light chain kinase by a protein kinase activated by cyclic AMP, which, in turn, is produced in response to β-adrenoreceptor activation.

namely the transport of Na^+ (inward) and Ca^{2+} (outward). Any reduction in the Na^+ gradient (due to a rise in the internal Na^+ concentration following decreased activity of the Na^+-K^+ pump) would hinder the outward transport of Ca^{2+} through this carrier mechanism, thus increasing the intracellular Ca^{2+} concentration.

Any or all of these three mechanisms may operate to increase intracellular Ca^{2+}, to cause an increase in vascular tone, in peripheral resistance, and hence in arterial pressure (Fig. 2). Inhibition of the Na^+,K^+-ATPase lowers the efficiency of the Na^+-K^+ pump, allows the extracellular accumulation of K^+, with an increase in membrane excitability and an activation of voltage-dependent Ca^{2+} channels. Sympathetic overactivity will activate smooth muscle, at least partly through receptor-operated Ca^{2+} channels. Lastly, Na^+-K^+ pump failure will allow the intracellular accumulation of Na^+, a slowing of Na^+-Ca^{2+} countertransport, and a rise in intracellular Ca^{2+}. Once again, let it be said that these are highly speculative schemes.

The mechanisms by which intracellular Ca^{2+} activate smooth muscle contraction are discussed by W. Gevers (Chapter 6, *this volume*). One postulated sequence of events (Fig. 1) follows (1,25): Ca^{2+} in the cell binds with a 16,500 dalton Ca^{2+}-binding protein (calmodulin) and the Ca^{2+}-calmodulin complex activates myosin light chain kinase. This activated enzyme phosphorylates myosin, which results in contraction. Relaxation depends on the inactivation of myosin light chain kinase. This may be produced by protein kinase which is activated by cyclic AMP. An important trigger to cyclic AMP formation is the β_2-adrenoreceptor in the vascular smooth muscle cell membrane.

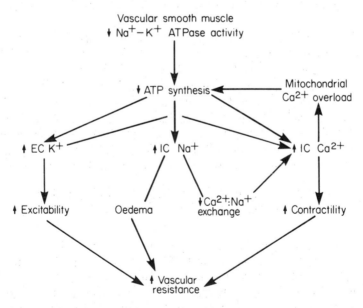

FIG. 2. Summary of the main features of the ionic hypothesis of vascular smooth muscle hypercontractility. Inhibition of Na^+,K^+-ATPase activity (e.g., by the "natriuretic hormone") allows an increase of intracellular Na^+ and of extracellular K^+. Na^+ will alter the transmembrane osmotic gradient to retain water in the cell, and will inhibit Ca^{2+}-Na^+ countertransport causing a rise in intracellular Ca^{2+}. Extracellular K^+ will increase the electrical excitability of the membrane and will open voltage-operated Ca^{2+} channels.

There are some experimental findings which are not in accord with this theory. For example, de Mendonca et al. (16) have found a decrease in another Na^+-K^+ transport system in red blood cells from hypertensive patients. This is not the Na^+-K^+ pump, because this system cannot be inhibited by ouabain which is specific to Na^+,K^+-ATPase. Also, there is no direct evidence that the vascular smooth muscle membrane of hypertensive patients shares the electrolyte abnormality which has been demonstrated in their red blood cells, nor that such smooth muscle contains a higher concentration of free intracellular Ca^{2+} than that of normotensive subjects. However, rats with experimental hypertension have increased arteriolar smooth muscle Ca^{2+} transport (52), and drugs which specifically reduce the influx of Ca^{2+} into the cell through the cell membrane, and from bound sites within the cell, have a vasodilator antihypertensive action. It might also be predicted that the degree of blood pressure reduction brought about by Ca^{2+} antagonists be directly related to the magnitude of the pretreatment blood pressure, and, generally, this has been found to be the case.

What has not been established with certainty in vascular smooth muscle is the relative contribution of Ca^{2+} channels which are opened by a rise in the extracellular K^+ and, by implication, by action potentials (voltage-dependent channels), and those which are switched on by norepinephrine, acetylcholine, 5-hydroxytryptamine, histamine, ergotamine, and angiotensin II (neurotransmitter or receptor-operated channels). Also, what is not clear is the interrelationship between the two types of channel or the role of the release of Ca^{2+} from intracellular organelles such as the sarcoplasmic reticulum and the mitochondria.

Lastly, there is controversy over the intracellular action of Ca^{2+} in initiating interactions between the contractile proteins of vascular smooth muscle. The Ca^{2+}-calmodulin, myosin light chain kinase, myosin-phosphate sequence (1,25), calcium-leiotonin regulation of contraction (18), and the concept of myosin phosphorylation being necessary for cross-bridge cycling, but not for actin-myosin "latch" cross-bridging (2) are all different models of Ca^{2+} interactions with smooth muscle contractile proteins. Regardless of which of these Ca^{2+}-activated mechanisms proves more important in vascular smooth muscle, it is agreed that *an increase in cytostolic Ca^{2+} concentration represents the signal that initiates the contractile process in vascular smooth muscle.*

CLINICAL STUDIES OF CALCIUM CHANNEL BLOCKERS IN HYPERTENSION

The ability of Ca^{2+} channel blockers to relax vascular smooth muscle and, therefore, to decrease peripheral vascular resistance makes them potentially useful antihypertensive drugs (29). However, their use in the treatment of arterial hypertension has not yet been fully established, and the number of good clinical trials is quite small. Most studies have been performed on nifedipine and verapamil, with a few on diltiazem and tiapamil.

Acute Therapy

Nifedipine is antihypertensive at doses ranging from 5 to 30 mg (4,38,48). The effect is dose-related (34) and the higher the blood pressure or the total peripheral resistance before treatment, the greater the fall in blood pressure (19,24). Normotensive patients do not drop their blood pressure in response to nifedipine. Treatment of hypertension with 10 or 20 mg orally or sublingually drops blood pressure within 15 to 20 min (23,34). This rapid onset of action makes nifedipine a drug which is eminently suitable for the emergency treatment of hypertension (6,24,34). The extent of the blood pressure fall in these patients was 21 to 35% (6,30) and was seen 30 min after the oral administration of the 10 mg capsule. This acute reduction in blood pressure was often (5,34,49), but not always (12,30), accompanied by an increase in heart rate, probably mediated by a baroreceptor reflex stimulation. Magometschnigg et al. (39) have shown that the higher the pretreatment blood pressure, the less the increase in heart rate following therapy with nifedipine. This could be explained on the basis of a very high blood pressure causing some degree of cardiac insufficiency. Unloading of the heart, in these circumstances, may reduce the tachycardia of heart failure, or at least limit the reflex tachycardia caused by the antihypertensive drug (29).

Nifedipine increases urinary volume and urinary Na^+ secretion (27), in contrast to many other types of vasodilator drugs (28). Plasma renin activity and plasma norepinephrine concentration usually increase in response to 10 mg or more of nifedipine (5,11,12). However, plasma aldosterone does not change (33,49). In one study, nifedipine was shown to be an inhibitor of the angiotensin II-mediated release of aldosterone (42).

Intravenous verapamil also decreases blood pressure (7). Oral verapamil (160 mg) has no effect on blood pressure of normotensive subjects, but lowers blood pressure of hypertensive patients with no change in heart rate and plasma renin activity (13). In a small pilot study (10) 1 mg/kg loading dose followed by 50 μg/kg/min infusion of tiapamil lowered both blood pressure and heart rate significantly in 6 male patients with Grade 1 (WHO) essential hypertension. In an oral study, patients received 6 mg/kg tiapamil which significantly reduced blood pressure, but had no effect on heart rate or on PR interval. The effect was somewhat short-acting: the blood pressure effect lasted about 1 to 2 hr.

Chronic Therapy

Nifedipine is an effective antihypertensive drug at total daily doses of 15 to 60 mg. The acute effect, coming on within 15 to 20 min, is sustained for weeks during subsequent chronic therapy (L. Opie and L. Jee, Chapter 31, *this volume*). There is no clear-cut dose relationship (33,38). Discontinuation of therapy was followed by a slow increase in blood pressure which came back to pretreatment level within 2 days (24,44). In most studies, heart rate tended to remain unchanged or decreased (19,38,43) and may be explained on the basis of resetting of the baroreflex mechanism. Nifedipine did not produce postural hypertension and tolerance did not develop (12,19,44). There was no change in body weight suggesting the absence of Na^+ and fluid retention (24,32,44). Plasma volume was measured in one study on 18 patients treated with nifedipine and found to be unchanged after a year (24). Also, in contrast to other vasodilators, long-term treatment with nifedipine did not result in any consistent increase in plasma renin activity (12,33,38). However plasma renin was increased by nifedipine in one study (14) in which nifedipine was found to be as effective an antihypertensive drug as prazosin in a double-blind cross-over trial.

Verapamil is also effective as an antihypertensive in total daily doses of 240 to 720 mg in patients with mild to moderate essential hypertension (WHO stage I and II) (3,13,22,31,35,36,37,41). As with nifedipine, there was a direct correlation between pretreatment value and the fall in blood pressure, and there was no effect on blood pressure of normotensive subjects (13). In one study, the antihypertensive effect was said to wane after 7 weeks of treatment (31), but this could not be confirmed in a later study over one year (37). There is a wide individual variation in the response to verapamil explained on the basis of a high first-pass metabolism (41). As with nifedipine, heart rate tends to remain unchanged or even to decrease after long-term use of the drug (35,37,41).

Other Calcium Antagonists

Perhexiline has not been adequately tested in hypertension, but has serious adverse effects including peripheral neuropathy, raised intracranial pressure, disturbances of liver function, dizziness, nausea, and ataxia.

Prenylamine is widely used as an antianginal agent, but recent publications have given more emphasis to its tendency to cause arrhythmias (47) especially in the presence of hypokalemia and heart failure, and especially in patients taking β-blockers. Other Ca^{2+} channel blockers which are potent inhibitors of vascular smooth muscle tone are *lidoflazine* (51), *cinnarizine,* and *flunarizine* (21), but there is no information on their use in hypertension.

Practical Implications

Since the use of Ca^{2+} channel blockers in hypertension is still new, their indications, efficacy in different types and grades of hypertension, side-effects, and interactions with other drugs are all questions that require further investigation. From the available evidence it is likely that:

1. The dihydropyridines, such as nifedipine, nisoldipine, and nitrendipine, are as effective in the therapy of hypertension as verapamil, but, in the doses used, they have less effect than verapamil on atrioventricular conduction.

2. To date, nifedipine in hypertension has been more thoroughly researched than any other Ca^{2+} channel blocker and should be used in preference to other

dihydropyridines. Where there is cerebrovascular insufficiency, nimodipine (26), when it becomes available, may be the drug of choice; however, its antihypertensive efficacy has not yet been established.

3. Tiapamil is a promising drug for the treatment of hypertension and of superventricular arrhythmias; it, therefore, resembles verapamil in its pharmacologic profile, but its use may be limited by its short duration of action.

4. Nifedipine seems to be devoid of serious side-effects, however, minor problems include flushing, headache, and fluid retention.

5. Nifedipine has been used safely with diuretics and with propranolol (4,15). On the other hand, verapamil produces significant negative inotropic and chronotropic effects in patients treated with β-blockers; combination therapy should be used with great caution, if at all (45). The long-term effects of other Ca^{2+} antagonist/β-blocker combinations remain to be documented. We also have very little data on the interactions of Ca^{2+} antagonists, including nifedipine, with α_1-blockers (e.g., prazosin), vasodilators (e.g., hydralazine), α_2-agonists (e.g., clonidine), angiotensin-converting enzyme inhibitors (e.g., captopril), or other commonly used antihypertensive agents. Until experience in this area accumulates, it is best to use nifedipine as monotherapy, or in combination only with diuretics and/or β-blockers.

6. In a canine model of renovascular hypertension, nifedipine has hemodynamic effects similar to hydralazine, that is, it decreases peripheral resistance, lowers systolic and diastolic arterial pressures, increases cardiac output, and causes a reflex tachycardia and increase in plasma renin activity. In contrast to hydralazine, however, nifedipine also reduces coronary vascular resistance, thereby increasing coronary blood flow, and also decreases myocardial O_2 consumption. Therefore, nifedipine, with or without a β-blocker, may be the drug of first choice in the therapy of hypertension with stable angina, and should be used as first therapy, without the β-blocker, in hypertension with vasospastic angina.

7. There is accumulating evidence that nifedipine is safe and effective in treating accelerated hypertension; 10 mg sublingually, or 20 mg orally, brings blood pressure down to reasonable, but not hypotensive, levels in 15 to 60 min.

8. It is not inconceivable that our current concepts of stepped-care therapy for hypertension will be radically revised in the near future. Diuretics and β-blockers are not harmless drugs. The hypokalemia, hyperuricemia, impotence (46), and impairment of glucose tolerance (17) of thiazide diuretics; and the peripheral vasoconstriction, negative inotropy, reduction of effort tolerance, and bronchoconstriction of β-blockers may become unacceptable at a time when newer antihypertensive drugs, such as Ca^{2+} channel blockers, and newer α-blockers, have a much less potentially serious side-effect profile.

SUMMARY

This chapter summarizes the possible mechanisms of increasing intracellular Ca^{2+} and the action of Ca^{2+} on contractile proteins in vascular smooth muscle.

Inhibition of Na^+,K^+-ATPase activity increases intracellular Na^+ and extracellular K^+. Na^+ inhibits Ca^{2+}-Na^+ countertransport causing a rise in intracellular Ca^{2+}. Ca^{2+} antagonists reduce Ca^{2+} influx, and therefore vascular smooth muscle tone. Ca^{2+} channel blockers are effective antihypertensive agents in both acute and chronic therapy with a low incidence of side-effects. Ca^{2+} antagonists of the dihydropyridine group decrease peripheral resistance, systolic and diastolic arterial pressures, and coronary vascular resistance. They may be used, with safety, with diuretics and/or β-adrenoreceptor blocking drugs.

REFERENCES

1. Adelstein, R. S., and Hathaway, D. R. (1979): *Am. J. Cardiol.*, 44:783–787.
2. Aksoy, M. O., Murphy, R. A., and Kamm, K. E. (1982): *Am. J. Physiol.*, 242:C109–C116.
3. Anavekar, S. N., Christophidis, N., Louis, W. J., and Doyle, A. E. (1981): *J. Cardiovasc. Pharmacol.*, 3:287–292.
4. Aoki, K., Yoshida, T., Kato, S., Tazumi, K., Sato, I., Takikawa, K., and Hotta, K. (1976): *Jpn. Heart J.*, 17:479–483.
5. Aoki, K., Kondo, S., Mochizuki, A., Yoshida, T., Kato, S., Kato, K., and Takikawa, K. (1978): *Am. Heart J.*, 96:218–226.
6. Bartorelli, C., Magrini, F., Moruzzi, P., Olivart, M. T., Polese, A., Fiorentini, C., and Guazzi, M. (1978): *Clin. Sci. Mol. Med.*, 55:291S–292S.
7. Bender, F. (1970): *Drug Res.*, 20:1310.
8. Blaustein, M. P. (1977): *Am. J. Physiol.*, 232:C165–C173.
9. Bolton, T. B. (1979): *Physiol. Rev.*, 59:607–718.
10. Chu, D. (1981): In: *Proceedings of the 1st International Symposium on Tiapamil,* Lausanne, p. 8 (Abstracts).
11. Corea, L., Miele, N., Bentivoglio, M., Boschett, E., Agabiti-Rosei, E., and Muresan, G. (1979): *Clin. Sci.,* (Suppl. 5) 57:115S–117S.
12. Corea, L., Alunni, G., Bentivoglio, M., Boschetti, E., Cosmi, F., Giaimo, M. D., Miele, N., and Motolese, M. (1980): *Acta Ther.,* 6:177–182.
13. Corea, L., Bentivoglio, M., Agabiti-Rosei, E., Muiesan, L., Alicandri, C. L., and Muiesan, G. (1981): *Acta Ther.,* 7:107–111.
14. Corea, L., Bentivoglio, M., Cosmi, F., Alunni, G., and Carnovali, M. (1981): *Curr. Ther. Res.,* 30:708–717.
15. Dargie, H., Rowland, E., and Krikler, D. (1981): *Br. Heart J.,* 46:8–16.
16. De Mendonca, M., Grichois, M. L., Garay, R. P., Sassrd, J., Ben-Ishay, D., and Meyer, P. (1980): *Proc. Natl. Acad. Sci. USA,* 77:4283–4286.
17. Dollery, C. T. (1981): *Clin. Sci.,* 61:431S–420S.
18. Ebashi, S. (1980): *Proc. R. Soc. Lond. (Biol.),* 207:259–286.
19. Ekelund, L.-G., Orö, L. (1979): *Clin. Cardiol.,* 2:203–211.
20. Godfraind, T. (1981): In: *New Perspectives on Calcium Antagonists,* edited by G. B. Weiss, pp. 95–107. American Physiological Society, Bethesda, Maryland.
21. Godfraind, T. (1981): *Fed. Proc.,* 40:2866–2871.
22. Gould, B. A., Mann, S., Kieso, H., Subramanian, V. B., and Raftery, E. (1982): *Circulation,* 65:22–27.
23. Guazzi, M. D., Olivari, M. T., Polese, A., Fiorentini, C., Magrini, F., and Moruzzi, P. (1977): *Clin. Pharmacol. Ther.,* 22:528–532.
24. Guazzi, M. D., Fiorentini, C., Olivari, M. T., Bartorelli, A., Necchi, G., and Polese, A. (1980): *Circulation,* 61:913.
25. Hartshorne, D. J. (1980): *Chest,* 78:140–149.
26. Kazda, S., and Towart, R. (1982): *Acta Neurochir.,* 63:259–265.
27. Klütsch, K., Schmidt, P., and Grosswendt, J. (1972): *Drug Res.,* 22:377–380.
28. Koch-Weser, J. (1974): *Arch. Int. Med.,* 133:1017–1027.
29. Krebs, R., Graefe, K.-H., and Ziegler, R. (1982): *Clin. Exp. Hypertens.,* A4(1–2):271–284.

30. Kuwajima, I., Ueda, K., Kamata, C., Matsushita, S., Kuramoto, K., Murakami, M., and Hata, Y. (1978): *Jpn. Heart J.,* 19:455–467.
31. Lederballe Pedersen, O. (1978): *Eur. J. Clin. Pharmacol.,* 13:21–24.
32. Lederballe Pedersen, O., and Mikkelsen, E. (1978): *Eur. J. Clin. Pharmacol.,* 14:375–381.
33. Lederballe Pedersen, O., Mikkelsen, E., Christensen, N. J., Kornerup, H. J., and Pedersen, E. B. (1979): *Eur. J. Clin. Pharmacol.,* 15:235–239.
34. Lederballe Pedersen, O., Christensen, N. J., and Rämsch, K. D. (1980): *J. Cardiovasc. Pharmacol.,* 2:357–366.
35. Leeuw, P. W., De Smont, A. J. P. M., Willemse, P. J., and Birkenhäger, W. H. (1981): In: *Calcium Antagonism in Cardiovascular Therapy,* edited by A. Zanchetti and D. M. Krikler, pp. 233–238. Exerpta Medica, Amsterdam.
36. Leonetti, G., Pasotti, C., Ferrari, G. P., and Zanchetti, A. (1981): In: *Calcium Antagonism in Cardiovascular Therapy,* edited by A. Zanchetti and D. M. Krikler, pp. 260–266. Excerpta Medica, Amsterdam.
37. Lewis, G. R., Morley, K. D., and Maslowski, A. H. (1979): *NZ Med. J.,* 9:62–64.
38. MacGregor, G. A., Markandu, N. D., Bayliss, J., Brown, M. J., and Roulston, J. E. (1981): In: *Proceedings of the 8th Scientific Meeting of the International Society of Hypertension,* Milan, Abstract No. 264.
39. Magometschnigg, D., Rameis, H., and Sertl, K. (1981): In: *Proceedings of the 8th Scientific Meeting of the International Society of Hypertension,* Milan, Abstract No. 266.
40. Meisheri, K. D., Hwang, O., and van Breemen, C. (1981): *J. Membr. Biol.,* 59:19–25.
41. Midtbø, K., and Hals, O. (1980): *Curr. Ther. Res.,* 27:830–834.
42. Millar, J. A., McLean, K., and Reid, J. L. (1981): *Clin. Sci.,* 61:65S–68S.
43. Murakami, M., Murakami, F., Takekoshi, N., Tsuchiya, M., Kin, T., Onoe, T., Takeuchi, N., Funatsu, T., Hara, S., Ishise, S., Mifune, J., and Maeda, M. (1972): *Jpn. Heart J.,* 13:128–135.
44. Olivari, M. T., Bartorelli, C., Polese, A., Fiorentini, C., Moruzzi, P., and Guazzi, M. D. (1979): *Circulation,* 59:1056–1062.
45. Packer, M., Meller, J., Medina, M., Smith, H., Holt, J., Guererro, J., Todd, G. D., McAllister, R. G., Jr., and Gorlin, R. (1982): *Circulation,* 65:660–668.
46. Peart, W. S. (1981): *Clin. Sci.,* 61:403S–411S.
47. Puritz, R., Hendersen, M. A., Baker, S. N., and Chamberlain, D. A. (1977): *Br. Med. J.,* 11:608–609.
48. Takekoshi, N., Murakami, E., Murakami, H., Matsui, S., Masuya, K., Nomura, M., Fujita, S., Tsuji, S., Chatani, T., Emoto, J., Tsugawa, T., Emoto, J., Tsuguwa, H., and Hashimoto, A. (1981): *Jpn. Circ. J.,* 45:852–860.
49. Thibonnier, M., Bonnet, F., and Corvol, P. (1980): *Eur. J. Clin. Pharmacol.,* 17:161–164.
50. Van Breemen, C., Mangel, A., Fahim, M., and Meisheri, K. (1982): *Am. J. Cardiol.,* 49:507–510.
51. Vanhoutte, P. M. (1981): In: *New Perspectives on Calcium Antagonists,* edited by G. B. Weiss, pp. 109–121. American Physiological Society, Bethesda, Maryland.
52. Wei, J. W., Janis, R. A., and Daniel, E. E. (1977): *Blood Vessels,* 14:55–64.

Calcium Antagonists and Cardiovascular Disease, edited by L. H. Opie. Raven Press, New York © 1984.

Chapter 31

Nifedipine: Expanding Indications in Hypertension

Lionel H. Opie and Larry D. Jee

Hypertension Clinic, Groote Schuur Hospital, and MRC-UCT Ischaemic Heart Disease Research Unit, Department of Medicine, University of Cape Town, South Africa

Ca^{2+}-antagonist agents have not generally been regarded as antihypertensive agents, although widely recognized as having a major effect on vascular smooth muscle. Recent emphasis on the role of increased peripheral vascular resistance in the pathogenesis of hypertension (F. Bühler et al., Chapter 29, *this volume*) has made the use of vasodilators correspondingly more logical therapy in hypertension, especially because β-adrenergic receptor blocking agents are known to increase peripheral vascular resistance. Of the existing vasodilators, prazosin has the disadvantage of possible first-dose syncope and the development of tolerance (1), whereas hydralazine causes a reflex tachycardia and prolonged therapy may result in lupus erythematosus. Minoxidil and diazoxide, though recognized as powerful vasodilator agents, have serious side-effects which severely limit their use in chronic therapy.

Accordingly, it has been suggested that there should be a major role for Ca^{2+} antagonists in the therapy of hypertension (7). The agent of choice should be powerfully active on peripheral vascular smooth muscle with neither any major depressant effect on myocardial contractility, nor on the sinus or atrioventricular nodes. This chapter summarizes the hypotensive properties of nifedipine (Adalat, Bayer) as clinically tested at Groote Schuur Hospital, Cape Town.

NIFEDIPINE FOR HYPERTENSION AND ANGINA

Nifedipine was originally seen to be a "cardioactive" agent, largely used in the therapy of angina pectoris (3). In the Hypertension Clinic of Groote Schuur Hospital, a study was made of a group of hypertensive patients with co-existing angina pectoris; the problem was persisting angina of effort despite apparently reasonable control of the blood pressure. On adding nifedipine to atenolol, there was an additive hypotensive effect which, in one patient with an already well-controlled blood pressure, led to an adverse reaction with excessive hypotension (6). In other patients, elevated blood pressures were reduced to near-normal by nifedipine (e.g., Adalat, 10 mg twice daily) and the effect sustained for 6 weeks. Side-effects of nifedipine were negligible—facial flushing and an increased prominence of varicose veins. The antianginal effect of added nifedipine in this group of β-blocked patients was not marked, probably because higher doses are required for the nifedipine effect to be evident when combined with β-blockade (4). However, the definite added antihypertensive effect led to the use of nifedipine in other patients with hypertension without accompanying angina pectoris.

NIFEDIPINE FOR HYPERTENSION IMPERFECTLY CONTROLLED BY β-ADRENOCEPTOR BLOCKADE

Next, nifedipine (10 mg b.d.) was used in patients with hypertension without angina who were already receiving the β-adrenoceptor cardioselective agent atenolol, but were imperfectly controlled. Again an added hypotensive effect was obtained. In the course of these investigations, it was noted that the hypotensive effect of nifedipine was very rapid in onset, within minutes, and sustained for hours.

RAPID HYPOTENSIVE EFFECT OF NIFEDIPINE

In the next series of studies, nifedipine was given sublingually (10 mg) to a series of more than 50 hypertensive patients who were poorly controlled (Fig. 1). The majority of these patients were receiving therapy with a variety of other agents, usually including β-adrenoceptor antagonist therapy. However, some patients were untreated. In all, with two exceptions, nifedipine 5 to 20 mg as a single sublingual dose (usually 10 mg) reduced blood pressure acutely. There was little tachycardia, and few or no side-effects. We noted that sustained therapy with nifedipine apparently led to a sustained antihypertensive effect. Therefore, the predictive value of acute testing with nifedipine was investigated.

PREDICTIVE VALUE OF ACUTE NIFEDIPINE TESTING

In this series of patients, acute administration of nifedipine was followed by prolonged therapy for 4 to 8 weeks (5). The degree of the acute fall in blood pressure was a good predictor of the chronic effect, irrespective of the initial treatment. In a few individual patients, a minor initial response was followed by a better sustained response, or vice versa. However, there was no evidence of tolerance with repeat acute testing. This finding supports other work which emphasizes that the antihypertensive effect of nifedipine is maintained during chronic treatment without the necessity of increasing the dosage (2).

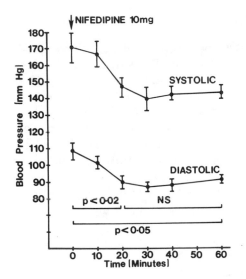

FIG. 1. Pilot study of acute blood pressure response to sublingual nifedipine in patients already receiving simultaneous β-blocker therapy (atenolol). Mean values of 14 patients. (From ref. 5.)

NIFEDIPINE FOR HYPERTENSIVE PATIENTS WITH CARDIOMEGALY OR HEART FAILURE

Concern has been raised about the possible adverse negative inotropic effect of nifedipine and other Ca^{2+} antagonist agents. We studied a group of patients with radiologically increased cardiothoracic ratio taken as an index of cardiomegaly. The ejection fraction was determined by standard multiple gated blood pool radionuclide techniques; in the majority of cases, values were high-normal except in a few patients with overt clinical heart failure. Acute nifedipine either left the ejection fraction unchanged or increased it slightly; the overall effect was a small but significant increase. This held even in patients receiving β-adrenoceptor blockade. We concluded that radiological cardiomegaly and even overt heart failure in hypertensive patients were not contraindications to therapy with nifedipine.

NIFEDIPINE FOR REFRACTORY HYPERTENSION

In a number of patients, the hypertension was apparently refractory and treated by a large number of agents. Even in these patients, nifedipine gave an adequate acute response, with a sustained effect, thereby avoiding agents with undesirable side-effects such as minoxidil, or intravenous agents such as labetalol or diazoxide (5).

SIDE-EFFECTS

In all our studies, side-effects have been few and frequently relatively trivial, such as facial flushing or minor degrees of ankle edema (the mechanism of the latter effect is not clear). In a few patients, lightheadedness and postural syncope have been associated with an excess hypotensive effect. In none were there serious side-effects such as those reported for β-adrenoceptor antagonists (bronchoconstriction with occasional near-fatality in asthmatics; heart failure; excess bradycardia). Thus the major side-effect of lightheadedness is, in fact, predictable by the blood pressure response which is, in turn, predictable by acute testing. Nevertheless, because of this possible effect, we have been careful not to test the effect of acute nifedipine in the standard dose of 10 mg in patients with past cerebrovascular accidents, rather using nifedipine 5 mg.

DRUG INTERACTIONS

The major problem of possible interactions with β-adrenoceptor antagonists is examined in a subsequent chapter; we hold that adverse interaction is rare in contrast to beneficial possibility of the vasodilating effect of nifedipine attenuating some of the adverse consequences of β-blockade, such as peripheral vasoconstriction. One new drug interaction has emerged—an additive acute hypotensive with prazosin. We were first alerted to this in a patient with refractory hypertension and unstable angina pectoris, already receiving prazosin 10 mg twice daily, in whom acute therapy with nifedipine and prazosin caused acute hypotension. Subsequently, three other similar patients have been recorded. Our current practice is: (a) in patients already receiving prazosin, the acute test is conducted with nifedipine 5 mg instead of the standard 10 mg capsule; and (b) in patients already receiving nifedipine, prazosin is added acutely as 1 or 2 mg with careful testing for postural hypotension.

NIFEDIPINE—CURRENT PRACTICE

Based on our experience with over 100 patients over 3½ years, we regard nifedipine as an extremely reliable antihypertensive agent. Acute testing can predict the chronic effect and help fix the appropriate dose. Not only is nifedipine effective in patients with mild to moderate hypertension, but it is convenient and safe to administer to patients with apparently refractory hypertension. We do not hesitate to give nifedipine to patients with radiological cardiomegaly, even in hypertensive cardiac failure. Nifedipine, as a vasodilator, has substantial advantages over hydralazine which may well be replaced by nifedipine in clinical practice. Caution is required when adding nifedipine dosages to patients already receiving prazosin.

NIFEDIPINE—OUTSTANDING QUESTIONS

Three groups of patients require specific evaluation with nifedipine. First, are those untreated patients presenting with mild to moderate hypertension for the first time likely to benefit from nifedipine as first-line therapy? Here an appropriate trial would compare nifedipine with a β-blocker as first-line therapy. Second, patients with hypertension and renal failure need specific evaluation for the possible effect of nifedipine on renal function. Third, long-term studies over years are required to assess if nifedipine is able to prevent myocardial infarction in patients with hypertension.

REFERENCES

1. Graham, R. M., Thornell, I. R., Gain, J. M., Bagnoli, C., Oates, H. F., and Stokes, G. S. (1976): *Br. Med. J.*, 2:1293–1294.
2. Krebs, R., Graefe, K.-H., and Ziegler, R. (1982): *Clin. Exp. Hypertens.*, A4(1–2):271–284.
3. Kroneberg, G. (1973): *1st International Nifedipine "Adalat" Symposium*, edited by K. Hashimoto, E. Kimura, and T. Kobayashi. University of Tokyo Press, Tokyo.
4. Lynch, P., Dargie, H., Krikler, S., and Krikler, D. (1980): *Br. Med. J.*, 280:184–187.
5. Opie, L. H., Jee, L., and White, D. (1982): *Am. Heart J.*, 104:606–612.
6. Opie, L. H., and White, D. A. (1980): *Br. Med. J.*, 281:1462–1464.
7. Pedersen, O. L. (1981): *Acta Pharmacol. Toxicol.*, 49(Suppl. 11):5–31.

Calcium Antagonists and Cardiovascular Disease, edited by L. H. Opie.
Raven Press, New York © 1984.

Chapter 32

Nifedipine for Hypertension and Angina Pectoris: Interactions During Combination Therapy

Larry D. Jee and Lionel H. Opie

Hypertension Clinic, Groote Schuur Hospital, and MRC-UCT Ischaemic Heart Disease Research Unit, Department of Medicine, University of Cape Town, South Africa

The most widely studied combination therapy involving nifedipine is undoubtedly the use of this drug with β-adrenoceptor antagonist agents. Even before the antihypertensive effect of nifedipine was widely recognized, the potential for the combination of the two drugs arose from their primary common indication, namely the treatment of angina pectoris (21). Prominent amongst the early reports on the combination were descriptions of well demonstrated adverse interactions, usually typified by symptoms of cardiac failure (1,2,27,30). Included in these descriptions was a report from our group (24). The cause of most of these adverse interactions was never clearly shown, and the literature concerning them usually took the form of case reports describing individual patients or small groups.

INTERACTION OF CALCIUM ANTAGONISTS WITH β-ADRENOCEPTOR BLOCKADE

In order better to understand the interaction between Ca^{2+} antagonists and β-adrenoreceptor blockade, it is appropriate to consider briefly the effects of each on the cardiovascular system. These are summarized in Table 1.

Effects of Calcium Antagonists on the Cardiovascular System

The effects of the Ca^{2+} antagonists on the cardiovascular system are evident over a broad spectrum, from the conducting tissue of the heart to the peripheral vasculature. Nifedipine, diltiazem, and verapamil all have depressant effects on isolated sinoatrial tissue, causing a decrease in the frequency of spontaneous firing, the amplitude and rate of rise of the action potential, and the slope of

TABLE 1. *Contraindications and side-effects of β-adrenoceptor blocking agents and calcium antagonists*

Effects	β-blockade	Nifedipine
Contraindications	Bronchospasm Heart failure Heart block Bradycardia Peripheral vascular disease	Pregnancy Previous adverse reactions
Side-effects	Exacerbation of above Tiredness Disturbance of serum lipid balance	Facial flushing Headache and dizziness Palpitations Gastrointestinal disturbance (tends to settle with continued treatment)

the diastolic depolarization (12). All three drugs at therapeutic concentrations also delay conduction through the atrioventricular node.

Differences emerge when these effects are studied under clinical conditions—due, apparently, to enhanced reflex sympathetic discharge as a result of the enhanced hypotensive action of nifedipine (12,13). In this setting, nifedipine enhances rather than inhibits atrioventricular conduction, whereas the inhibiting action of verapamil and diltiazem is maintained (12).

In the myocardium, nifedipine removes Ca^{2+} ions from the membrane surface Ca^{2+} pool, and blocks the so-called "slow channels" to the influx of Ca^{2+} (14). This makes available fewer Ca^{2+} ions in the sarcoplasmic reticulum and mitochondria. Normally, these ions activate myofibril ATPase, which, by splitting ATP, liberate energy which is used to achieve activation of the contractile process via actin and myosin. By reducing the number of Ca^{2+} ions available for this process, nifedipine tends to accomplish electromechanical uncoupling, reflected by diminished myocardial contractility. In the case of nifedipine, this direct negative inotropic effect is overcome by the cardiovascular compensations resulting from vasodilation.

The electromechanical uncoupling effect of the Ca^{2+} antagonists results also in dilatation of vascular smooth muscle (17). Quantitative differences with respect to site of action occur between nifedipine, diltiazem, and verapamil. Thus, nifedipine has a stronger peripheral vasodilating action than the other two drugs, whereas diltiazem preferentially dilates the coronary vasculature (17).

Effects of β-Adrenoceptor Blockade on the Cardiovascular System

β-Adrenoceptor antagonists (β-blockers) exert their effects on the cardiovascular system (and at other sites) by means of competitive inhibition of catecholamines on the β-receptors. Stimulation of the β-receptors by catecholamines usually activates the adenyl cyclase, which allows the reaction forming cyclic AMP from ATP to proceed. The cyclic AMP thus produced is the intracellular messenger of β-stimulation and is responsible for the physiological effects of such stimulation on the heart (22), which include an increase in the rate of discharge of the sinoatrial node and an increase in the force and speed of myocardial contraction. Thus, β-blockers would inhibit all these actions and cause a reduction in heart rate, and a decrease of the rate and strength of contraction.

Both large and small coronary arteries have convincingly been shown to contain β-receptors which mediate vasodilatation (28). The vasoconstriction which follows β-adrenoceptor blockade (28) results in a diminished O_2 supply to the myocardium, but the associated decreases in heart rate, contractility, afterload, and O_2 wastage, reduce the O_2 demand to a far greater degree (21). These moderating effects do not occur in the periphery, and the cold extremities often associated with the use of β-blockers are probably the result of reflex α-stimulation which causes peripheral vasoconstriction (29).

ACTIONS OF THE COMBINATION OF CALCIUM ANTAGONISTS AND β-ADRENOCEPTOR ANTAGONISTS

From the above descriptions, the theoretical consequences of combined Ca^{2+} antagonist and β-blocker therapy are apparent (Fig. 1). The final effect on the sinoatrial and atrioventricular nodes and on myocardial contractility would be the result of the effects of both agents. In the case of nifedipine, the overall effect is one of increased heart rate and left ventricular ejection fraction (32). Verapamil, in contrast, causes a decrease in heart rate and ejection fraction,

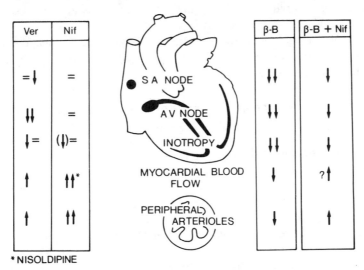

FIG. 1. Effect of Ca^{2+} antagonists and β-blockade alone and in combination on cardiovascular system. Ver, verapamil; Nif, nifedipine.

when added to treatment with propranolol (32). The coronary vessels per se would be affected only by the Ca^{2+} antagonists, and the effects on the peripheral vasculature would be the net result of the opposing vasoconstrictive influence of the β-blockers, and vasodilatory effects of the Ca^{2+} antagonists.

Since the Ca^{2+} antagonists, particularly nifedipine, cause reflex sympathetic stimulation (12) and the β-blockers blunt the sympathetic response, it is theoretically possible that the combination would give rise to adverse interactions. That this does not occur in practice is borne out by the increasing number of reports describing beneficial responses when β-blockers and Ca^{2+} antagonists are combined in patients with angina of effort (7,25,26), exercise-induced ST-segment elevation (22), Prinzmetal's angina (3,6,20), angina at rest (20), hypertension (4,8,11,22), and hypertrophic obstructive cardiomyopathy (16).

Other Protective Mechanisms Possibly Operating After Administration of Calcium Antagonists

A second protective mechanism which may be at work was described by Schwartz's group in dog experiments (19), namely that there may be a withdrawal of parasympathetic tone, an effect most marked with nifedipine and least marked with verapamil, with diltiazem having an intermediate effect. The mode of modification of parasympathetic tone, and whether the phenomenon occurs in man is still open to investigation. Yet, an indirect parasympathetic effect of Ca^{2+}-antagonist agents is a useful clinical concept.

A third mechanism, whereby the intrinsic negative inotropic effect of Ca^{2+} antagonists is counteracted, is the reduction of myocardial O_2 demand by afterload reduction (9) which might be even more marked in the presence of β-adrenergic blockade (not yet tested in man).

Thus, there are three potential mechanisms to counter the negative inotropic effect, and two possible mechanisms to counter the potential negative chronotropic effect of Ca^{2+} antagonists.

CLINICAL APPLICATIONS OF THE COMBINATION OF NIFEDIPINE AND β-ADRENERGIC BLOCKADE

The combination of nifedipine and β-blockade has enjoyed widespread application in cardiovascular disease.

Angina of Effort

The most widely reported condition for which the combination of nifedipine and β-blockade has been used is effort-induced angina pectoris. Patients with effort-induced angina had better exercise tolerance on both nifedipine and acebutolol than on either drug alone, with nifedipine appearing to make the major contribution (7). Another study, also with acebutolol and nifedipine, demonstrated improved hemodynamics after acute administration of both drugs, when compared to either drug alone (26). In patients with severe exertional angina pectoris, propranolol combined with nifedipine decreased the number of episodes of ST depression and tended, with higher doses, to limit the number of episodes of angina (18). A further study describes the benefit with respect to exercise capacity, onset of symptoms, relief of ST depression, and maximal heart rate when nifedipine is added to existing therapy with atenolol (5). The combination of verapamil and propranolol gave better exercise tolerance and improved ST-segment depression when compared to either drug alone (31).

Exercise-Induced ST-Segment Elevation

We reported a case of interest which was noted during a study assessing the effects of nifedipine on hypertension, when added to existing β-blockade. The patient concerned developed ST-segment elevation and ventricular tachycardia (23) on exercise, while treated with atenolol plus a diuretic. Nifedipine was added to her regime, and besides additional blood pressure control, she was able to exercise beyond her earlier limits without developing ST elevation or arrhythmias of any description.

Angina Due to Coronary Artery Spasm

Prinzmetal's angina, caused by coronary artery spasm, appears to be one disease which, at present, is better treated by Ca^{2+} antagonism than by any other regime. We are not aware of published data where nifedipine and β-blockade are used together to treat the condition. Delahaye et al. (6) describe a trial wherein patients who manifest coronary artery spasm during catheterization respond significantly better to nifedipine than to β-blockade. In similar patients who showed no coronary artery spasm on catheterization, the frequency or severity of attacks was not significantly different, whether treated with β-blockade or nifedipine. Another study relates better control of symptoms in patients with coronary artery spasm when treated with nifedipine, after a wide variety of medications, including β-blockade with propranolol, had failed to provide adequate control of symptoms (3).

Angina at Rest

Studies on the pathogenesis of angina at rest or unstable angina have failed to demonstrate the cause of this condition in all cases, although coronary artery spasm does occur in some of these patients (15). Nevertheless, patients with this condition have also been beneficially treated with nifedipine and β-blockade. Moses et al. (20) abolished angina at rest in 14 of 19 patients, and improved symptoms in another 2 patients by adding nifedipine to existing propranolol and nitrate treatment. Another group of patients showed a significant reduction in ischemia-related events (bypass surgery, myocardial infarction, and death) when nifedipine compared to placebo was added to propranolol and nitrate therapy (10).

Hypertrophic Obstructive Cardiomyopathy

A recent study (16) has demonstrated that in hypertrophic cardiomyopathy, treatment with nifedipine and propranolol offers hemodynamic advantages over treatment with nifedipine alone. The combination could thus be useful treatment in this group of patients as well.

Combination Therapy for Hypertension

The bulk of our early experience with nifedipine and β-blockade concerns the antihypertensive action of nifedipine. We have found that nifedipine added to β-blockade (usually by atenolol) brings about additional falls in blood pressure rapidly and maintains these falls over a period of months, at least. Follow-up studies are continuing. Similar findings have been made by other workers: A trial assessing the antihypertensive effects of nifedipine showed a greater fall in blood pressure after nifedipine and propranolol, than after nifedipine alone (4). Another study on severe hypertensives showed added hypotensive effect when propranolol was added to existing therapy with nifedipine (11). Further work demonstrated added antihypertensive effects when nifedipine was combined with metoprolol, compared to either drug alone (8).

The hypothesis that the presence of β-blockade would blunt the sympathetic response to nifedipine, and so permit a greater fall in blood pressure after treatment, is denied by a study carried out by our group. This study compared the fall in blood pressure after nifedipine in two groups of patients with severe hypertension: one untreated and one receiving β-blockade. There was no difference in the magnitude of the fall in blood pressure between the two groups: Those doses of β-blockade accepted to be clinically effective (in this case atenolol 100 mg daily) did not change the response of the patients to nifedipine, when compared to untreated patients with similarly elevated blood pressures.

Contraindications and Side-Effects

Nifedipine has, at present, no contraindications other than its use in pregnancy and the occurrence of previous adverse reactions to the drug. In general, side-effects are mild and include dizziness, facial flushing, headache, pedal edema, and occasionally palpitations and gastrointestinal disturbances. In contrast, β-adrenoceptor blocking agents have a host of contraindications (21) of which the most important are probably bronchospasm, heart failure, bradycardia, heart block, and peripheral vascular disease. Side-effects cover a similar spectrum (see Table 1).

INTERACTION OF NIFEDIPINE WITH α-ADRENOCEPTOR
ANTAGONISTS

A second and, at present, less well documented interaction is that between nifedipine and α-blockade by prazosin. This combination has produced variable results in our clinic. Most patients appear to tolerate the combination well, although in some isolated cases, the addition of nifedipine to preexisting therapy with prazosin has resulted in precipitous falls in blood pressure, with a marked orthostatic element. Of 16 patients who were receiving prazosin at the time of treatment with nifedipine, 3 showed reactions which were judged to be excessive. In most patients treated, nifedipine caused considerable falls in blood pressure, yet the concept of an "excessive response" is difficult to define. We used as our definition, a marked fall in blood pressure with simultaneous symptoms suggestive of impaired organ perfusion, such as initiation or aggravation of chest pain, dizziness, or syncope.

The reaction appears to occur when the two medications are taken within 2 hr of each other. We observed it only when nifedipine had been administered after prazosin, rather than when prazosin had been added after pretreatment with nifedipine. That the interaction can be reproducible is borne out by the fact that it was provoked three times in the same patient, under similar conditions.

Until the mechanism and frequency of this reaction is better documented, we recommend that if nifedipine is to be added to the regime of a patient already receiving prazosin, an initial small dose (5 mg) be given under monitored conditions, to detect any severe interaction which may occur. Treatment of such interactions consists of placing the patient in the head-down position and observing until the blood pressure rises. Further pharmacological intervention has not been necessary in our experience.

SUMMARY

The interaction of nifedipine and β-adrenergic blockade is in most cases a beneficial one, with improvement in angina symptoms, exercise tolerance, and blood pressure control. In the treatment of angina pectoris, coronary vasodilation by nifedipine improves myocardial perfusion and relieves ischemia. Spontaneous and exercise-induced ST-segment elevations respond well to nifedipine. Mild negative inotropy (with diminished myocardial O_2 consumption) is compensated for by peripheral vasodilatation, with decreased total peripheral resistance and improved cardiac output. When added to the negative chronotropic and inotropic effects of β-adrenergic blockade, these actions help to improve symptoms of chest pain and permit improved exercise tolerance.

Patients with hypertension derive most benefit from the peripheral vasodilation which follows treatment with nifedipine. This causes falls in systolic and diastolic pressures. The presence of β-adrenergic blockade has additive hypotensive effects, and the combination is usually tolerated well, even though the reflex sympathetic response to nifedipine may be blunted by β-adrenergic blockade. It is possible that other compensatory mechanisms are invoked by nifedipine.

The possible interaction of nifedipine with prazosin are, at present, largely unknown but warrant careful further observation.

REFERENCES

1. Anastassiades, C. J. (1980): *Br. Med. J.,* 281:1251.
2. Anastassiades, C. J. (1982): *Br. Med. J.,* 284:506.
3. Antman, E., Muller, J., Goldberg, S., et al. (1980): *N. Engl. J. Med.,* 302:1269–1273.
4. Aoki, K., Kondo, S., Yoshida, T., et al. (1978): *Am. Heart J.,* 96:218–228.
5. Broustet, J. P., Rumeau, P., and Guern, P. (1980): *Eur. Heart J.,* 1:59–64.
6. Delahaye, J. P., Touboul, P., and Cassagnes, J. (1979): In: *Proceedings of the 4th International Adalat Symposium,* edited by P. Peuch and R. Krebs, 87–94. Excerpta Medica, Amsterdam.
7. De Ponti, C., De Biase, A. M., Pirelli, S., et al. (1981): *Cardiology,* 68:195–199.
8. Ekelund, L.-G., Eckelund, C., and Rössner, S. (1982): *Acta. Med. Scand.,* 212:71–75.
9. Ferlinz, J., Easthope, J. L., and Aronow, W. S. (1979): *Circulation,* 59:313–319.
10. Gerstenblith, G., Onyang, P., Achuff, S. C., et al. (1982): *N. Engl. J. Med.,* 306:885–889.
11. Imai, Y., Abe, K., Otsuka, Y., et al. (1980): *Drug Res.,* 30:674–678.
12. Kawai, C., Konishi, T., and Matsuyama, E. (1981): *Circulation,* 63:1035.
13. Konishi, T., Yui, Y., Matsuyama, E., et al. (1979): In: *Proceedings of the 4th International Adalat Symposium,* edited by P. Peuch and R. Krebs, pp. 236–240. Excerpta Medica, Amsterdam.
14. Kroneberg, G., and Krebs, R. (1979): In: *Proceedings of the 4th International Adalat Symposium,* edited by P. Peuch and R. Krebs, pp. 14–24. Excerpta Medica, Amsterdam.
15. L'Abbate, E., and Maseri, A. (1979): In: *Proceedings of the 4th International Adalat Symposium,* edited by P. Peuch and R. Krebs pp. 81–86. Excerpta Medica, Amsterdam.
16. Landmark, K., Sire, S., Thanlow, E., et al. (1982): *Br. Heart J.,* 48:19–26.
17. Low, R. I., Tadeka, P., Mason, D. T., and DeMaria, A. N. (1982): *Am. J. Cardiol.,* 49:547–553.
18. Lynch, P., Dargie, H., Krikler, D., et al. (1980): *Br. Med. J.,* 280:184–187.
19. Millard, R. W., Lathrop, D. A., Grupp, O., et al. (1982): *Am. J. Cardiol.,* 49:499–506.
20. Moses, J. W., Wertheimer, J. H., Bodenheimer, M. M., et al. (1981): *Ann. Int. Med.,* 94:425–429.
21. Opie, L. H. (1980): *Drugs and the Heart.* The Lancet, London.
22. Opie, L. H. (1982): *Cardiovasc. Res.,* 16:483–507.
23. Opie, L. H., Jee, L., and White, D. (1982): *Am. Heart J.,* 104:606–612.
24. Opie, L. H., and White, D. A. (1980): *Br. Med. J.,* 281:1462–1464.
25. Packer, M., Leon, M. B., Bonow, R. O., Kieval, J., Rosing, D. R., and Subramanian, V. B. (1982): *Am. J. Cardiol.,* 50:903–912.
26. Pfisterer, M., Müller-Brand, J., and Burkart, F. (1982): *Am. J. Cardiol.,* 49:1259–1266.
27. Robson, R. H., and Vishwanath, M. C. (1982): *Br. Med. J.,* 284:104.
28. Ross, G. (1976): *Circ. Res.,* 39:461–465.
29. Simpson, W. T. (1977): *Postgrad. Med. J.,* 53:162–167.
30. Staffurth, J. S., and Emergy, P. (1981): *Br. Med. J.,* 282:225.
31. Subramanian, B., Bowles, M. J., Davies, A. B., and Raftery, E. B. (1982): *Am. J. Cardiol.,* 49:125–132.
32. Winniford, M. D., Markham, R. V., Firth, B. G., Nicol, P., and Hillis, L. D. (1982): *Am. J. Cardiol.,* 50:704–710.

Review Article

Pederson, O. L. (1981): *Acta Pharmacol. Toxicol.,* 49(Suppl. 11):5–31.

Calcium Antagonists and Cardiovascular Disease, edited by L. H. Opie.
Raven Press, New York © 1984.

Chapter 33

Calcium Antagonists: New Vistas in Theoretical Basis and Clinical Use

Rolf Krebs

*Bayer AG, Pharma Forschungzentrum, Ressort Medizin,
D5600-Wuppertal 1, Federal Republic of Germany*

The intensive investigation of Ca^{2+}-antagonistic drugs has shown that they not only differ in chemical structure, but also in their pharmacological and clinical effects (13,15,21,22). The basis for this is their differing potency and tissue specificity, but it is now even doubtful if they share a common site of action at the cellular level (22). As evidence exists that the source of cytoplasmic Ca^{2+} may be both tissue- and stimulus-dependent, the possibility exists for antagonism or interference with the regulation of Ca^{2+} at several different sites at the cellular membrane. The interaction of Ca^{2+} with myofibrils and the accumulation or release of Ca^{2+} at the sarcoplasmic reticulum or the mitochondria are not directly affected by these drugs. However, because the therapeutic effect in patients with angina pectoris as well as hypertension is improved clinically with prolonged treatment duration, the indication may be that the size of the intracellular Ca^{2+} compartments is indirectly affected.

There are some newer results which do not fit into the concept that all Ca^{2+} antagonists act, exclusively and simply, by a specific and competitive blockade of the slow inward channels for Ca^{2+}.

ELECTROPHYSIOLOGY

Because reentrant supraventricular tachyarrhythmias can be effectively terminated by verapamil, but not by nifedipine (21), sophisticated investigations into the electrophysiological properties of both the drugs (Table 1) were stimulated. Using the voltage-clamp technique, it has been shown that the influence of verapamil on some electrophysiological parameters is, in clear contrast to nifedipine, rate-dependent (13,21,22). The depression of the slow inward current by nifedipine was found to be clearly dose-dependent, whereas that of verapamil

TABLE 1. *Electrophysiologic properties of nifedipine and verapamil*

Drug (dosage)	Slow inward (Ca²⁺) current channel		Fast inward (Na⁺) current	Channel reactivation	K⁺ outward current	Rate dependency
	Number	Kinetics				
Nifedipine (10^{-7}–10^{-5} M)	+	−	−	−	Increased	−
Verapamil (10^{-7}–10^{-6} M)	+	+	+ᵃ	Delayed	Decreased	+

ᵃ At high concentration.

was predominantly dependent on frequency and markedly enhanced by prolonged incubation. From these experiments, the conclusion was drawn that both verapamil and nifedipine reduce the number of operating slow inward channels. However, in contrast to nifedipine, verapamil has, additionally, an influence on the kinetics of the still operating channels with the result that the activation and, more predominantly, the recovery from inactivation is slowed down by verapamil, but not by nifedipine. Furthermore, verapamil and gallopamil, but not nifedipine, have been found to reduce K⁺ outward current under certain circumstances. The effects of diltiazem on the monophasic action potential resembles that of verapamil. This similarity is confirmed because both verapamil and diltiazem, in contrast to nifedipine, exert fast-channel blocking effects at high concentrations. As a result, in the clinical situation, verapamil and diltiazem may delay atrioventricular conduction (13,21,25). In humans, the effective and functional refractory periods of the atrioventricular node are increased by diltiazem and verapamil, but decreased by nifedipine (21).

RECEPTOR BINDING

There is evidence that dihydropyridine compounds have a common binding site, but completely different from other Ca²⁺-antagonistic drugs (28). Whereas verapamil binds to the lipoproteins of the inner surface of the plasmalemma, a binding to the Ca²⁺ regulatory protein, calmodulin, has been shown for the dihydropyridine felodipine (3). The Ca²⁺ binding at the calmodulin molecule, which is usually 4 moles Ca²⁺ at 1 mole calmodulin, is reduced to 3 moles Ca²⁺. By reducing the releasable Ca²⁺ fraction in vascular smooth muscle, relaxation occurs. Additionally, a reduction of Ca²⁺ in the membrane may influence electrophysiological parameters by diminishing membrane capacity.

INTRACELLULAR CALCIUM EXCHANGE

As the Ca²⁺ entering the cell per beat undergoes exchange with intracellularly released Ca²⁺, it is possible by using radiolabeled Ca²⁺ to study the influence of drugs on the free intracellular Ca^{2+} concentration, which directly determines cellular activity. Using this technique would also give information concerning the exchangeability of Ca^{2+} from intracellularly located Ca^{2+} compartments. Unfortunately, investigations into the intracellular Ca^{2+} exchange are very limited so far. On cardiac tissue, it has been demonstrated that organic Ca^{2+} antagonists, in contrast to La^{3+}, do not impair $^{45}Ca^{2+}$ uptake in concentrations which totally block mechanical activity (4). In rabbit aortic smooth muscle, Weiss et al. (27) demonstrated that neither nitrendipine nor gallopamil blocked norepinephrine-induced contractions and $^{45}Ca^{2+}$ uptake, but both had a strong blocking effect on K^+-induced contractions as well as the accompanying $^{45}Ca^{2+}$ uptake. An inhibition of Ca^{2+} uptake by vascular smooth muscle has also been shown for gallopamil and SKF 525 A as well as for cinnarizine. Although this would mean that only potential-dependent Ca^{2+} channels are inhibited by organic Ca^{2+} antagonists, the effect of these drugs on the receptor-operated Ca^{2+} channel is still under discussion, as Flaim and Craven (9) have shown that diltiazem and verapamil inhibit norepinephrine-stimulated $^{45}Ca^{2+}$ uptake in rabbit aorta. However, differences between the drugs seem to exist also with regard to $^{45}Ca^{2+}$ exchange: La^{3+}-resistant Ca^{2+} uptake into heart and vessel tissue was not influenced by nifedipine and verapamil but even enhanced by diltiazem (4). $^{45}Ca^{2+}$ efflux from the mesenteric vein of rabbits has been found to be increased by nifedipine, but to be unaffected by verapamil and diltiazem (4). Clearly, more studies are needed before definite conclusions as to the effect of Ca^{2+} antagonists on intracellular Ca^{2+} compartments can be drawn.

MEMBRANE TRANSPORT

From their experiments on the action of diltiazem, Flaim et al. (10) concluded that this drug stimulates the Na,K-ATPase. This has also been shown for nitrendipine and nimodipine. By reducing the intracellular Na^+ concentration, more binding sites for Ca^{2+} at the carrier would be available. As a consequence, either the sequestration or efflux of Ca^{2+} would be increased. This was supported by the finding that diltiazem stimulates the efflux of Na^+ from equilibrated rings of rabbit aortic smooth muscle. Whereas diltiazem was found to stimulate O_2 consumption rate by approximately 40%, verapamil inhibited the rate by 18%, and nifedipine had no significant effect. This also supports the idea that Ca^{2+} antagonists differ in their mode of action. This is further confirmed by the fact that reperfusion arrhythmias in dogs are strongly suppressed by verapamil, but hardly affected by nifedipine. In this effect, diltiazem resembles verapamil. A clear difference between nifedipine and verapamil has also been shown concerning their effects on rat vas deferens, as well as on hemodynamics and regional myocardial perfusion (13,25).

TISSUE SPECIFICITY

Experimental and clinical investigations indicate the existence of a difference between Ca^{2+} antagonists concerning their tissue specificity which could open the possibility of developing more specialized drugs. By infusing verapamil intraarterially, a decreasing sensitivity could be shown from the femoral artery, to coronary arteries, and renal artery or aorta, respectively. These regional vascular sensitivities indicate that different vascular smooth muscles have a variable dependence upon membrane Ca^{2+} flux to maintain their tonus. An intracellularly releasable Ca^{2+} pool that is relatively insensitive to Ca^{2+} channel antagonists has been suggested to explain these differences in sensitivity. Differences in the reaction of various structures are confirmed because the contractility of the heart and its conduction system (especially atrioventricular conduction) in animal experiments, as well as in humans, is affected by nifedipine only when the drug is applied in a dose or a concentration exceeding the therapeutic range by more than 10, but can be affected by verapamil within its therapeutic dose range (1,13). The resultant advantage of verapamil is its high effectiveness in blocking reentrant tachyarrhythmias, something which makes it the drug of choice for these conditions. On the other hand, the failure of nifedipine to precipitate atrioventricular block permits its combination with drugs like β-receptor blockers and digitalis compounds (13,25). In accordance with the concept of differing tissue and organ sensitivity is the result that the Ca^{2+}-dependent release of norepinephrine from sympathetic nerve endings is not inhibited at therapeutic plasma concentrations by either nifedipine or verapamil. This, together with the finding in peripheral arteries that Ca^{2+}-antagonistic drugs do not specifically block the α-adrenergic effects of norepinephrine or phenylephrine at therapeutic concentrations may be the basis for the fact that postural hypotension in humans has so far been reported for neither drug. Moreover, contractions of the basilar artery induced by serotonin, norepinephrine, phenylephrine, and histamine are blocked by the dihydropyridine compound, nimodipine, very effectively, whereas its effects on the same stimulation of the femoral artery are small. Therefore, it has been concluded that this drug has a preferential effect on cerebral blood vessels.

One of the approaches for the development of Ca^{2+}-antagonistic drugs in the future may be to select compounds with a high specificity for selected target organs. The development of the dihydropyridine compound, nisoldipine, may serve as an example. Pharmacologically, it differs from nifedipine in that it has a much more selective effect on venous smooth muscle *in vitro* (16). In contrast to nifedipine, for which the portal vein is the least sensitive structure of all vessels tested, the portal vein is the most sensitive structure affected by nisoldipine. The effect on heart muscle tissue is, for both drugs, in the same molar concentration range. Therefore, the dose-response curves on vessel structures and heart muscle are close together for nifedipine, but differ greatly in the molar concentration range for nisoldipine. Nisoldipine seems to be the first Ca^{2+} antagonist for which an effect on the venous system at therapeutic concentrations has been demonstrated. Moreover, it has been found to be the most powerful drug in preventing and relieving coronary vasospasms due to thromboxane.

Recent results indicate that not all the effects of Ca^{2+} antagonists can be explained solely by their effect on vascular smooth muscle and the resulting consequences in hemodynamics. Under various experimental conditions, as well as in man, it has been shown that myocardial cell structure and function tends to be preserved by Ca^{2+} antagonists, even under extreme ischemia when the heart is disconnected from the circulation (5,22). This seems to apply to other organs, such as kidney, brain, pancreas, and liver, as well. On this basis, a wide range of possible new indications is open for clinical exploration. More detailed exploration of the mechanism of action of Ca^{2+} antagonists on the cellular basis is necessary also to understand the reasons for differences seen between acute and chronic effects of these drugs, as well as to explain their cytoprotective properties.

INDICATIONS CURRENTLY UNDER CLINICAL INVESTIGATION

For nifedipine, an improvement in clinical efficacy with prolonged treatment has been shown for angina pectoris and hypertension. As pharmacokinetic parameters do not differ when acute and 2-week administrations are compared, the most likely explanation is a change in pharmacodynamics. However, the hypothesis has still to be proven that the acute effect of Ca^{2+}-antagonists induces, intracellularly, a reduction in compartmentally bound Ca^{2+}, which would reduce the amount of Ca^{2+} that can be released on a stimulus of the same strength.

The well-known importance of Ca^{2+} in the regulation of cellular activity in numerous organs and the resulting physiopathologic consequence has stimulated investigations into the potential therapeutic effectiveness of Ca^{2+} antagonists in many cardiovascular (Table 2), but also noncardiovascular (Table 3) diseases. It can be assumed that the number of diseases studied will increase.

Angina pectoris, including angina on effort, variant angina, and unstable angina, can be considered well covered indications for the Ca^{2+} antagonists, diltiazem, nifedipine, and verapamil (13,15,23,25). Also available are studies with

TABLE 2. *Calcium antagonists: Cardiovascular indications currently under clinical investigation*

Myocardial infarction
  Acute treatment
  Prevention
Arrhythmias
Congestive heart failure
Systemic arterial hypertension
Pulmonary hypertension
Protection against ischemic damage (e.g., cardiac surgery)
Atherogenesis
Hypertrophic cardiomyopathy
Aortic insufficiency
Disturbances in cerebral perfusion (stroke, subarachnoid hemorrhage)
Raynauds's disease

TABLE 3. *Calcium antagonists: Noncardiovascular indications currently under clinical investigation*

Bronchial asthma
Spasm—intestine, gallbladder, ureter, achalasia
Irritable bladder
Premature labor
Dysmenorrhea
Ergotism
Increase of antitumor activity of vinca alkaloides and adriamycin
Duchenne muscular dystrophy

nifedipine and verapamil in hypertension, which demonstrate that not only chronic hypertension, but also hypertensive crisis, can be effectively controlled by these drugs (15,18,25). Independent of the cause, verapamil is regarded as drug of choice for the treatment of reentrant supraventricular tachycardia, whereas nifedipine exhibits no antiarrhythmic effects (1,13,15,25).

The presence of particular Ca^{2+}-antagonistic substances has stimulated the study of further cardiac (Table 2), as well as noncardiac indications (Table 3), because of the great significance of Ca^{2+} in the pathophysiology of numerous diseases.

The basis for all the indications currently undergoing clinical investigation is the relaxation of the smooth muscle induced by Ca^{2+} antagonists. The main effect resulting from this on the cardiovascular system is the reduction of afterload which creates, in turn, relief of cardiac requirements for O_2, and thus a reduction in O_2 consumption. However, in addition, the O_2 transport to the ischemic myocardium is also increased. Coronary spasms are prevented or abolished, and an increase in poststenotic blood flow can be confirmed even with arteriosclerotically altered vessel walls. Independent of these hemodynamic effects, the Ca^{2+} antagonists also have a direct protective action on myocardial cells endangered by ischemia.

ACUTE MYOCARDIAL INFARCTION

A consequence of these promising pharmacological effects was, of course, that numerous investigators studied, both experimentally and clinically, the influence of Ca^{2+} antagonists on acute myocardial infarction. It was possible to determine a reduction of the size of experimentally induced infarctions in the dog model with nifedipine and verapamil, but, as yet, this has not been studied with diltiazem. Because they could not find a reduction in infarction size in their investigations with nifedipine on baboons, Geary and colleagues (12) were led to the conclusion that an effect may be dependent on the presence of collaterals, which, in contrast to baboons, are very pronounced in dogs. Since, however, the action of Ca^{2+} antagonists on infarction size depends on peripheral vasodilation and, therefore, on the administered dose (25), it might be the excessively high dose of 30 μg/kg/hr which Geary et al. (12) used in their experiments which prevented a reduction of infarction size. As yet, verapamil has not been used clinically in acute myocardial infarction, possibly because, in the animal experiments, a distinct limitation of the infarction could only be found with doses which caused disturbances of atrioventricular conduction or a selective impairment of contractility in the acute ischemic myocardium.

In the clinical investigations carried out with nifedipine on acute myocardial infarction, the action of 10 to 20 mg of the drug was investigated starting not earlier than 2 days after occurrence of the infarction. A simultaneous fall in peripheral resistance and, so far as was measured, a rise in stroke volume and cardiac output were found. Heart rate rose only mildly, if at all. The best results were obtained with patients who exhibited no serious cardiac insufficiency or whose pain was refractory to nitrates and β-blockers. At present, the longest period of treatment averaged 5.4 months (26). If no intense cardiac insufficiency persisted, raised pulmonary arterial pressure and pulmonary wedge pressure were reduced. A worsening of the hemodynamic situation did, nevertheless, occur in 2 patients with serious cardiac insufficiency. The only investigation comparing the acute effects of nifedipine and diltiazem (6) showed statistically significant differences in peripheral resistance, heart rate, and cardiac index. Peripheral resistance, which fell significantly with nifedipine, showed no change with diltiazem. Cardiac index rose with nifedipine and fell with diltiazem. Heart rate remained practically unchanged by nifedipine (79–82 beats/min), but sank distinctly under diltiazem from 89 to 77 beats/min. It will take some time before the currently running, larger studies can answer the question as to whether the relatively favorable acute effects of nifedipine result in a reduction in cardiac insufficiency, sudden deaths, and the occurrence of reinfarctions. Nifedipine can, nevertheless, be recommended now in patients with myocardial infarction whose persistent cardiac pain is refractory to nitrates and β-blockers (26). However, care should be taken in patients with cardiac insufficiency of the most severe degree.

CONGESTIVE HEART FAILURE

The concept of treating heart failure with vasodilators results from the knowledge that through elimination of excessive vasoconstriction, the workload of the heart is reduced, and an increase in volume output by the heart with an advantageous distribution of blood flow and blood volume occurs. The results which have been published are all concerned with acute investigations with nifedipine, using doses of 10 to 20 mg as capsules, in which the substance exhibits a high invasion rate. As expected, peripheral resistance is reduced and the heart, therefore, relieved. If the volume output of the heart was previously reduced, it increased. Cardiac index, ejection fraction, and stroke-volume index are raised and heart rate generally remains unchanged. On the other hand, left ventricular end-diastolic pressure (17), pulmonary arterial, and pulmonary wedge pressures all fall. A reduction in plasma volume was determined after only 24 hr (20). The cause of this was established as an increase in water and Na^+ excretion, whereas K^+ excretion was unchanged (20). An increase in water and Na^+ excretion, while K^+ concentration remained unchanged, something which has already been observed in hypertensive patients under treatment with dihydropyridines (18), leads one to suspect a direct influence on kidney function because the total excretion of K^+ should also be raised when renal perfusion increases. The available results are encouraging, but must be confirmed in investigations of longer duration.

HYPERTROPHIC CARDIOMYOPATHY

The present studies show that the Ca^{2+} antagonists, verapamil and nifedipine, offer an effective alternative to the treatment of hypertrophic cardiomyopathy with β-blockers. Their effect improves with the duration of treatment. Left ventricular outflow obstruction and heart size are reduced, and the work capacity of the patient is increased. The greater efficacy of verapamil hypothesized from a historical comparison to propranolol could not be confirmed for patients without angina pectoris when it was directly compared with nifedipine. Nifedipine and verapamil were, however, clearly superior to β-blockers in those patients who exhibited anginal attacks. As with the β-receptor blockers, progressive development of the disease was also observed under continuous therapy with verapamil. Whether the very high verapamil doses used (up to 720 mg/day), which led to some serious side-effects, were strictly necessary is contested. In any case, a comparison of 320 and 480 mg/day verapamil showed no differences in efficacy. Since the effect clearly improves with the duration of treatment, investigations of longer duration with verapamil in patients with hypertrophic cardiomyopathy, using smaller doses, are indicated. For nifedipine, favorable effects have been described in a dose range between 40 and 80 mg/day.

PULMONARY HYPERTENSION

As yet, relatively few patients with pulmonary hypertension have been treated with Ca^{2+} antagonists (19,24). Main diseases studied were primary pulmonary hypertension, congenital heart diseases, pulmonary fibrosis, or hypoxically caused pulmonary vasoconstriction. Pulmonary arterial pressure falls from an elevated initial value under all substances, sometimes markedly. The effects of verapamil in comparison to diltiazem and nifedipine are, however, classified much lower. In addition, verapamil can lead to a fall in cardiac output (24) due to its—compared to nifedipine and diltiazem—much more marked negative-inotropic effect. Therefore, it even can cause lung edema, especially if heart function is already impaired and the drug is given intravenously. On the other hand, an increase was observed with nifedipine and diltiazem in cardiac output in all investigations, even when administered orally. Nifedipine maintains its full effect in patients with pulmonary hypertension continuously treated over 4 months (19). For a final conclusion on the effectiveness of Ca^{2+} antagonists in pulmonary hypertension, further intensive exploration is still necessary.

AORTIC INSUFFICIENCY

Recently, a clinically favorable action of nifedipine after acute sublingual administration of 20 mg in 12 patients with severe isolated aortic insufficiency was reported (8). In these patients, left ventricular end-diastolic pressure, average aortic pressure, and peripheral resistance fell, while cardiac index was increased by 24%. The higher the peripheral resistance before commencement of treatment, the more the regurgitant fraction was reduced. The latter did, however, rise in one patient who had an extraordinarily low initial peripheral resistance. Left ventricular function was unaffected, and O_2 consumption even decreased.

MYOCARDIAL PRESERVATION

Numerous experimental investigations show that Ca^{2+} antagonists enhance the ischemic tolerance of the heart and moderate the deleterious effects of massive Ca^{2+} influx in the reperfusion phase after a circulation stop (1,13,22,25). This effect was recently exploited using nifedipine in 38 high-risk patients with poor ventricular function, who had to undergo heart surgery. The usual cardioplegic solution contained an additional 0.2 $\mu g/ml$ nifedipine. Notable results were that stroke work and other heart indices returned quickly to nearly normal values after the operation. As a result, an intraaortal balloon pump had to be used by a factor of 3, less frequently in comparison to 40 similar patients. The distinct reduction in the liberation of CPK-MB isoenzyme makes the protective effect which took place under nifedipine clearly recognizable (5). A further study, just completed, confirms these results. Both studies show such a marked improvement in cardioplegia concerning protection of myocardial tissue and function that further exploration can be expected to establish routine use of nifedipine in cardioplegia.

ATHEROGENESIS

It must surely be worthwhile to establish if the influence on atherogenesis found in animals with nifedipine and verapamil (11,14) can also be detected in humans. In rats, a distinct reduction in the calcification occurring after vitamin D_3 was measured. The $^{45}Ca^{2+}$ uptake by the vessels, as well as the absolute Ca^{2+} content of the latter, were reduced by about 90% (11). Henry and Bentley (14) were able to reduce aortic lesions on the intima surface from 40% in the control group to 17% under nifedipine treatment in cholesterol-fed rabbits.

Total plasma cholesterol remained unchanged. The strength of both effects, as well as the possible species differences, should not prevent the investigation of more tolerable doses in humans, in spite of the high doses administered in the animal experiments (verapamil 2 × 30 mg/kg subcutaneously, or 2 × 100 mg/kg orally; nifedipine 16 mg/kg).

NONCARDIOVASCULAR INDICATIONS

The interest in clinical exploration of the potential therapeutic effectiveness of Ca²⁺ antagonists in noncardiovascular diseases has included, above all, pulmonology, gastroenterology, urology, and gynecology.

The investigations in bronchial asthma have, as yet, not been able to demonstrate convincing therapeutic effects under either nifedipine or verapamil. They have, however, shown that Ca²⁺ antagonists in contrast to, e.g., β-receptor blockers, do not impair lung function and, in particular, respiratory tract resistance. Preliminary investigations in achalasia (2) produced excellent and long-lasting results in this disease. This is also the case in dysmenorrhea, delay in premature labor, ureter colic, detrusor hyperreflexia in prostatic adenoma patients, neurogenic upsets of bladder evacuation, and, in particular, irritable bladder. The last-mentioned investigations were all carried out with nifedipine. The dose was between 10 and 20 mg, mostly 3 times daily. A study in Duchenne's muscular dystrophy (7) using verapamil had to be discontinued, in spite of relatively good clinical effect, because of the danger of severe conduction disturbances (13,21,23,25). Two children, receiving 2 × 40 mg/day verapamil, suddenly developed disorders in atrioventricular conduction after 8 and 18 weeks treatment, respectively. The full value of a Ca²⁺-antagonistic therapy could not be established because of the impossibility of further increasing the dose.

FUTURE ASPECTS

After recognition of the importance of the Ca²⁺ antagonists has taken place by the medical community, we certainly can expect a further development of new compounds on the basis of better understood differences in pharmacologic mechanisms of the already existing drugs. It is not speculative forecasting that at the end of this decade we will have Ca²⁺-antagonistic drugs being more selective both for different target organs and clinical indications. Consequently, the appearance of side-effects, which are already tolerable for some of the drugs used at present, will be reduced even more. Without any doubt, many more diseases will be explored and finally treated with these compounds.

REFERENCES

1. Antman, E. M., Stone, P. H., Muller, J. E., and Braunwald, E. (1980): *Ann. Intern. Med.*, 93:875–885.

2. Berger, K., and McCallum, R. W. (1982): *Ann. Intern. Med.*, 96:61–62.
3. Boström, S. -L., Ljung, B., Mardh, S., Forsen, S., and Thulini, E. (1981): *Nature*, 292:777–778.
4. Church, J., and Zsoter, T. T. (1980): *Can. J. Physiol. Pharmacol.*, 58:254–264.
5. Clark, R. R., Christlieb, J. Y., Ferguson, T. B., Weldon, C. S., Marbarger, J. P., Sobel, B. E., Roberts, R., Henry, P. D., Ludbrook, P. A., Biello, D., and Clark, B. K. (1981): *Ann. Surgery*, 193:719–732.
6. Debaisieux, J. -C., Theroux, P., Waters, D. D., Mizgala, H. F., and Bourassa, M. G. (1979): *Circulation*, 60:82.
7. Emery, A. E. H., Skinner, R., Howden, L. C., and Matthews, M. B. (1982): *Lancet*, I:559.
8. Fioretti, P., Benussi, B., Scardi, S., Klugmann, S., Brower, R. W., and Camerini, F. (1982): *Am. J. Cardiol.*, 49:1728–1732.
9. Flaim, S. F., and Craven, R. A. (1981): *Pharmacology*, 22:286–293.
10. Flaim, S. F., Irwin, J. M., Ratz, P. H., and Swigart, S. C. (1982): *Am. J. Cardiol.*, 49:511–518.
11. Frey, M., Keidel, J., and Fleckenstein, A. (1980): In: *Calcium-Antagonismus*, edited by A. Fleckenstein, and H. Roskamm, pp. 258–264. Springer, Berlin.
12. Geary, G. G., Smith, G. T., Suehiro, G. T., and McNamara, J. -J. (1982): *Am. J. Cardiol.*, 49:331–338.
13. Henry, P. D. (1980): *Am. J. Cardiol.*, 46:1047–1058.
14. Henry, P. D., and Bentley, K. I. (1981): *J. Clin. Invest.*, 68:1366–1369.
15. Karlsberg, R. P. (1982): *Arch. Intern. Med.*, 142:452–455.
16. Kazda, S., Garthoff, B., Meyer, H., Schlossmann, K., Stoepel, K., Towart, R., Vater, W., and Wehinger, E. (1980): *Arzneim. Forsch.*, 30:2144–2162.
17. Klugmann, S., Salvi, C., and Camerini, F. (1980): *Br. Heart J.*, 43:440–446.
18. Krebs, R., Graefe, K. -H., and Ziegler, R. (1982): *Clin. Exp. Hypertens.*, 4:271–284.
19. McLeod, A. A., Wise, J. P., Daly, K., and Jewitt, D. E. (1981): *Circulation*, 64(Suppl. IV):180.
20. Mollaioli, M., Cosmi, F., Aini, M., Conti, G., Corbacelli, C., and Gazzini, M. (1981): *Clin. Eur.*, XX:3–11.
21. Mitchell, L. B., Schroeder, J. S., and Mason, J. W. (1982): *Am. J. Cardiol.*, 49:629–635.
22. Nayler, W. G., and Grinwald, P. (1981): *Fed. Proc.*, 40:2855–2861.
23. Opie, L. H. (1980): *Lancet*, II:806–810.
24. Simonneau, G., Escourrou, P., Duroux, P., and Lockhart, A. (1981): *N. Engl. J. Med.*, 304:1582–1585.
25. Stone, P. H., Antman, E. M., Muller, J. E., and Braunwald, E. (1980): *Ann. Intern. Med.*, 93:886–904.
26. Stone, P. A., and Muller, J. E. (1981): *Am. J. Cardiol.*, 47:490.
27. Weiss, G. B., Hatano, K., and Stull, J. T. (1981): *Blood Vessels*, 18:230.
28. Williams, L. T., and Tremble, P. (1982): *J. Clin. Invest.*, 70:209–212.

Calcium Antagonists and Cardiovascular Disease, edited by L. H. Opie.
Raven Press, New York © 1984.

Chapter 34

Calcium Channel Blocking Drugs: What Now?

Arnold Schwartz

Department of Pharmacology & Cell Biophysics, University of Cincinnati, Cincinnati, Ohio 45267

In tracing the history of pharmacology to the present, there have been a number of milestones that are clearly consistent with the acquisition of new fundamental biological information. We remember, for example, the excitement generated by the introduction of the concept of α- and β-adrenergic receptors by Raymond Ahlquist, the more recent subdivision of both the α- and β-receptors, the concept of an H_1 and H_2 histamine receptor and, of course, the development of selective, and even specific, drugs that interact with sites to produce dramatic pharmacological effects. During the last decade, we saw the introduction of relatively selective β-adrenergic blocking agents, first for the treatment of certain types of hypertension and stable angina pectoris, and within recent years, for a very wide spectrum of disease entities. This is not so surprising when one considers the importance of the nervous system and the widespread presence of adrenergic receptors.

Within the past 10 years, our knowledge in the area of excitation-contraction-relaxation coupling in heart muscle has increased significantly, so that we now have a fundamental understanding of how Ca^{2+} links these processes and how the cardiac cell may be regulated even on a beat-to-beat level. While progress has been slower in vascular smooth muscle, nevertheless, recent exciting developments have provided considerable information on a fundamental level. Thus, it is not surprising that pharmacological agents should emerge which appear to have relatively selective effects on the movement of Ca^{2+}. Indeed, perhaps the oldest cardiovascular drug, digitalis, is known to increase the availability of cellular Ca^{2+}, thereby producing a powerful stimulant action on the heart. One could almost think of digitalis as a type of "ionophilic" prototype. In this regard, then, we can imagine that an inhibition of the movements of Ca^{2+} might yield interesting and potentially important effects. A drug of this type might be called "ionophobic." Such action would lead to very important potential beneficial therapeutic actions.

There is no question that the cardiovascular drugs of the 1980s will fall into the classification of "calcium antagonists." We owe a significant debt of gratitude to Professor Albrecht Fleckenstein for providing us with the excitement of this new class of drugs. As is the case with the development of all new classes of drugs, the situation has become much more complex than originally thought. There is no question that we are dealing with chemical structures that are not only different on paper, but even in a space-filling mode (Fig. 1). Accordingly, the fact that these agents share certain effects is interesting, but the fact that they do have qualitative and quantitative differences should not be surprising (1,2).

In the United States, there are three drugs on the market which have been labeled Ca^{2+} channel blocking drugs, or Ca^{2+} antagonists. These are verapamil, nifedipine, and diltiazem. These agents have been approved for the treatment of variant (spasm) angina, as well as for stable angina pectoris. In addition, intravenous verapamil has been approved for the treatment of certain supraventricular cardiac arrhythmias. We, of course, realize that this approval is based on quantitative clinical data. Those of us who deal with experimental animals, however, also recognize the potential for these drugs in a variety of clinical situations is extremely high. Again, the reason is quite clear, namely that Ca^{2+} is the most important ionic link between processes involving excitation and biological responses. The drugs certainly interact with vascular smooth muscle and produce relaxation, hence the potential for treating certain types of hypertension is high. If, in some way, a "spasm" or change in contractile tone is involved in certain types of refractory migraine headaches, one could imagine that these drugs could be useful in that condition and, indeed, preliminary evidence supports this contention. For some years, alterations of Ca^{2+} metabolism in skeletal muscle associated with some types of muscular dystrophy has been an attractive hypothesis, and if so, again, one could imagine that these drugs might be useful in that debilitating illness. Preliminary evidence in this regard is encouraging. It is possible that some of the Ca^{2+} antagonists might inhibit the process of atherogenesis without altering serum cholesterol, but by somehow inhibiting the formation of free cholesterol and cholesteryl esters inside the vascular smooth muscle cell. Again, preliminary evidence is supportive of this concept.

As we continue to increase our knowledge base in this extremely important pharmacological area, I can predict the synthesis of countless numbers of chemical structures that will end up being selective for specific areas, such as cerebral blood vessels, peripheral blood vessels, secretory tissues, bronchiolar muscle, gastrointestinal muscle, uterine muscle, etc., so that these substances will surely find significant use in diseases which have been difficult to treat. Among these are certain allergies, stroke, dysmenorrhea, perhaps peptic ulcer, and certain endocrine disorders. Moreover, extending our receptor horizons from the cell membrane, where most of the available Ca^{2+} antagonists appear to act at the present, to the interior of the cell, we can predict the development of drugs that inhibit Ca^{2+} delivery to the contractile proteins and/or extrusion of Ca^{2+};

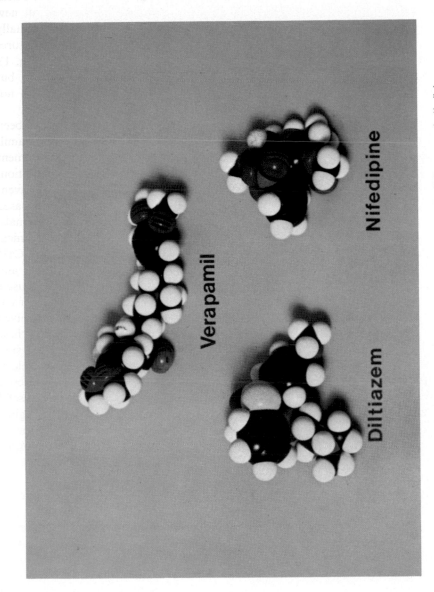

FIG. 1. Space-filling models of the calcium antagonists verapamil, diltiazem, and nifedipine.

and these agents too, would have profound effects on a variety of processes.

We must keep in mind that the drugs we are dealing with are extraordinarily complex, that we are not dealing with a single class of drugs, and that when we do alter Ca^{2+}, we are manipulating perhaps the most fundamental component of life's processes. Even with the limited number of Ca^{2+} antagonists available at the present time, the complexities of their effects and the difficulties of interpretation are clearly demonstrated by examining the very recent [³H]nitrendipine- and nimodipine-binding data. The nifedipine-like drugs clearly inhibit the binding in a single site process, the verapamil-like drugs only inhibit the binding to about 50%, and diltiazem either has no effect or actually stimulates the binding (1,3).

My prediction is that the age of "calcium antagonists" will dominate cardiovascular pharmacology and perhaps other areas of pharmacology for years to come, and from the continued and hopefully increased basic and clinical activities, we will see emerge from these studies drugs that have highly selective actions and extraordinarily important clinical benefits.

REFERENCES

1. DePover, A., Matlib, M. A., Lee, S. W., Dube, G. P., Grupp, I. L., Grupp, G., and Schwartz, A. (1982): *Biochem. Biophys. Res. Commun.,* 108:110–117.
2. Schwartz, A. (1982): *Am. J. Cardiol.,* 49:497–636.
3. Schwartz, A., and Taira, N. (1983): *Circ. Res.,* 52:I1–I181.

Subject Index